Congenital Lower Limb Deficiencies

Editor
Ali Kalamchi

Congenital Lower Limb Deficiencies

Springer-Verlag
New York Berlin Heidelberg
London Paris Tokyo Hong Kong

Ali Kalamchi, M.D., F.A.C.S., F.R.C.S.
Limestone Medical Center, Suite 209,
Wilmington, DE 19808, USA

Library of Congress Cataloging-in-Publication Data
Congenital lower limb deficiencies/edited by Ali Kalamchi.
p. cm.
Includes index.
1. Extremities, Lower—Abnormalities. I. Kalamchi, Ali.
[DNLM: 1. Leg—abnormalities. WE 850 C749]
RD779.C66 1989
617.3'98043—dc20
DNLM/DLC
for Library of Congress 89-11551

Typeset by TCSystems, Inc., Shippensburg, Pennsylvania.
Printed and bound by Arcata Graphics/Halliday, West Hanover, Massachusetts.
Printed in the United States of America.

9 8 7 6 5 4 3 2 1

ISBN 0-387-96968-3 Springer-Verlag New York Berlin Heidelberg
ISBN 3-540-96968-3 Springer-Verlag Berlin Heidelberg New York

Dedicated to the children with lower limb defects and their caring families.

Preface

This book was produced in response to the need for a single source reference guide for complex, but rare, congenital deficiencies of the lower limb.

For orthopedists and other medical specialists, the text presents a comprehensive review of traditionally acceptable methods of treating patients who present with major lower limb congenital defects.

The diagnosis of each type of defect is discussed with a special section on the natural history of each deficiency which will aid in conferences that we conduct with anxious parents soon after the child is born. Also discussed are differential diagnoses with a comprehensive review of associated complications of which the treating physicians should be aware.

Many chapters include overall reviews of the management of conditions with emphasis on the timing of surgery and selection of a prosthesis for different age groups.

The contributing editors share their wealth of experience in dealing with these conditions and convey their preference of management of each condition.

I would like to express my sincerest thanks to my colleagues, the contributing editors who worked tirelessly with us to meet the editorial goal of this mission. They have been generous with their time, expertise, and illustrations.

I am grateful to my publishers for their belief in the concept and their patience and professionalism during the preparation and publication process.

Ali Kalamchi, M.D.

Contents

Contributors

J. Richard Bowen, M.D., Director, Department of Orthopaedics, Alfred I. duPont Institute, Wilmington, Delaware 19899

In Ho Choi, M.D., Orthopaedic Fellow, Alfred I. duPont Institute, Wilmington, Delaware 19899

Morris S. Dixon, Jr., M.D., Associate Professor, Department of Pediatrics, Case Western Reserve University School of Medicine, Cleveland, Ohio; Associate Medical Director, Rainbow Children's Center at Lakewood Hospital, Lakewood, Ohio 44107

Robert E. Eilert, M.D., Chief, Children's Orthopaedics, Denver, Colorado; Assistant Clinical Professor, Department of Orthopaedic Surgery, University of Colorado Health Sciences Center, Denver, Colorado; Chairman, Department of Orthopaedic Surgery and Rehabilitation, The Children's Hospital, Denver, Colorado 80218

Ali Kalamchi, M.D., Orthopaedic Surgeon, Medical Center of Delaware, A. I. DuPont Institute, Wilmington, Delaware 19899

J. Ivan Krajbich, M.D., B.Sc. F.R.C.S., Hospital for Sick Children, Division of Orthopaedic Surgery, Toronto, Ontario M5G 1X8 Canada

Alfred E. Kritter, M.D., Clinical Professor of Orthopaedics, Medical College of Wisconsin, Waukesha, Wisconsin 53186

S. Jay Kumar, M.D., Assistant Professor of Orthopaedic Surgery, Jefferson University, Philadelphia, Pennsylvania; Orthopaedic Surgeon, Alfred I. DuPont Institute, Wilmington, Delaware; Director, Prosthetic Clinic, Alfred I. DuPont Institute, Wilmington, Deleware 19899

Jon P. Leimkuehler, B.B.A., C.P.O.; President, Union Orthotics and Prosthetics Company, Pittsburgh, Pennsylvania 15201

John A. Ogden, M.D., Professor of Surgery and Rehabilitation Professor of Pediatrics, University of South Florida College of Medicine, Tampa, Florida; Chief of Staff, Shriner's Hospital for Crippled Children, Tampa, Florida 33612

Alan Peoples, M.Ed., P.T., Associate Director Blue Hen Physical Therapy, Incorporated, Newark, Delaware 19711

Peter D. Pizzutillo, M.D., Associate Professor, Director, Division of Pediatric Orthopaedics, Department of Orhtopaedic Surgery, Jefferson Medical College of Thomas Jefferson University, Philadelphia, Pennsylvania

Thomas L. Schmidt, M.D., Associate Professor, School of Medicine, University of Missouri at Kansas City, Kansas City, Missouri; Director, Pediatric Orthopaedic Surgery, Children's Mercy Hospital, Kansas City, Missouri 64108

Charles I. Scott, Jr., M.D., Director, Department of Medical Genetics, Alfred I. DuPont Institute, Wilmington, Delaware 19899-0269

George Harman Thompson, M.D., Department of Orthopaedic Surgery, Cleveland Metropolitan General Hospital, Cleveland, Ohio 44109

Introduction

The selection of the proper regimen of management of the patient with a congenital defect of the lower limb is often difficult because such conditions are rare and because there is little organized information regarding these defects. This text, prepared by individuals who have an interest in, and a great deal of experience with, the care of such children, addresses both these concerns.

The organization of the text is not a chance happening, but reflects the approach that should be used in managing children with these problems. There are three aspects to the general evaluation of the child. First, the development of the lower extremity must be appreciated in order to understand the abnormality in development that has taken place. Then the deformity must be categorized as to whether it is an inherited problem or whether it occurred on a chance basis in order to counsel the patient and his, or her, family. Moreover, it is imperative to know if the defect is part of a particular syndrome. Next a complete evaluation of the individual should be carried out looking for the abnormalities of other organ systems which may accompany syndromes.

The second section of the text deals with the management of specific deformities. The chapters in this section have been prepared by pediatric orthopaedic surgeons who have had a major interest in the care of children with these problems for a number of years, and the chapters reflect the philosophy of planning a long-term program of management for these children. This program should be developed as early as possible, and be based on the clinical and radiographic finding. The classifications of the deformities presented in these chapters, while they may differ from standard classifications, are intended to aid in the selection of the proper program of management for these children.

The final section deals with specific types of treatment. This is the proper location for this material, since no specific modality of therapy should be undertaken until the child has been evaluated, the family counseled, and the deformity completely understood by the physician.

Finally, it must be mentioned that the proper care of a child with a congenital defect of the lower extremity requires a team approach. Only when the skills of the geneticist, the pediatrician, the orthopedist, the therapist, and the prosthetist are combined will the child receive optimal care.

Henry R. Cowell, M.D., Ph.D.

Section I—General

1
Development of the Lower Limb

JOHN A. OGDEN

Evaluation of the developing lower limb—whether dealing with the multitude of skeletal dysplasias, the highly variable deficiency and duplication situations of congenital deformities, or the manifestations of acquired, traumatic, metabolic, or infectious problems—requires an adequate understanding of developmental chondro-osseous biology. The musculoskeletal and neurovascular components of the leg undergo not only basic differentiation processes, but also specific steps leading to the discrete morphology of the various regions. Major alterations in the initial differentiation will result in focal deficiencies such as absence of the proximal femur or tibial hemimelia. The considerable morphologic variation in these and other hemimelic disorders suggests variable susceptibility to the etiologic factors. Subsequent intrauterine conditions also may affect development, leading to disorders such as tibial pseudarthrosis or amputation from amniotic band syndrome.

The prenatal development of the lower limb has been detailed by numerous authors.* O'Rahilly and Gardner presented the most detailed summaries of the literature concerning early development of the limbs, basing appearance of the various skeletal and neuromuscular components upon stages of development.[42–44] These stages are summarized in Table 1.1.

The two basic types of osseous tissue formation—membranous and endochondral—refer *only* to the primary prenatal development of each individual structural unit, whether maxilla, femur, or metatarsal. Subsequent growth of any particular bone after its initial differentiation involves discrete, juxtaposed, and interspersed areas of each basic pattern within the same bone.[26,27,37,38] Endochondral-derived bones have concomitant membranous ossification by appositional bone growth from the periosteum (Fig. 1.1). In fact, such membranous-derived periosteal bone eventually makes up the mature diaphyseal cortex, with endochondral bone being progressively replaced.[37,38]

---

* References 1, 4, 6, 7, 10–15, 47–49.

TABLE 1. Developmental stages of lower limb components.[a]

Feature	Developmental stage
Limb bud	13
Apical ectodermal ridge	15–18
Footplate	16
Mesenchymal skeleton	16
Mesenchymal hip	15–18
Mesenchymal femur/tibia/fibia	17
Cartilaginons femur	17–18
Chondrifying tibia	17–18
Chondrifying fibula	17–18
Chondrifying metatarsus	18–19
Chondrifying tarsus	18–19
Toe rays	18
Chondrifying hip	19
Chondrifying phalanges	19–23
Interzone, hip and knee	19–21
Interzone, ankle	21–23
Ossification in fibula and tibia	22–23
Ossification in fibula	23
Cavitation, hip and knee	23
Cavitation, ankle	23

[a] Modified from O'Rahilly and Gardner.[44]

Membranous Bone Formation

Primary membranous bone formation occurs when small groups of cells elaborate a fibrous, extracellular matrix that is calcified and ossified to form primary trabecula. Ossification then spreads outward from this primary ossification center to cover relatively large areas. The trabecular orientation is relatively random when first formed, but becomes responsive to internal and external mechanical stress factors that initiate early remodeling.

All skeletal elements of the leg are involved in secondary membranous ossification. The diaphyseal cortex of each developing tubular bone is progressively formed (modeled) by the periosteum and modified (remodeled) by changing the woven trabecular bone to more dense cortical bone, which, in turn, is further refined (remodeled) by the formation of osteon systems. This peripheral periosteal process of membrane-derived ossification is extensive and rapid in some types of fracture healing, as in reactive osteogenesis of osteomyelitis, although the rate declines with increasing skeletal age. The replacement process may also be seen when portions of the developing metaphysis or diaphysis are removed for use as bone grafts. The membranous periosteal bone is mechanically "weak" when first formed and must be progressively strengthened to meet biologic demands (i.e., walking), a process that necessitates histomorphologic changes.[9]

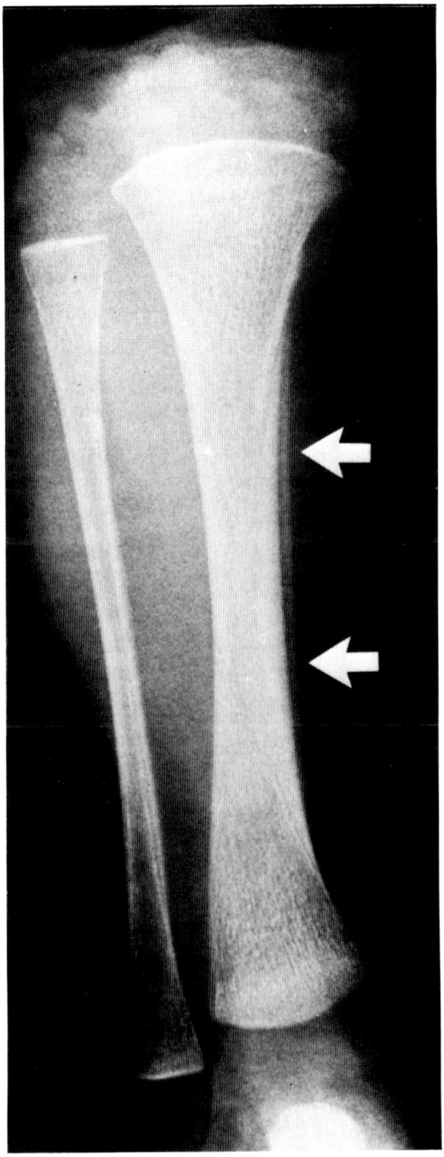

FIGURE 1.1. Subperiosteal new bone formation (*arrows*) along medial side of tibia in a newborn. This may have been due to birth trauma in this neonate who died approximately 2 weeks after birth.

Endochondral Ossification

Endochondral ossification is the primary formation process of the appendicular skeletal components and may recur in selected areas of established bone as part of fracture repair through the formation and maturation of callus. Succinctly, this type of bone formation is the staged, synchronous replacement of mesenchymal tissue by cartilaginous tissue

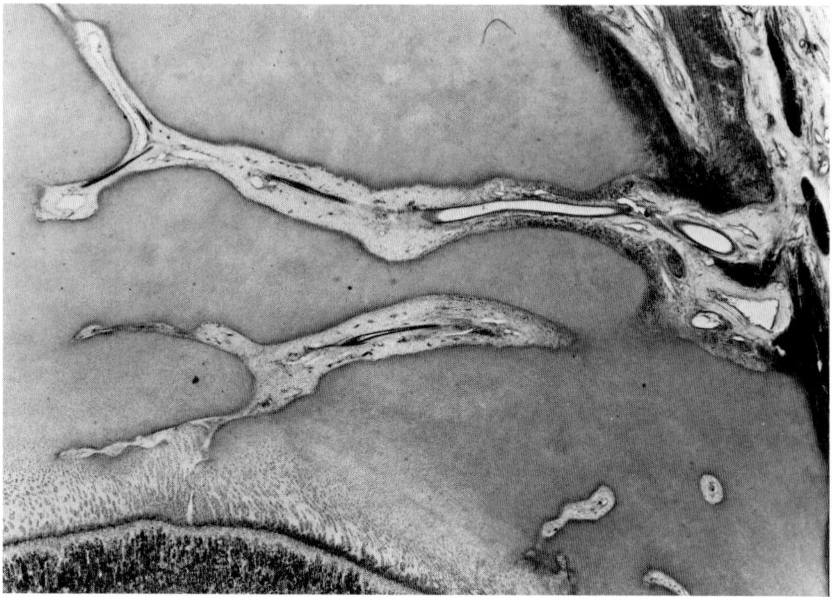

FIGURE 1.2. Penetrating cartilage canals entering an unossified proximal femoral chondroepiphysis. These vessels distribute throughout the epiphysis and also selectively supply the germinal zone of the physis.

and the subsequent replacement of the cartilaginous model by osseous tissue.

Once the initial ossification center has formed, expansile ossification progresses rapidly toward each end. The bone first formed is a loose trabecular network that fuses with the multilayered periosteal shell.[2] Initially, the endochondral ossification process extends at approximately equal rates toward each end of the bone. Postnatally, however, there are significant differences in the rates of physeal growth at each end of a given bone (e.g., 40% of the leg length is contributed by the distal femoral growth plate compared with 20% from the proximal femoral growth plate).

Once the physis is morphologically established (usually after 70% to 80% of the initial cartilaginous anlage has been replaced by primary ossification), the periosteal ring stops further extension toward the epiphysis and remains level with the zone of hypertrophic cartilage (with which it continues growth in an integrated fashion), although it may extend further as osteoid tissue to reach the germinal zone. This periphyseal bone collar may be referred to as the fibro-osseous ring of Lacroix. The cellular association of periosteal ring, peripheral physis, and fibrovascular tissue is referred to as the zone of Ranvier, which is an

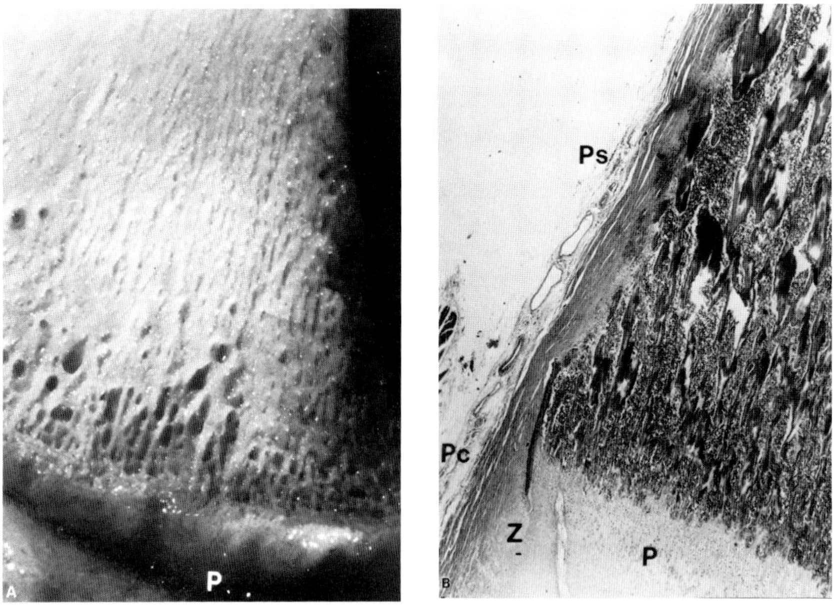

FIGURE 1.3. **A:** Distal femur from a 10-year-old. Note that the dense diaphyseal cortex (*top*) becomes progressively porous, reaching a maximum porosity near the physis (P). **B:** Histologic sections from 2-month-old infant. Note how the periosteum (Ps) blends into the metaphyseal fenestrations. Pc = perichondrium, P = physis, Z = zone of Ranvier.

important area of diametric (latitudinal) expansion of the physis and a source of vascular ingrowth (Fig. 1.2).

As the individual bone elongates and widens in the metaphysis by the normal process of endochondral ossification, extensive remodeling begins. When the endochondral trabecular bone and the membranous bone collar initially unite, they form a shaft of relatively uniform diameter. However, the metaphysis must progressively widen to accomodate the diametrically expanding physis and epiphysis. Active remodeling occurs in two areas of the metaphysis—central and peripheral. Bone modeling and remodeling is so active that the metaphyseal cortex is relatively porous (Fig. 1.3). This porous bone is a factor in susceptibility of the immature skeleton to torus fracture and also allows spontaneous "decompression" of a metaphyseal focus of osteomyelitis into the subperiosteal space. As the skeleton matures, especially around and after the stage of physeal closure, the metaphyseal cortex progressively "solidifies" with osteon bone.[16] The central part of the metaphysis also remodels, with the primary spongiosa being replaced by secondary spongiosa.[34]

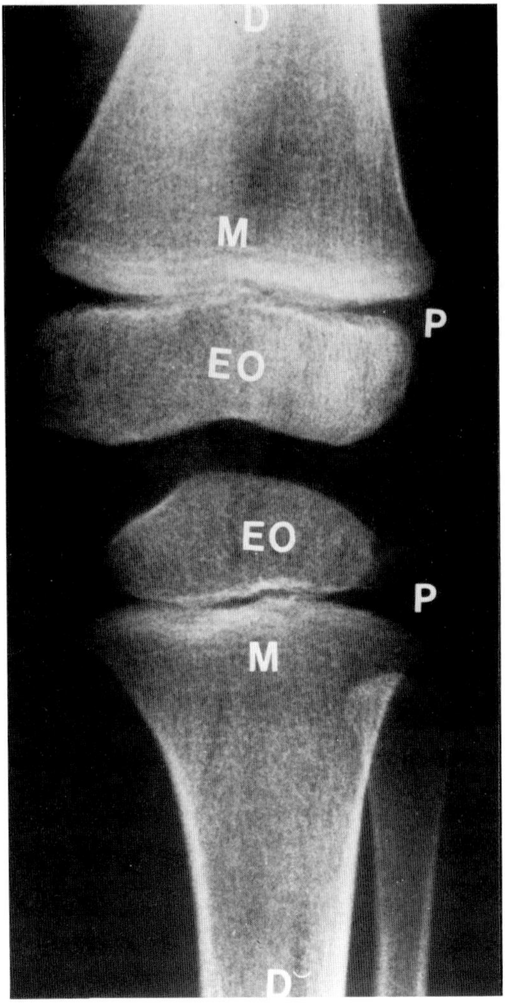

FIGURE 1.4. Anatomic regions of developing bone in the radiograph of the knee of a 7-year-old. D = diaphysis, M = metaphysis, P = physis, EO = epiphyseal ossification center.

Skeletal Components

The major long bones may be divided into distinct anatomic areas—epiphysis, physis, metaphysis, and diaphysis (Fig. 1.4). The four regions originate and become modified as a result of the basic endochondral ossification process.

Diaphysis

The diaphysis comprises the major portion of each long bone. It is a product of periosteal, membranous osseous tissue apposition on the original endochondral model. At birth, the diaphysis comprises laminar (fetal, woven) bone characteristically lacking in haversian systems (osteons). The neonatal femoral diaphysis appears to be the only area exhibiting any significant change from the fetal osseous state to the more mature bone with the osteon system (lamellar bone). Mature, lamellar bone with intrinsic, but constantly remodeling osteonal patterns progressively becomes the dominant feature (Fig. 1.5). The active remodeling osteon is referred to as a bone metabolic unit or bone-modeling unit and is the mechanism of response within the cortex to physiologic and biomechanical conditions throughout life.

The developing bone in a neonate or young child is extremely vascular. When analyzed in cross section it appears much less dense than the maturing bone of older children, adolescents, and adults. Subsequent growth leads to increased complexity of the haversian systems and the elaboration of increasing amounts of extracellular matrix, causing a relative decrease in cross-sectional porosity and an increase in hardness.[5,9,29,33]

Metaphysis

The metaphysis is the variably contoured flare at each end of the diaphysis. The major characteristics are decreased thickness of the cortical bone and increased trabecular bone in the secondary spongiosa. Extensive endochondral modeling centrally and peripherally initially forms the primary spongiosa, which is then transformed (remodeled) into more mature secondary spongiosa, a process that involves osteolytic, osteoclastic, and osteoblastic activity. The metaphyses exhibit considerable bone turnover compared with other regions of the bone, a factor undoubtedly responsible for the increased uptake of radionuclides during bone scans. The metaphysis, because of the high rate of bone modeling and remodeling, appears most susceptible to the development of lesions such as fibrous cortical defects.[17,18,29,45]

Like the diaphysis, the metaphyseal cortex changes with time. Relative to the confluent diaphysis, the metaphyseal cortex is thinner and has greater porosity or trabecular fenestration (Fig. 1.3). These cortical fenestrations contain fibrovascular soft-tissue elements interconnecting the metaphyseal marrow spaces with the subperiosteal region. The metaphyseal cortex exhibits greater fenestration near the physis than the diaphysis, with which it gradually blends as an increasingly thicker, dense bone. As longitudinal growth continues, cortical fenestration becomes a less dominant feature, and the overall width of the cortex increases, creating a greater morphologic transition between the juxtaphyseal and juxtadiaphyseal cortices.

The metaphysis is the site of extensive osseous modeling and remodeling, both peripherally and centrally. The metaphyseal cortex is fenestrated, modified trabecular bone on which the periosteum elaborates

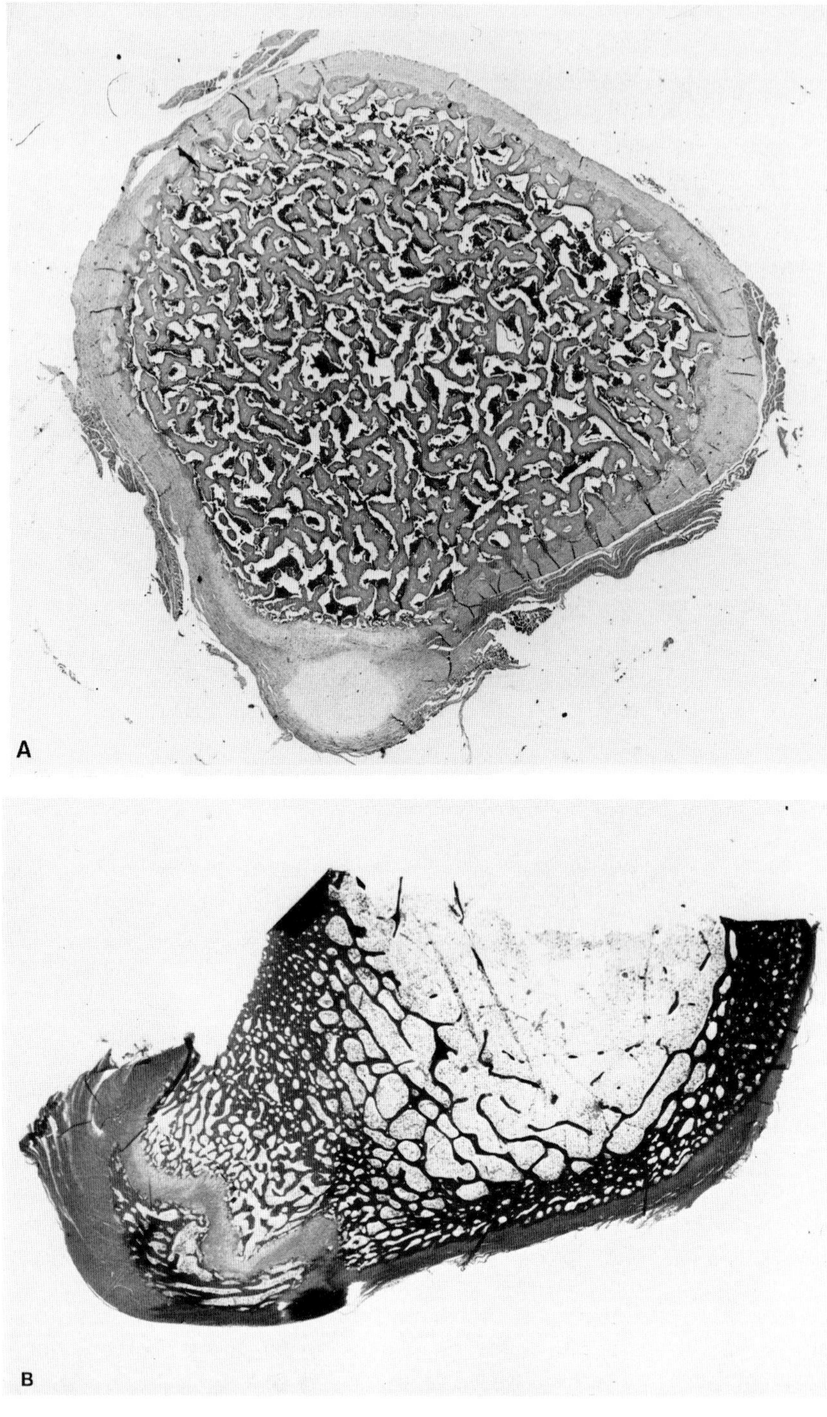

FIGURE 1.5. Transverse sections of the proximal femur at the level of the lesser trochanter in a neonate **(A),** 12-year-old **(B),** and 15-year-old.

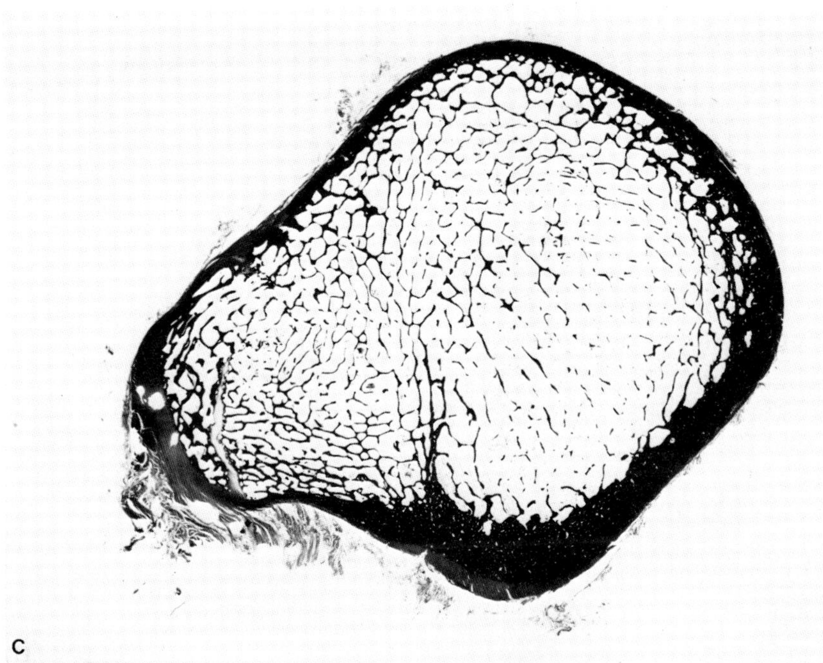

FIGURE 1.5 (*Continued*) **(C).** Note there is little cortical bone in the neonate, with progressive thickening and development of osteon patterns.

membranous bone to progressively thicken the cortex. Similar endosteal bone formation occurs. As this metaphyseal region thickens, the trabecular bone is progressively invaded by diaphyseal osteon systems, not unlike osteons traversing the fracture site in primary bone healing. This converts peripheral trabecular (woven) bone to lamellar (osteon) bone, which has different biomechanical capacities, and thus progressively transforms metaphyseal cortex into diaphyseal cortex as longitudinal growth continues.

Many leg bones exhibit transversely oriented, dense trabecular patterns in the metaphysis (Fig. 1.6). These usually duplicate the appropriate contiguous physeal contour. They may appear after trauma, particularly when the child has been immobilized (e.g., traction for femoral fracture), and also may appear following generalized illnesses or even localized processes within the bone (e.g., osteomyelitis). They represent a temporary slowdown of normal longitudinal growth rates during the postinjury period or illness and often are referred to as Harris growth arrest lines. Because of the slowdown, the trabeculae of the primary spongiosa become more transversely than longitudinally oriented when initially formed, creating a temporary thickening in the primary spongiosa adja-

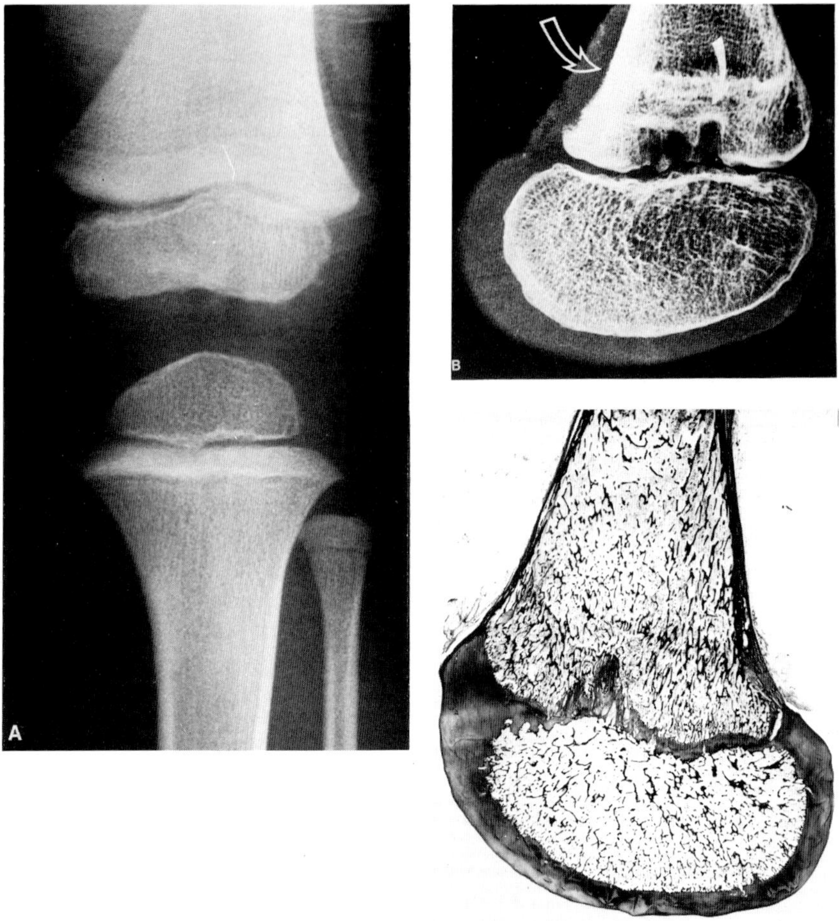

FIGURE 1.6 **A:** Dense metaphyseal bone from slowdown of growth in child undergoing treatment for leukemia. **B:** Radiograph of radioopaque Harris line (*open arrow* and physeal irregularity (*solid arrow*). **C:** Histologic section from patient shown in **B.**

cent to the physis. Once normal longitudinal growth rates resume, longitudinal trabecular orientation is restored. The thickened, transverse osseous plate is "left behind" as the bone continues to elongate and is gradually remodeled as primary spongiosa becomes secondary spongiosa.

Epiphysis

At birth, with the exception of the distal femur, each epiphysis is a completely cartilaginous structure at the end of each long bone. This includes the small longitudinal bones of the hands and feet. Such a

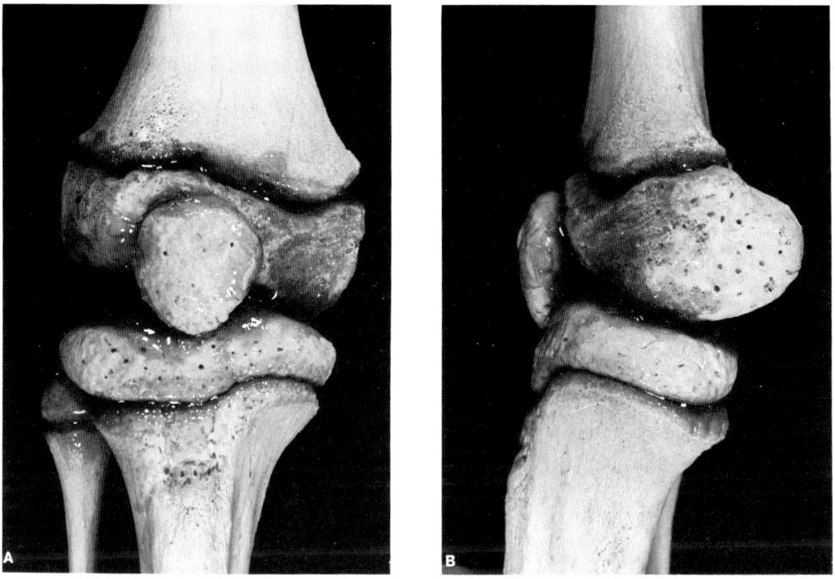

FIGURE 1.7 Anteroposterior **(A)** and lateral **(B)** views of the secondary ossification center (at approximately 6 years of age) in an osseous preparation. Note how the subchondral bone is relatively smooth and has multiple pores through which the vessels necessary for chondro-osseous nutrition traverse.

cartilaginous structure is referred to as the chondroepiphysis; the corresponding ossifying structure is termed the chondro-osseous epiphysis. At a time characteristic for each chondroepiphysis, a secondary center of ossification forms and enlarges until the cartilaginous model has been virtually completely replaced by bone at skeletal maturity (only articular cartilage will remain). With the exception of the distal femur, all secondary (epiphyseal) ossification centers appear postnatally.

As the ossification center expands, it undergoes structural modifications (Fig. 1.7). Particularly, the region adjacent to the physis forms a distinct subchondral plate parallel to the metaphysis, creating the roentgenographically characteristic lucent physeal line. Certain chondroepiphyses exhibit variations in the appearance and enlargement of the ossification centers, factors that must be considered in the appropriate diagnosis of biologic variation rather than congenital variation or traumatic response.

The ossification center imparts increasing rigidity to the more resilient epiphyseal cartilage as the secondary osseous tissue expands. The secondary ossification center progressively enlarges in a pattern reasonably characteristic for each epiphysis.

The appearances of the secondary ossification centers are often variable when comparing one side of the skeleton with the other, and one must be very careful in the evaluation of symmetry versus asymmetry. This process is related to biomechanics, and there often is increased maturation (i.e., ossification) in the epiphyses of the dominant side compared with the nondominant side.

The external surface of an epiphysis is comprised of either articular cartilage or periochondrium. Muscle fibers, tendons, and ligaments attach directly into the perichondrium, which is densely contiguous with the underlying hyaline cartilage. Again, this anatomic arrangement imparts susceptibility to certain types of injury, particularly epiphyseal and physeal fractures. The perichondrium contributes to continued centrifugal enlargement of the epiphysis. It also blends imperceptibly into the periosteum. This perichondrial-periosteal tissue continuity contributes to the biomechanical strength of the region.

Physis

The growth plate, or physis, is the essential mechanism of endochondral ossification. The primary function of the physis is rapid, integrated longitudinal and latitudinal growth.

Since the physeal cartilage remains radiolucent, except for the final stages of physiologic epiphysiodesis, the radiographic appearance often must be inferred from the metaphyseal contour, which follows the physeal contour. The changing size of the secondary ossification center more effectively demarcates the physeal contour on the epiphyseal (germinal layer) side. As this center of ossification enlarges centrifugally to approach the physis, the originally spherical shape of the ossification center flattens and gradually develops a contour paralleling the metaphyseal contour. Similar contouring also occurs as the ossification center approaches the lateral and subarticular regions of the epiphysis. The region of the ossification center juxtaposed to the physis forms a discrete subchondral bone plate through which the epiphyseal blood vessels penetrate to reach the physeal germinal zone.

From a macroscopic viewpoint there are two basic types of growth plates—discoid and spherical. Primary growth plates of the major long bones are discoid. They are characterized by a relatively planar area of rapidly differentiating and maturing cartilage that grades imperceptibly from the epiphyseal hyaline cartilage. Initially, most discoid physes are transversely planar, but with subsequent response to growth and biomechanical stresses, each physis assumes variable degrees of three-dimensional contouring, while retaining the basic planar nature. Additionally, small interdigitations of cartilage extend into the metaphyseal bone. These are termed mammillary processes. Contouring and mammillary processes appear to contribute to the intrinsic stability of the physis, particularly to shearing forces.

Discoid (planar) growth plates also may be found between the metaphysis and an apophysis, which has been defined as an epiphysis subjected primarily to tensile, rather than compressive forces. The tibial tuberosity is such a structure. However, instead of the normal columnar cytoarchitecture, such a tension-responsive structure is characterized by variable amounts of fibrocartilage that represent a microscopic structural adaption of the physis to the high tensile forces imparted by the quadriceps mechanism.

The spherical growth plate, which is the major growth mechanism of the epiphyseal ossification center, also is found in the small bones of the tarsus. By progressive centrifugal expansion, each spherical growth plate gradually assumes the contours of the cartilaginous anlage. Such enlargement of the secondary ossification center leads to juxtaposition of part of the spherical growth plate against the primary discoid physis, creating a bipolar growth zone. Similar bipolar growth zones are present in the acetabular triradiate cartilage and between the proximal tibial and tuberosity ossification centers.

The physis has a characteristic and essentially unchanging basic cytoarchitecture from early fetal life until skeletal maturation. Histologic differences among the various physes are a reflection of growth rates and biomechanical stresses. These variations include the relative numbers of cells in each zone, the overall height of the physis, peripheral differences in the zone of Ranvier, and specific cellular modifications, such as replacement of the zone of hypertrophic cartilage by a zone of fibrocartilage.

Normal Variations

The developing leg, especially the foot skeleton, is subject to considerable variation in the ossification patterns (Fig. 1.7). This is particularly prevalent in the secondary ossification centers and the tarsal bones. Such variation in either the pattern or degree of ossification may even vary from side to side and should make one cautious about the interpretation of symmetry when taking comparison views. Ossification centers do not become smooth until the late stages of chondro-osseous maturation. Regions such as the distal femur can be very irregular, an appearance that probably reflects rapidity of chondro-osseous transformation rather than any discrete response to altered biomechanics or a specific disease state.

Care also must be taken in the arbitrary assignment of the term "congenital variation." There is increasing acceptance that many of the lesions defined as osteochondroses actually may be chronic, stress-related, responses (i.e., the residual of microfractures). Osgood-Schlatter disease certainly fits such a category. Furthermore, disorders such as bipartite patella and accessory navicular, although usually being interpreted as congenital "variations," may be subject to injury, and when patients with such diagnostic findings happen to be acutely symptomatic in that region, the diagnosis of superimposed acute injury must be considered.[21,39] Bone scans showing increased radionuclide uptake can help distinguish the radiologic variation from the injured variation.

Maintenance and Repair

Cartilage and bone are dynamic, mechanically responsive tissues that constantly model and remodel, no matter what the degree of skeletal maturation. Initial responses to stresses occur at a microstructural level and represent either a direct cellular response, as in trabecular bone, or a combined cellular and vascular response, as in cortical bone. The ability to model and remodel requires active physiologic mechanisms. For joint cartilage the physiologic status is maintained through joint motion and fluid dynamics. For the osseous tissues, as well as hyaline epiphyseal cartilage, maintenance is extremely dependent on vascularity.

The developing osseous and cartilaginous components are both extremely vascular.[24,26,27,37,38] The periosteum contains multiple, small vessels that play a role in cortical osteogenesis and contribute to the increasingly complex haversian systems of the immature and mature diaphyseal cortices. The endosteal surfaces of the diaphysis and metaphyses receive blood through the nutrient artery, a major vessel that sends branches to each metaphysis and throughout the diaphysis. The epiphysis receives its blood supply from vessels that penetrate into and ramify through the cartilage and bone. The two major circulatory patterns—epiphyseal and metaphyseal vessels—appear to be functionally and anatomically separate, even after skeletal maturity is attained.

The epiphyseal circulation varies relative to the development and enlargement of the secondary center of ossification. Vessels initially enter the chondroepiphysis within specialized structures termed cartilage canals (Fig. 2). These canals ramify throughout the chondroepiphysis and send branches to the resting/germinal zones of the physis. These canals have several important functional and morphologic characteristics: (a) they supply discrete regions of the epiphysis and physis, with no significant intraepiphyseal anastomoses; (b) the mesenchymal tissue within and around the canals may serve as a source of chondroblastic cells for continued interstitial enlargement of the chondroepiphysis; and (c) the canals play an integral role in the formation of the secondary center of ossification.

The degree of vascularity to the skeleton changes significantly over time. In recent studies major changes in flow distribution patterns were found in the developing canine tibia and femur.[22,23,46] In particular, there was a dramatic quantitative decrease of tibial circulation commensurate with increasing skeletal maturation. If this also occurs in humans, which is quite likely, it would explain the increasing delay in fracture healing and the high incidence of nonunion characteristic of the tibia of an adult. A poor vascular response would impair the early, crucial stages of callus formation. Adequate vascularity is a major factor in fracture healing. These chronobiologic circulatory changes in distribution patterns also affect diagnostic tests such as radionuclide scans. Furthermore, there is a significant correlation between changing flow patterns and the likelihood of hematogenous osteomyelitis.

Regional Development

Pelvis

Each hemipelvis arises as a blastemal condensation that migrates posteriorly toward the somites to establish the sacroiliac articulation, as well as anteriorly to form the pelvic ring and establish anterior continuity at the symphysis pubis. The initial vascular invasion of the ilium occurs between the second and third month. Similar primary ossification centers develop in the ischium and pubis during the fifth to sixth months.[19,20,31] Failure to establish any one of these primary ossification centers would have a variable effect on the overall development of the hemipelvis. Failure of the initial anlagen to form the complete anterior pelvic ring may lead to abnormalities such as exstrophy of the bladder. Failure to adequately differentiate the caudal (lumbosacral) somites causes structural abnormalities of pelvic development, even though overall skeletal differentiation of the lower extremities may continue relatively unaffected. These major pelvic abnormalities lead to variable secondary deformities in the acetabulum, although the proximal femur may be relatively unaffected during the early stages of development.

After each of the three components has undergone the developmental stages of precartilage, cartilage, and primary ossification, a residual area of hyaline cartilage exists where the three anlagen are juxtaposed. This is the triradiate cartilage (Fig. 1.8). The two superior arms are between ilium and pubis anteriorly, and ilium and ischium posteriorly, while the third limb is located inferiorly between the pubis and ischium. The triradiate cartilage effectively divides the acetabulum into three sectors.

Functionally, the intricate interrelationships between acetabular and triradiate cartilage appear necessary to allow progressive expansion of the acetabular "concavity" to accommodate the proximal femoral "convexity." The three growth sectors—iliac, pubic, and ischial—are confluent with respective physeal regions of the acetabulum. Thus, the three physes appose each other through a common epiphysis—the triradiate hyaline

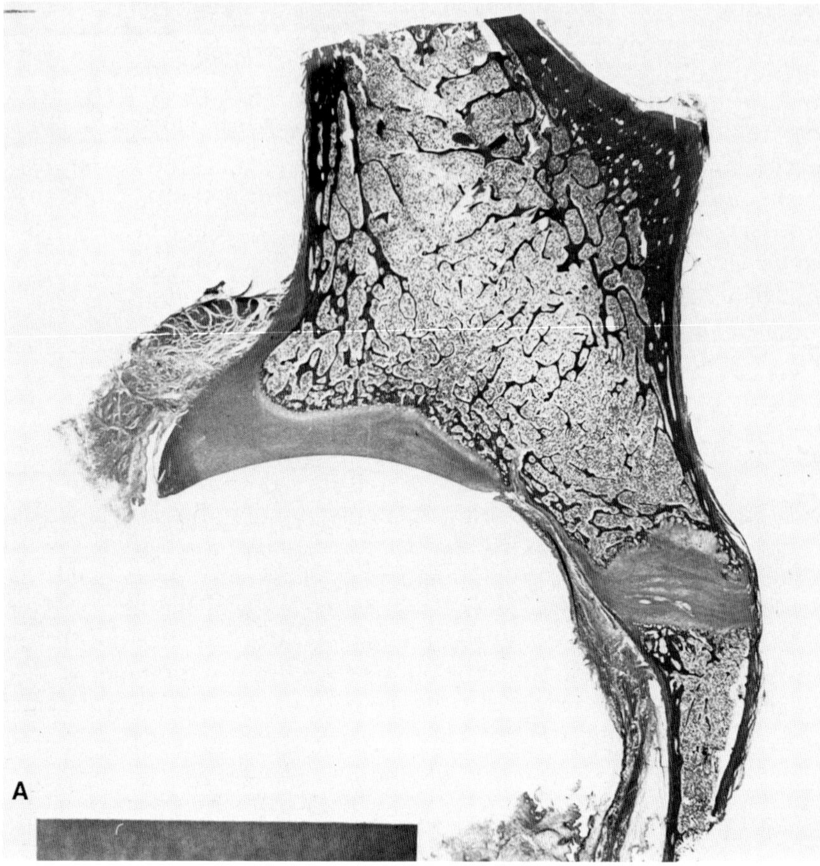

FIGURE 1.8 Acetabular development at 10 **(A)** and 15 **(B)** years. Note the arm of the triradiate cartilage in **A.**

and physeal cartilage. The bone adjacent to each physis is analogous to the metaphysis and thus represents bone capable of considerable remodeling, expecially above the lateral acetabular margin. Interstitial expansion of the physis and epiphysis (triradiate cartilage) may continue unimpeded. This allows progressive expansion of the acetabulum in response to proximal femoral growth. The major function of the triradiate-acetabular cartilage unit is to allow an increase in absolute size of the acetabulum while maintaining congruency between acetabulum and femoral head.

The labrum contributes significantly to overall acetabular depth and femoral head coverage. The component tissue of the labrum and contiguous transverse acetabular ligament is fibrocartilage, although the degree of cellularity and fibrous content change with time. Functionally, this tissue is biologically plastic and readily alters contour to accommodate

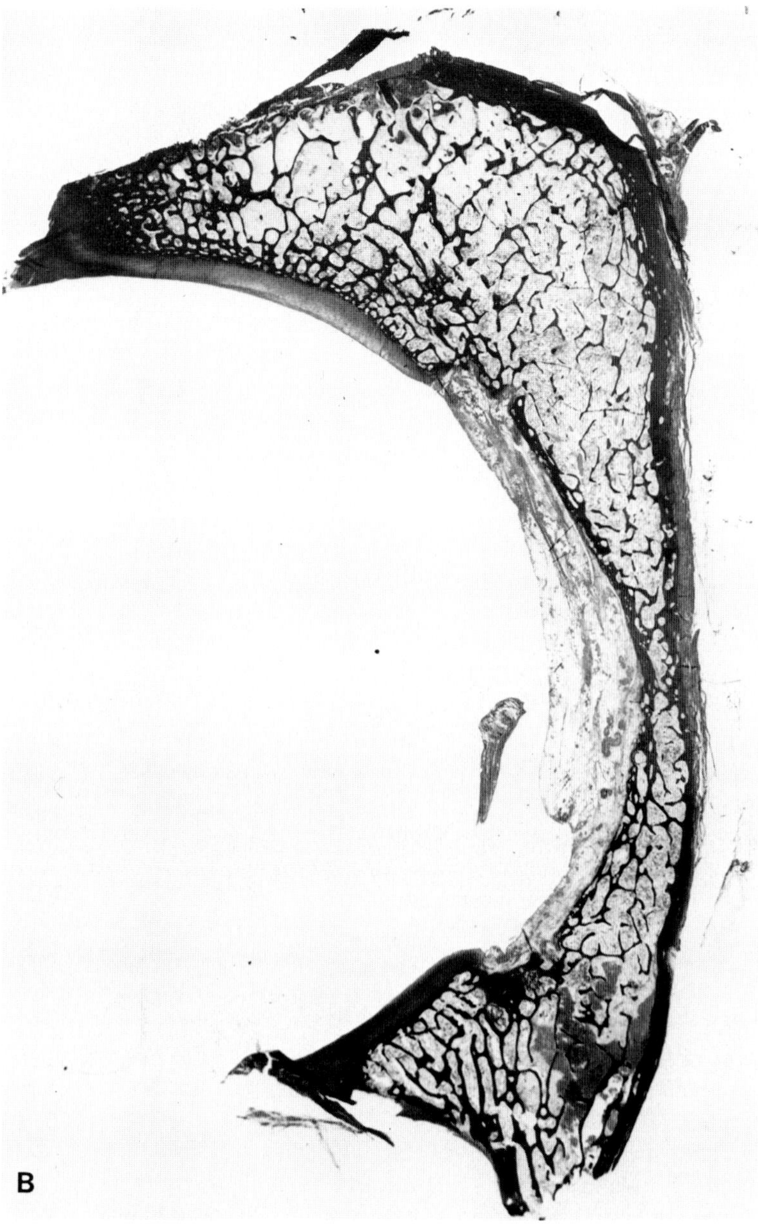

FIGURE 1.8 (*Continued*)

the changing size and shape of the proximal femur (elastic deformation). However, if an abnormal pressure is applied, the deformation may progressively worsen to the stage of plastic deformation, in which case spontaneous recovery of normal contour is slower to occur and, in severe cases, may never completely recur. This biologically pliable rim tissue appears to be one of the major factors in acetabular dysplasia of congenital hip disease. In many cases of mild, prenatal acetabular deformity, the only changes are concomitant deficiency of the fibrocartilaginous labrum anteriorly and minimal eversion of the labrum superiorly and/or posteriorly. In these instances, the hyaline/articular portion did not appear deformed. In more severely involved cases, the anterior labrum had almost completely disappeared.

Of the three osseous components, the ilium seems most subject to mechanical forces, whether normal or abnormal, during the last trimester. This is most evident at the lateral margin of the acetabulum, which is relatively transverse. This region of bone is above the combined physis of the superior two arms of the triradiate cartilage and the superior acetabular cartilage. However, as the fetal hip goes through the rapid enlargement associated with the last trimester, there is a gradual increase in acclivity of the osseous roof owing to a relatively increased growth rate of the more medial portion (i.e., the superior acetabulum). Undoubtedly, there is also a greater biomechanical stimulus to the lateral portion from the position of the femoral head within the acetabulum. The normally situated femoral head may cause enough "pressure" to slow down endochondral ossification rates over the acetabulum, relative to ossification rates in the triradiate cartilage. Progressively increased lateralization of the femoral head, as in a subluxation or even dislocation, could change this "pressure" from physiologic to pathologic and further retard development of the lateral region. In fact, since this is an actively remodeling metaphysis, such an eccentric femoral head might even stimulte osteolysis.

The osseous roof consists of both periosteal and endochondral bone (Fig. 1.8). The periosteal bone may project normally toward the physis of the triradiate cartilage along the inner table, but is less prominent laterally, where the fibrocartilaginous labrum is present.

A soft-tissue structure playing a significant role in the stability of the hip joint in the perinatal period of decreasing head coverage is the joint capsule. On the acetabular side, the capsule attaches to the metaphyseal portion of the ilium, pubis, and ischium, such that the fibrocartilaginous acetabular labrum and transverse acetabular ligament are intracapsular structures. The capsule inserts in the femur along the intertrochanteric region anteriorly and posteriorly. Because very little, if any, femoral neck develops prenatally, only the femoral head is contained within the capsule. The medial metaphysis, which will become a significant intracapsular structure postnatally, is an extracapsular structure for most of prenatal development.

Even during these early development stages, the capsule is a dense, fibrous structure anteriorly and less dense posteriorly. The zona orbicularis, a circumferential fibrous condensation, reinforces the retention of the femoral head by the soft tissues. These circular fibers play a major role prenatally, since the normal hip flexion position relaxes most of the longitudinal fibrous structures. In the third trimester, division of the capsule allows easier subluxation of the femoral head than during the second trimester. However, capsular division must include transection of the zona orbicularis and release of the "suction" effect for the lateral displacement to occur easily. In the normal full-term hip, if the capsule is divided completely circumferentially around the femoral head, the proximal femur may be dislocated only with difficulty. Further, if placed in the acetabulum, the suction effect is recreated immediately. It thus appears that one of the major roles of the soft-tissue restraints (i.e., capsule) is to allow sufficient tissue juxtaposition to create this suction affect, which definitely prevents significant displacement. Even if the hip is dislocated and subsequently relocated, and even if the ligamentum capitum femoris is also transected, it is difficult to redislocate the hip, as the suction affect is quickly reestablished, despite an open capsule, implying this physical affect is not due to joint pressure or fluid, per se, but rather to tissue (joint surface) congruency. As the joint structures become more congruent, this stabilizing affect seems to diminish.[28,40]

Proximal Femur

The initial shape of the femoral head is spherical. This basic shape is maintained throughout prenatal and postnatal development, although the overall contours change slightly. Particularly during the third trimester, increasing fetal size is accompanied by increasing restrictions to joint movement. This causes some mild changes in the biologically plastic femoral head, such that it may be variably molded "out-of-round." An ellipsoid shape is not uncommon. The plasticity of the femoral head (hyaline cartilage) is not as "fluid" as the acetabular labrum (fibrocartilage), so changes, whether normal variations or pathologic deformations, occur more slowly. Similarly, remodeling to restore sphericity also takes longer than restoration of the labral and acetabular contours.

When the first stage of rapid development of primary ossification center is complete, the capitum femoris, greater trochanter, and lesser trochanter are all coextensive cartilaginous structures. As ossification progresses proximally, the lesser trochanter becomes more precisely defined as a discrete structure. By full term, approximately 80% of the cartilaginous model is ossified. At this point, the common physis of the capitum femoris and greater trochanter is above the level of the lesser trochanter. The cell columns of the physis are parallel to the femoral shaft, and the overall contour is transverse to the longitudinal axis. In contrast, the physis of the lesser trochanter is parallel to the longitudinal axis, and the cell columns are perpendicular. Close inspection reveals a distinct continuity of both physeal and epiphyseal cartilage along the posterior intertrochanteric region. Even though the lesser trochanter

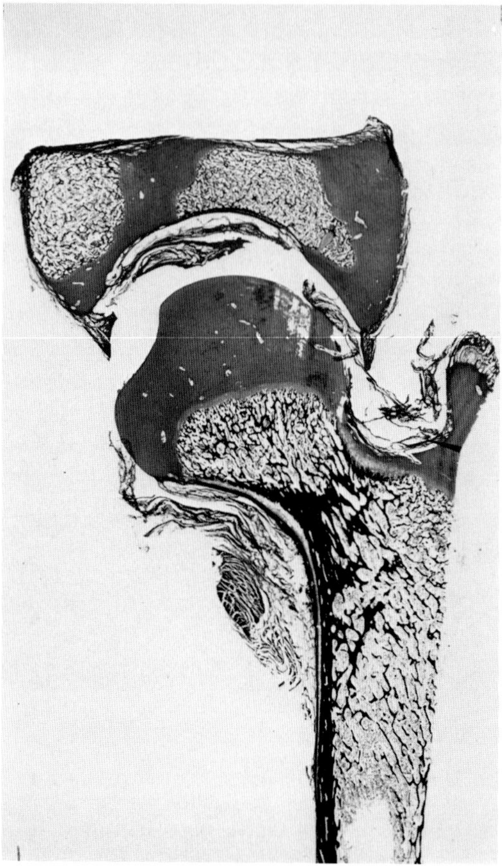

FIGURE 1.9 Acetabulum and proximal femur in a 6-month-old showing continuity of the cartilage along the developing femoral neck.

appears to be an independent structure, at the histologic level it is coextensive with the greater trochanter and capitum femoris. In fact, this histologic continuity with the greater trochanter remains throughout much of postnatal development and should be remembered whenever considering various proximal femoral osteotomies in the region. This continuity probably also plays a factor in the growth mechanisms and direction that lead to eventual physiologic "correction" of anteversion of the femoral neck.

Development of the characteristic femoral neck separating the capitum femoris and greater trochanter is a postnatal event (Fig. 1.9). These two areas are continguous during prenatal development and are grossly separated by the anterior and posterior intertrochanteric indentations, which should not be construed as a true femoral neck. Superiorly, a sulcus connects the anterior and posterior demarcations. The greater trochangeric tip is level with the femoral articular surface for much of the period. Toward term increased development of the femoral head estab-

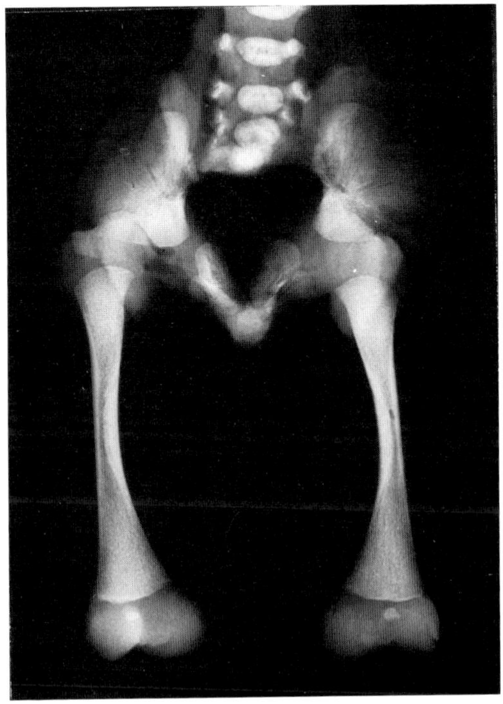

FIGURE 1.10 Radiograph from a neonate (stillborn) with a dysplastic right hip and normal left hip. Note the presence of secondary ossification in both distal femoral epiphyses.

lishes a slight articulotrochanteric difference. However, in some femurs, especially when there is dysplasia of the acetabulum, these two structures may be level, or the greater trochanter may even be higher, creating a relative coxa vara.

Anteversion, or femoral torsion, appears to be a highly variable entity. The commonly accepted angle at term is 35 degrees, with a range from 64 degrees of anteversion to 2 degrees of retroversion. The general consensus is that anteversion is maximal at birth and subsequently decreases throughout postnatal development to an adult norm of 15 degrees.

There has been an emphasis on structural interrelationships, biologic plasticity of the various types of cartilage, and responsiveness of metaphyseal bone to biomechanical forces. As long as the biomechanical factors are normal, then morphologic development also will be within normal ranges, although there will be a reasonable degree of structural variation, as might be expected in any biologic system.

The morphology during the neonatal stage shows a spherical femoral head, variable anteversion, and no osseous femoral neck. The trochanter is level with the femoral articular surface (Fig. 1.10). The normal morphology is thus characterized by very close proximity of the greater and lesser trochanters and capital femur and a neutral articulotrochanteric distance. However, in each ensuing developmental period, the articulotrochanteric distance becomes increasingly positive, commensurate with elongation of the femoral neck, which will progressively displace the capital femoral region of the physis away from the greater trochanteric region of the common physis. Because of the close proximity of these major regions of the proximal femur (capital femur and greater trochanter), marked abduction positions will bring the acetabular rim (labrum) directly into the posterior intertrochanteric region, where the primary vascular supply is found. Similar impingement of rim into the anterior intertrochanteric region can only be accomplished by extreme positions of internal rotation and adduction that are almost anatomically impossible.

The hip capsule attaches along the intertrochanteric region superiorly, anteriorly, and posteriorly just above the lesser trochanter. On the acetabular side, the capsule attaches into bone and hyaline cartilage just beyond the fibrocartilaginous labrum, making the rim, and its transverse acetabular ligament continuation, intracapsular structures. The capsule is loose during this period, allowing partial subluxation of the proximal femur. If the hip joint is fluid-filled, as in septic hip or reactive joint effusion (which are not uncommon complications in the neonatal period), capsular laxity allows the characteristic lateral displacement often used as a diagnostic sign during roentgenography. This capsular laxity also contributes to susceptibility to subluxation or even dislocation during the neonatal period by allowing static or dynamic muscle power, whether normal or unbalanced (e.g., myelomeningocele, beginning changes in cerebral palsy), to progressively displace the femoral head from its normal intra-articular relationship. Certain regions of the capsule, especially inferoposteriorly, exhibit contractures, rather than laxity, as a normal situation during the neonatal period. This is a direct consequence of the particular position in which the hip was held in utero, as well as the ability of the fetus to move in utero. These contractures, which are present in the inferior and posterior regions, predispose to externally rotating and adducting the hip, a possible factor in gradual anterolateral displacement, which may lead to subluxation or even dislocation in later stages of the first year of life. As the hip overcomes the intrauterine flexion contracture and becomes more extended, the ligamentum capitum femoris apparently plays a major role in preventing hip subluxation.

The labrum is an extremely pliable structure and may be easily deformed by chronic pressure from a subluxating or dislocated femoral head. Because of the inherent elasticity, it is not possible to acutely invert major portions of this structure experimentally and have them remain inverted. Upon release of the deforming pressure, the labrum immediately springs back to its normal anatomic position. The basic biomechanics of this rim structure therefore enhance the argument that congenital hip disease be considered a *progressive,* rather than acute, problem of the perinatal period.

The proximal femoral epiphysis is a completely cartilaginous structure with three discrete regions—capital femoral epiphysis, greater trochanteric epiphysis, and the intervening intraepiphyseal region. Underlying this unitary epiphysis is a transversely oriented growth plate. The most medial portion of this structure, as well as the juxtaposed metaphysis, are intracapsular structures. This anatomic position of the medial metaphysis explains intracapsular, rather than subperiosteal, decompression of proximal femoral osteomyelitis into the hip joint to create a concomitant septic hip (as is shown later, osteomyelitis characteristically affects the metaphysis directly under the capital femur during this age range).

Roentgenographic interpretation of the neonatal hip is difficult because of the cartilaginous structure and lack of orienting areas such as the capital femoral secondary ossification center. The triradiate cartilage is probably the most reliable reference point, especially when obtaining special radiographic views. The aforementioned capsular laxity also may allow hip motion, particularly during abduction positioning, to create an "air arthrogram" phenomenon. Familiarity with the normal roentgenographic anatomy of the neonatal hip can only lead to a better appreciation of normal versus abnormal angles and contours in the portions that are ossified and to a better realization that diagnosis of some types of congenital hip dysplasia are probably quite feasible with the use of roentgenography in the neonatal period.

Two major changes commence during the 3- to 6-month period: (1) beginning development of the femoral neck, with a more rapid growth of the medial side of the physis and metaphysis and (2) initial development of the capital femoral secondary ossification center. The hip continues to exhibit a significant degree of capsular laxity, allowing variable subluxation of the proximal femur if appropriate stresses are applied, or if there is excessive intra-articular fluid under pressure. As the femoral neck develops, more of the medial metaphysis becomes intracapsular, further increasing the likelihood of decompression of proximal femoral osteomyelitis into the hip joint. Growth of the acetabular labrum makes it a more evident structure with an increasingly important role in stabilizing the hip. There is continued susceptibility to vascular damage as the femoral neck develops. Since this is the period of initial appearance of the secondary ossification center, which depends upon an adequate blood supply derived primarily through the posterosuperior vessels, occlusion of the vessels by abduction treatment will seriously impair this stage of chondro-osseous transformation. As in the previous period, the structure most likely to cause selected vascular compression or occlusion is the acetabular labrum.

Radiographically, the secondary ossification center most commonly appears from 4 to 6 months. Delay in appearance should make one suspicious of vascular compromise only if the child were being treated for congenital hip disease, or some comparable situation, such as septic hip, where the hip required immobilization or had been treated with an open surgical procedure. However, delay in development also might suggest mild subluxation or muscle imbalance, as one of the factors that appears to stimulate ossification is adequate, appropriately directed, joint reaction forces. Certainly, the overall tendency to develop the secondary center is programmed genetically to appear approximately in this period; however, the preprogrammed direction of the cells capable of transforming cartilage into bone would seemingly require appropriate biomechanical stress. The osseous acetabular roof matures rapidly and should exhibit an acetabular index under 25 degrees by the end of this period. However, the soft-tissue components still extend the roof much further than is radiologically evident.

From 6 to 12 months the femoral neck continues elongation and establishes a discrete area defined as the capital femoral physis. Histologically, this region is developing a demarcation from the intraepiphyseal growth plate, establishing a certain degree of independence of the medial portion of the physis, a factor that will be important in the subsequent development of the femoral neck. Concomitant with elongation of the femoral neck, there is increasing separation of the capital femoral and greater trochanteric regions, although there is still a relatively large amount of hyaline cartilage in the intraepiphyseal region, which serves as a definite continuity between the two major developing regions of the proximal femoral epiphysis. As the neck develops, the superior articular surface of the capital femur gradually becomes more "proximal" than the greater trochanter, firmly establishing a positive articulotrochanteric distance. The secondary ossification center continues to mature as an enlarging spherical osseous mass (Fig. 1.11).

From 1 to 2 years the femoral neck continues to elongate, particularly leading to narrowing and lengthening of the intraepiphyseal hyaline cartilage zone, which makes this region decreasingly susceptible to direct vascular compression than during the previous developmental periods. The physis of the intraepiphyseal regions still contains a preponderance of columnated cells typical of compression—responsive growth plate cytoarchitecture. The increased growth of the medial physis leads to a more specific definition of the capital femoral physis. However, intraepiphyseal and trochanteric physes are still histologically indistinguishable. The secondary ossification center continues expansion and flattens where there is juxtaposition to the metaphysis, creating a hemispherical shape (rather than the original spherical appearance). This establishes a bipolar growth zone between the capital femoral ossification center and metaphysis. The capsule exhibits decreasing laxity so that subluxation becomes a less significant factor. The medial physis, in response to normal hip joint mechanics (joint reaction forces), is beginning to angulate as well as to develop mammillary processes, which give the physis an undulated

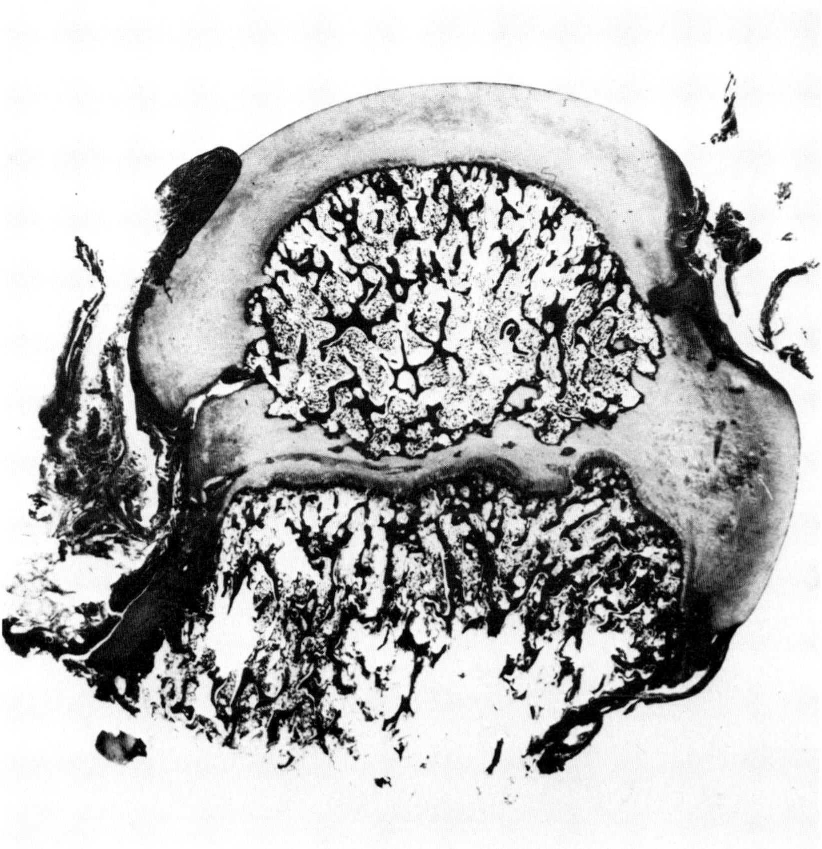

FIGURE 1.11 Secondary ossification center of the capitum femoris in a 10-month-old. Note the indentation of the fovea centralis and the large, solitary vessel supplying the capital femoral ossification center.

appearance. The processes probably increase resistance of the physis to shear stresses. The ligamentum capitum femoris enters a deepening fovea capitus.

From 3 to 10 years the secondary ossification center of the greater trochanter expands and is often associated with an additional ossification center near the proximal end of the remaining hyaline cartilage, which is comparable to the ossification pattern in the proximal tibial epiphysis and tibial tuberosity. This accessory secondary ossification center rapidly fuses with the main secondary center. The ossification of the capital femur enlarges in a hemispherical fashion, filling most of the epiphysis out to the metaphyseal margins. The area juxtaposed to the fovea capitus develops a distinct indentation in the ossification center. Interdigitating

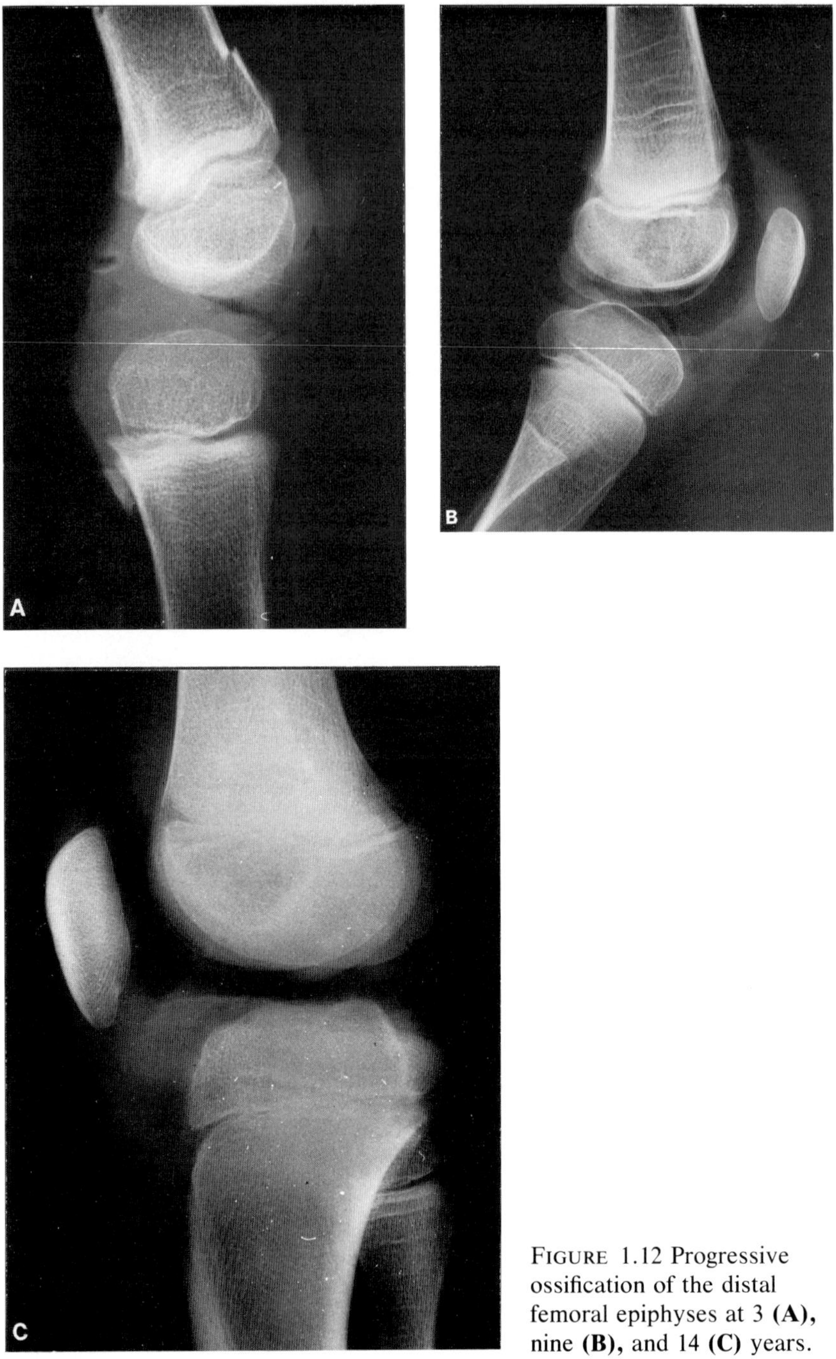

FIGURE 1.12 Progressive ossification of the distal femoral epiphyses at 3 **(A)**, nine **(B)**, and 14 **(C)** years.

mammillary processes continue to develop as discrete regions of the capital femoral physis. By the end of this stage of development, the proximal femur has formed the final anatomic contours of mild anteversion, functionally separate femoral head and trochanter (although still anatomically interconnected), and neck/shaft angle. Most subsequent growth through adolescence will comprise remodeling of trabecular patterns and integrated enlargement of capital femur and trochanter. By the end of this stage, the discrete trabecular arching patterns along the femoral neck are well established. The trabecular patterns show continuity of patterning as a stress response in both the capital femur and the femoral neck. Prior to this particular developmental stage, the patterning in the secondary ossification center of the capital femur had been seemingly indiscriminate and certainly not related to the beginning developmental patterns in the femoral neck and along the developing calcar femorale.

From 11 to 16 years there is a period of rapid growth of the femoral neck, which may be related to susceptibility to slipped capital femoral epiphysis and which ends with physiologic closure of the physis. Of the three active growth regions of the proximal femur, the capital femoral physis is the first to close. The closure process begins centrally, with increasing thickness of the subchondral bone plate of the epiphysis and similar thickening of the trabecular bone of the underlying metaphysis. Gradually, the growth plate cells become less functional, form occasional closures, rather than cell columns, and the entire plate begins to thicken. Similarly, as growth slows down, there is thickening of the subchondral region of the metaphysis, creating two dense osseous zones on either side of the cartilaginous growth plate. These dense osseous regions on either side of the attenuating physis begin to join by small bridges that gradually increase in size. This fusion progresses in a centrifugal fashion, incorporating the entire capital femoral physis and leading to a fusion between the epiphyseal ossification center and metaphysis. As this fusion is nearing completion in the capital femur, a similar process is just beginning in the greater trochanteric physis. Growth may continue, albeit slow, in the greater trochanter after cessation of capital femoral growth. In situations such as slipped capital femoral epiphysis, which is often associated with premature cessation of growth of the capital femoral physis, continued trochanteric growth may lead to loss of the articulotrochanteric distance; in the case of moderate to severe slips, it may contribute to the marked overgrowth of the trochanter (negative articulotrochanteric distance).

As the capital femoral ossification center progressively expands, the hyaline cartilage is completely replaced, leaving a thin layer of articular cartilage that is separated from the underlying maturing subchondral plate by the "tide" mark. This normal thinning of the cartilage may be misinterpreted radiographically as a pathologic narrowing of the joint

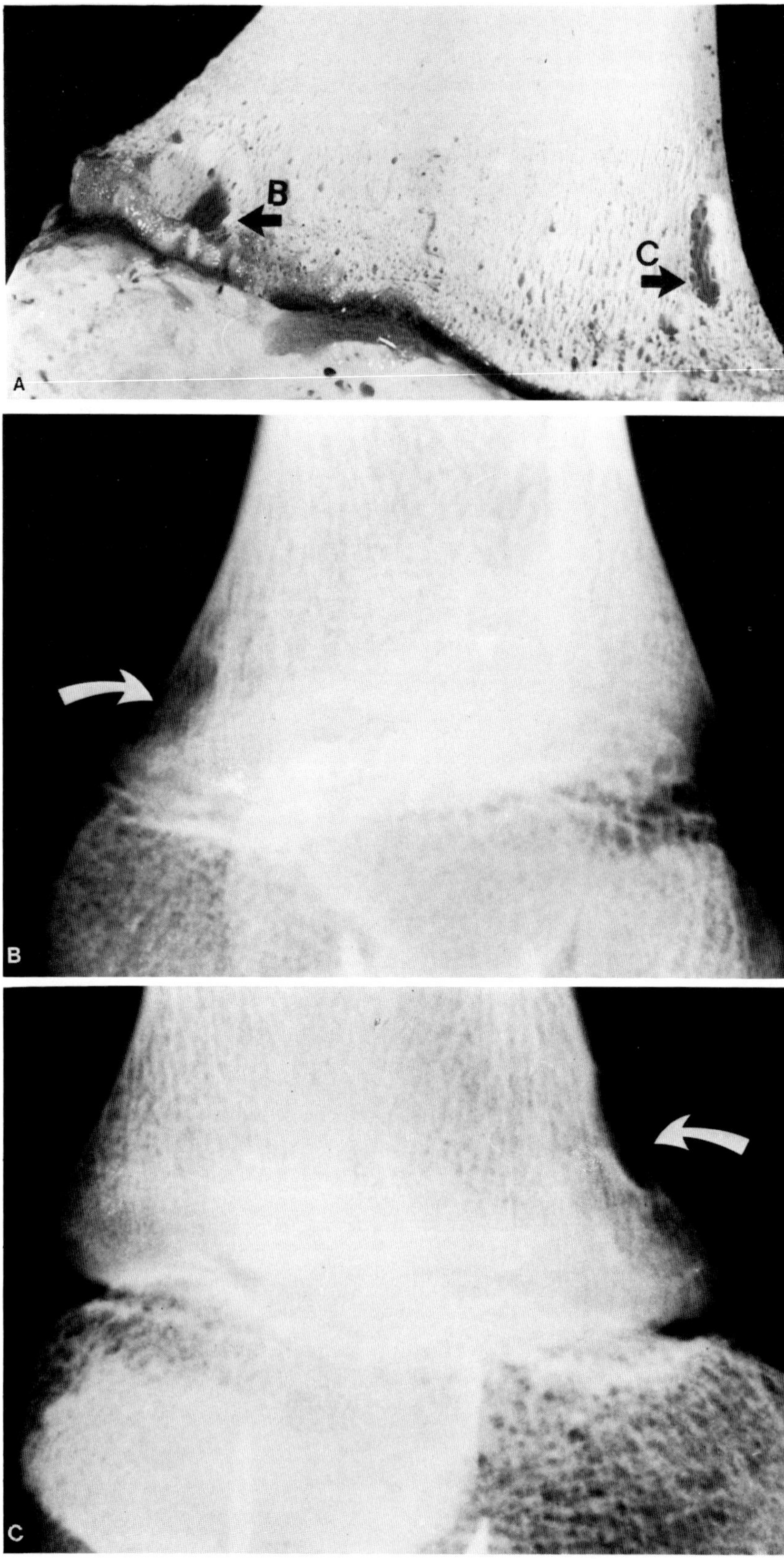

B
C
A
B
C

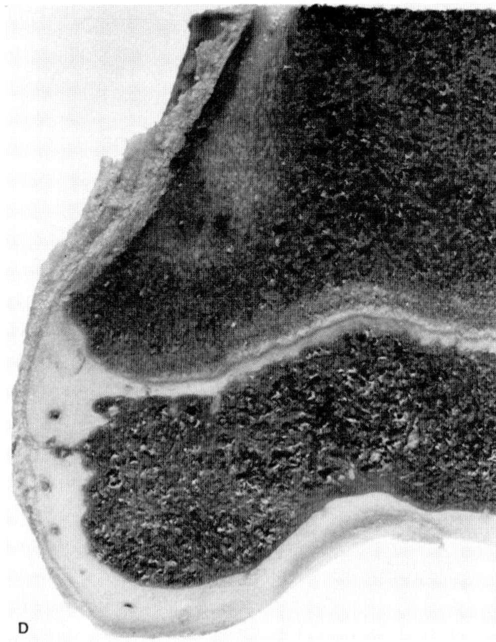

←

FIGURE 1.13 **A:** Osseous preparation of the distal femur in an 11-year-old showing two craterlike "defects" that appear radiographically as depicted in **B** and **C. D:** Slab section showing textural difference between trabecular bone and the fibrous cortical "defect."

space in diseases such as slipped capital femoral epiphysis and idiopathic cartilage necrosis.

Distal Femur

Distal femoral epiphyseal ossification is usually present at birth and is the only secondary center to begin formation (Fig. 1.10). Its presence in a radiograph is indicative of a full-term pregnancy. The initial secondary center is spherical and centrally located. Expansion and maturation then change it to a more elliptical shape and subsequently to a contour following the binodal epiphyseal contours.[3] The last area to ossify is the posterior portion of each condyle (Fig. 1.12). The physis develops a binodal contour in both coronal and sagittal planes, effectively becoming a quadrinodal structure. This occurs in midchildhood. Prior to that the physis is more transversely oriented. Peripheral lappet formation is evident within the first 18 months.

The distal femoral metaphysis is extremely fenestrated and, because of the significant amount of longitudinal growth, is constantly remodeling the cortex. This leads to a high incidence of modeling variations, the most common of which is the fibrous cortical defect. Simple irregularity of the medial metaphyseal cortex is also common (Fig. 1.13).

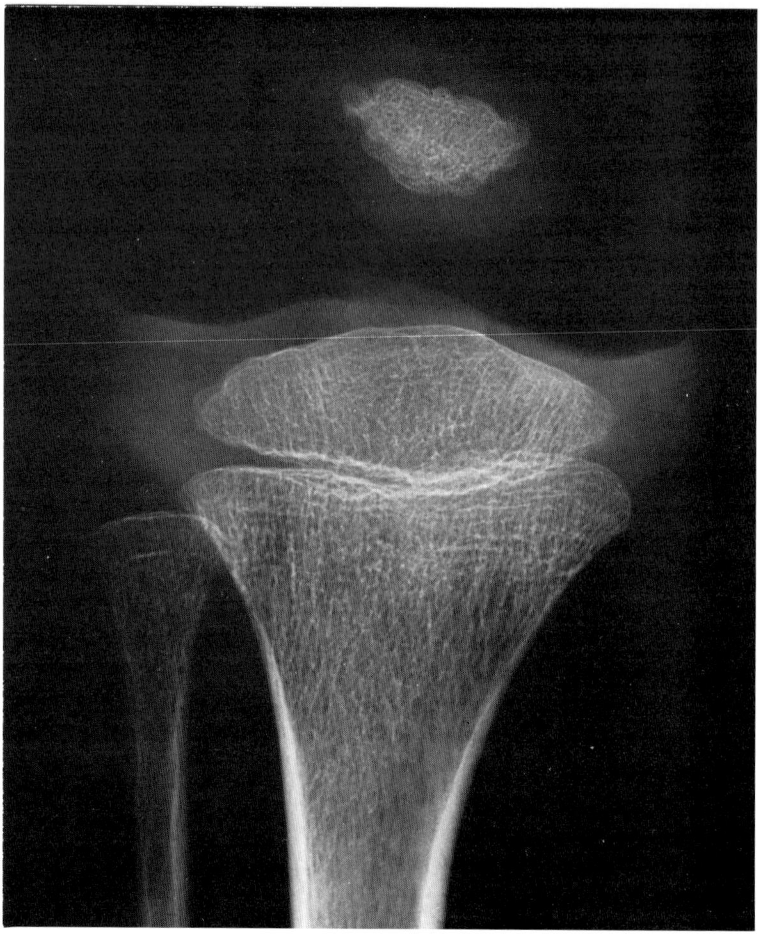

FIGURE 1.14 Irregular marginal ossification around patella.

Patella

The patella initially ossifies between 3 and 5 years, commencing as multiple foci that rapidly coalesce. As the patellar ossification center enlarges, the expanding margins may be irregular (Fig. 1.14) and associated with accessory ossification centers. These are most common superolaterally and may lead to the development of a bipartite patella, which has cartilaginous continuity despite the appearance of osseous discontinuity (Fig. 1.15). The patella expands to all cartilaginous contours during late adolescence when the epiphyseal ossification centers around the knee are also in the final stages of maturation (Fig. 1.16). The only cartilage not replaced is that occupying the superior two thirds of the articular surface (the lower one third is covered by the fat pad). The subchondral plate

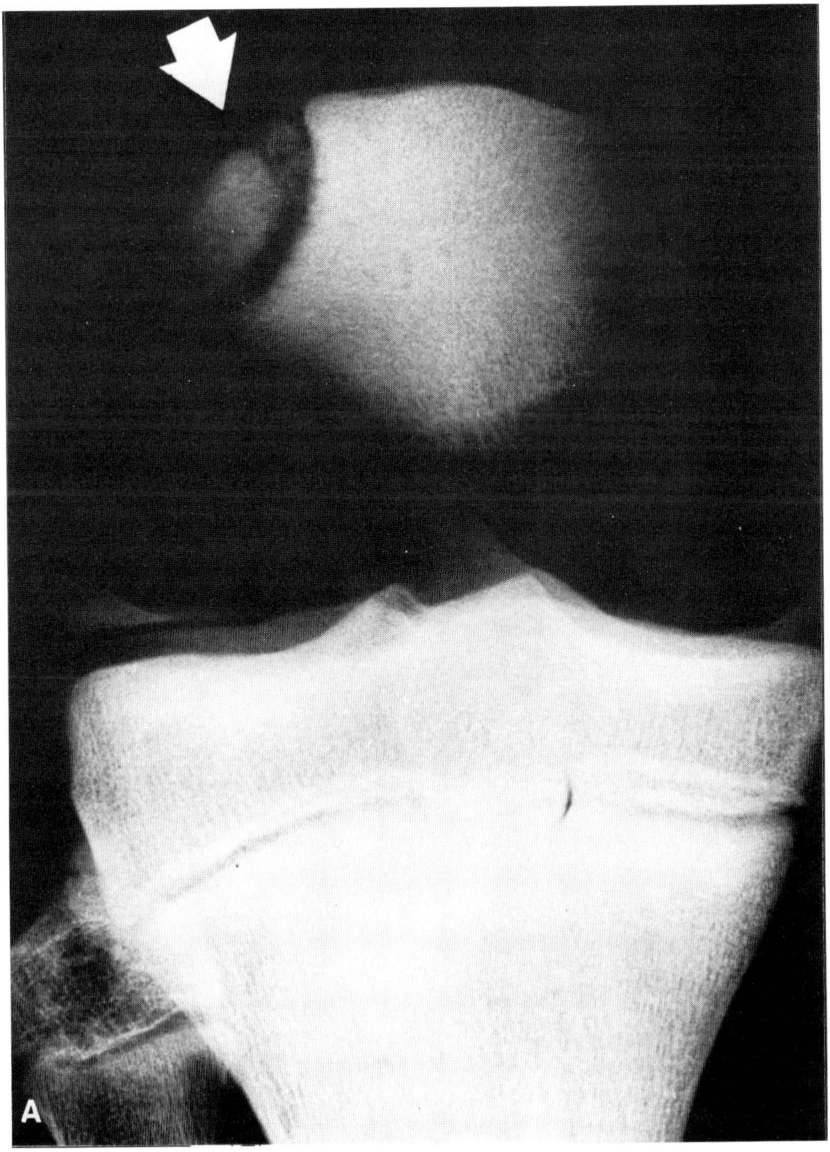

FIGURE 1.15 **A:** Specimen radiograph of bipartite patella (*arrow*) in an adolescent. **B:** Slab radiograph of specimen showing continuity of cartilage despite seeming osseous separation.

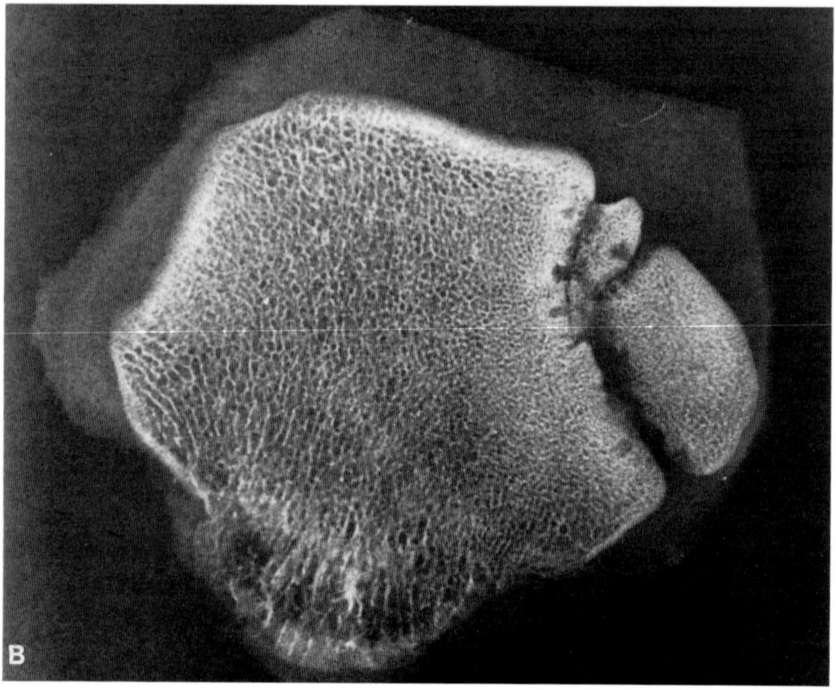

FIGURE 1.15 (*Continued*)

does not assume the actual articular contours until the late stages of osseous maturation, i.e., after 10 to 12 years. Accordingly, typical measurements such as medial and lateral angulation cannot be accurately done prior to the final stages of patellar ossification expansion and maturation.

Knee Joint

The articular contours of the knee joint remain virtually unchanged throughout postnatal skeletal development. Similarly, the various ligaments are the same, other than exhibiting a greater natural degree of laxity in early and midchildhood (Fig. 1.17). The menisci change from vascular structures to ones with only peripheral vascularity at maturation.[8] However, their basic shape, whether medial or lateral, is maintained throughout both prenatal and postnatal development. A discoid lateral meniscus is definitely an abnormal state and not an extreme normal variation of lateral meniscal development.

Proximal Tibia and Fibula

Proximal tibial ossification usually begins within the first 3 months following birth.[35] The initial secondary ossification is centrally located

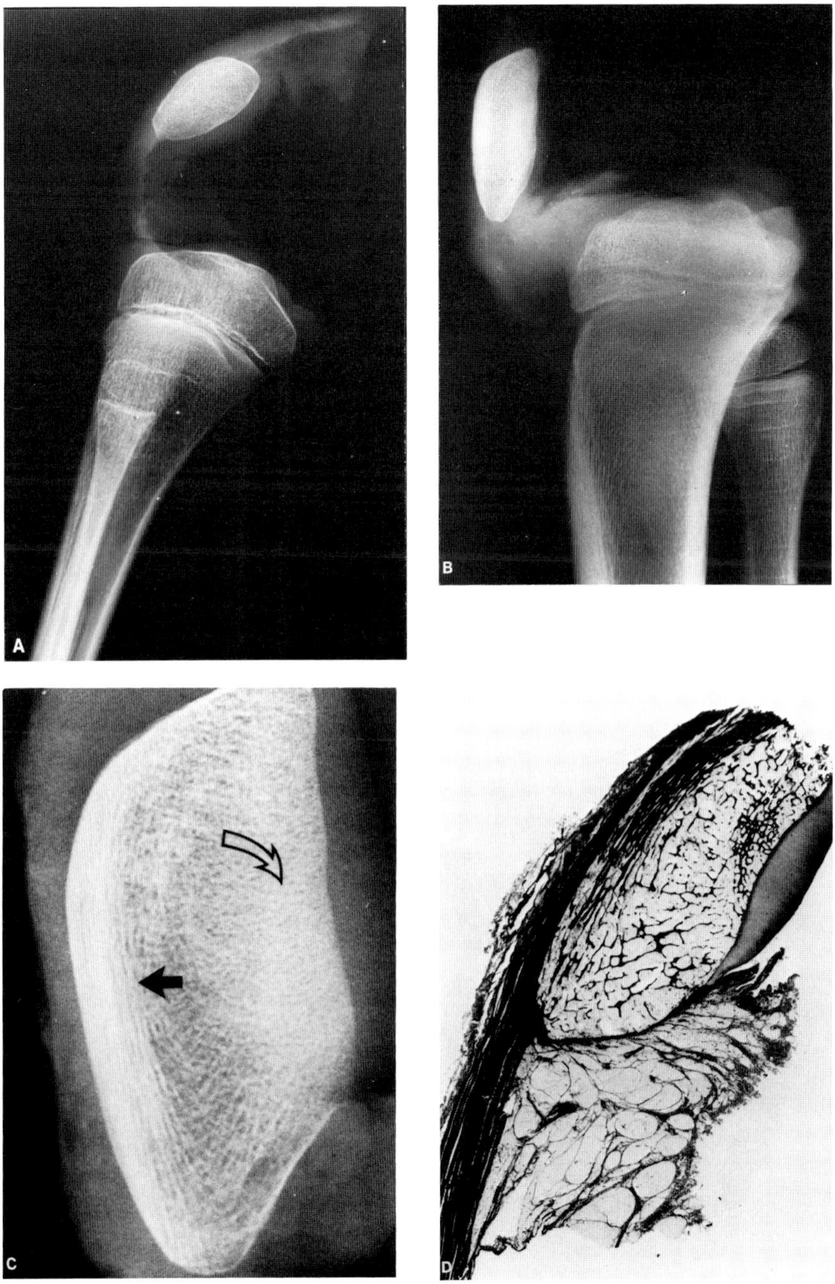

FIGURE 1.16 **A:** Radiograph of proximal tibia and patella from a 10-year-old. Note the patella is elliptical. **B:** Patella in a 15-year-old now exhibits a posterior contour that reflects the articular two thirds, nonarticular (inferior) one third of the mature patella. **C:** Specimen radiograph of patella from an adolescent showing compression (*open arrow*) and tension (*solid arrow*) responsive trabecular orientation. **D:** Histologic section of similar patella.

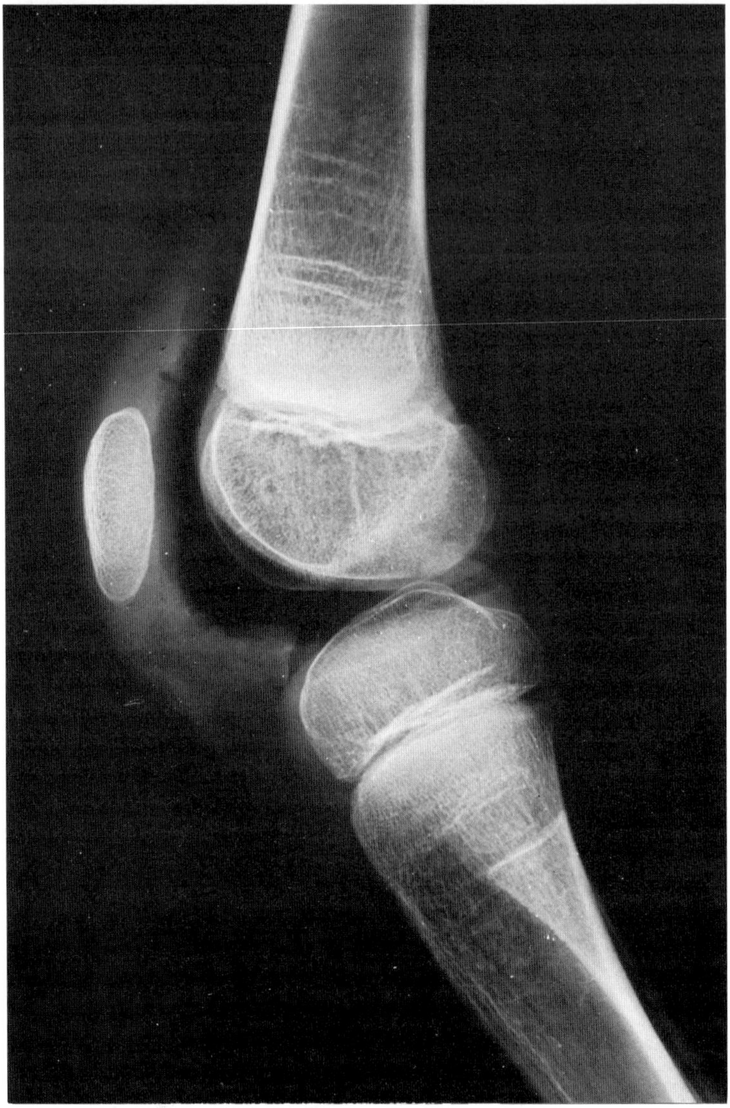

FIGURE 1.17 Lateral view of knee in a specimen from a 9-year-old boy. Air has been introduced into the joint to outline contours.

and spherical. Expansion and maturation then change the ossification center to a more elliptical shape. Variability in this expansion medially and laterally may create marginal irregularity in the first few years. Subsequently, ossificaton extends into the tibial spines as a single conical mass that eventually divides into two separate extensions (Figs. 1.18, 1.19). The physis remains relatively transverse throughout development, although contouring occurs under each tibial weight-bearing com-

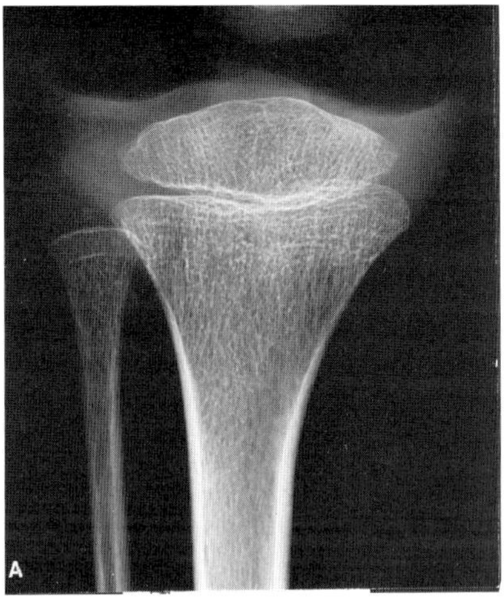

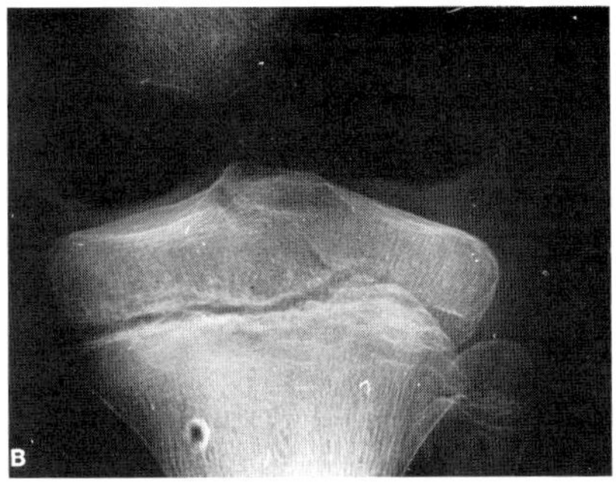

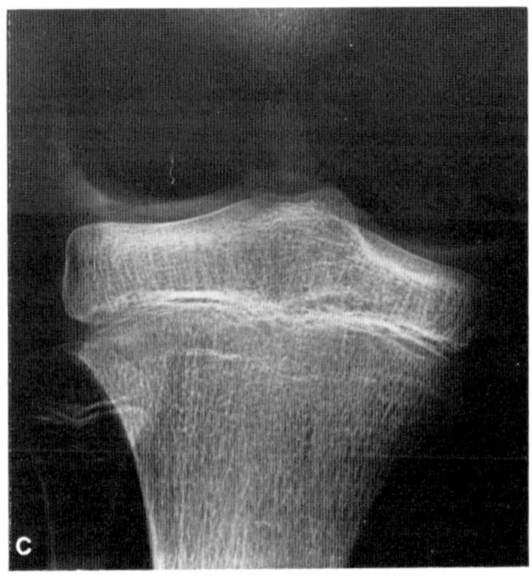

FIGURE 1.18 Progressive development of the proximal tibial ossification center at 7 **(A)**, 12 **(B)**, and 16 **(C)** years.

partment. Peripheral lappet formation appears within a few months. Anteriorly, there is an undulation at the site of the cartilaginous tibial tuberosity.

The proximal fibular physis begins as a transverse contour, but changes to one with peripheral lappet formation and multiple undulations. Secondary ossification begins just above the physis and extends proximally into the rest of the physis. However, the fibular styloid, similar to the ulnar styloid, does not ossify until late skeletal maturation. The proximal fibular physis usually is situated 5 to 10 mm distal to the tibial physis (Fig. 1.20).The tibiofibular joint morphology has considerable morphologic variation, and the joint may communicate with the knee joint.[25]

The angle of the proximal tibiofibular joint is undoubtedly a reflection of the amount of fibular rotation necessary to accommodate talar morphology during ankle flexion and extension.

Tibial Tuberosity

The tibial tuberosity develops by a concomitant and juxtaposed outgrowth of hyaline cartilage and ingrowth of fibrovascular tissue.[29,33] During the fetal period, this hyaline cartilage outgrowth is progressively

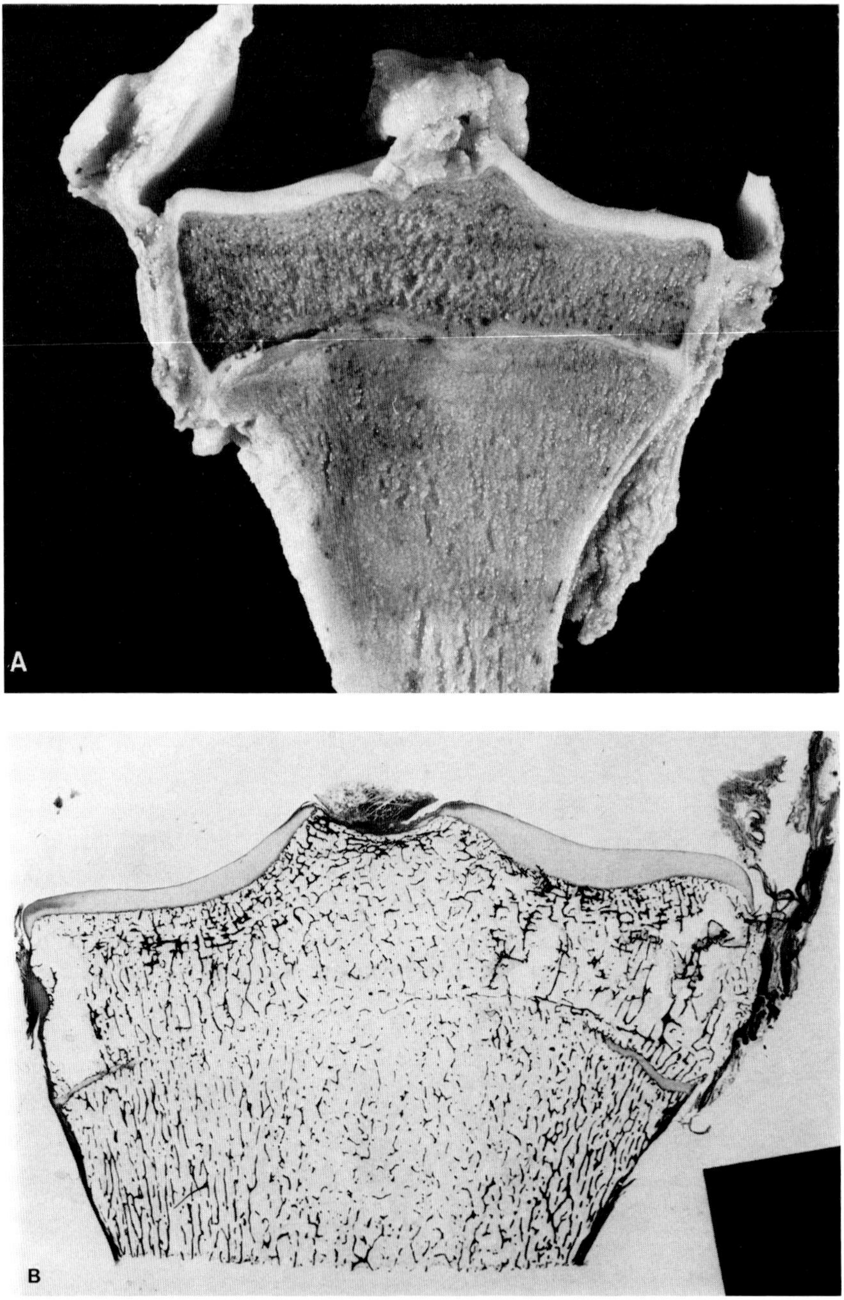

FIGURE 1.19 **A:** Slab section of proximal tibia at 15 years. **B:** Microscopic section of proximal tibia from a 17-year-old boy. This shows central closure, with peripheral physeal remnants.

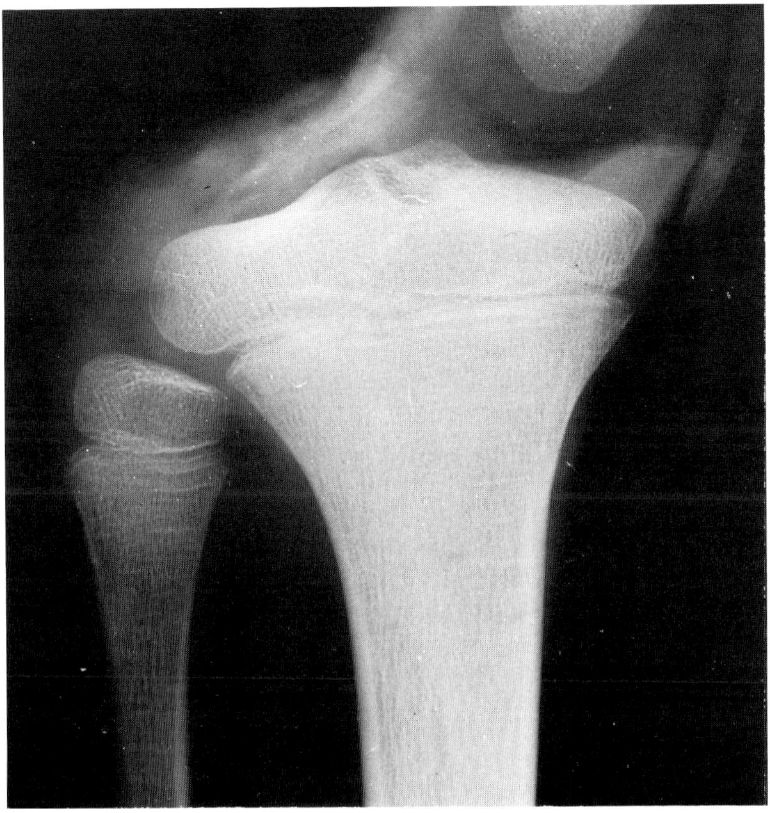

FIGURE 1.20 Relationship between the proximal fibula and tibula.

distally displaced to become situated adjacent to the anterior portion of the tibial metaphysis. About 4 to 6 months postnatally a growth plate develops under the tibial tuberosity. This growth plate shows structural adaptations that permit accommodation of large tensile stresses. The growth plate of the tibial tuberosity has three distinct regions: (1) a zone of endochondral bone formation, (2) a zone of intramembranous bone formation through fibrocartilage, and (3) a zone of intramembranous bone formation through fibrous tissue.

The tibial tuberosity begins ossification between 7 and 9 years as a distal focus.[36,41] This progressively enlarges proximally and anteriorly, while the main tibial ossification center concomitantly expands downward into the tuberosity (Fig. 1.21). A section of epiphyseal cartilage remains between these two ossification centers until close to physeal maturity. The anterior chondro-osseous region at the site of the patellar tendon attachment is a biomechanically susceptible region that may be acutely or chronically traumatized to create an Osgood-Schlatter lesion. The physis

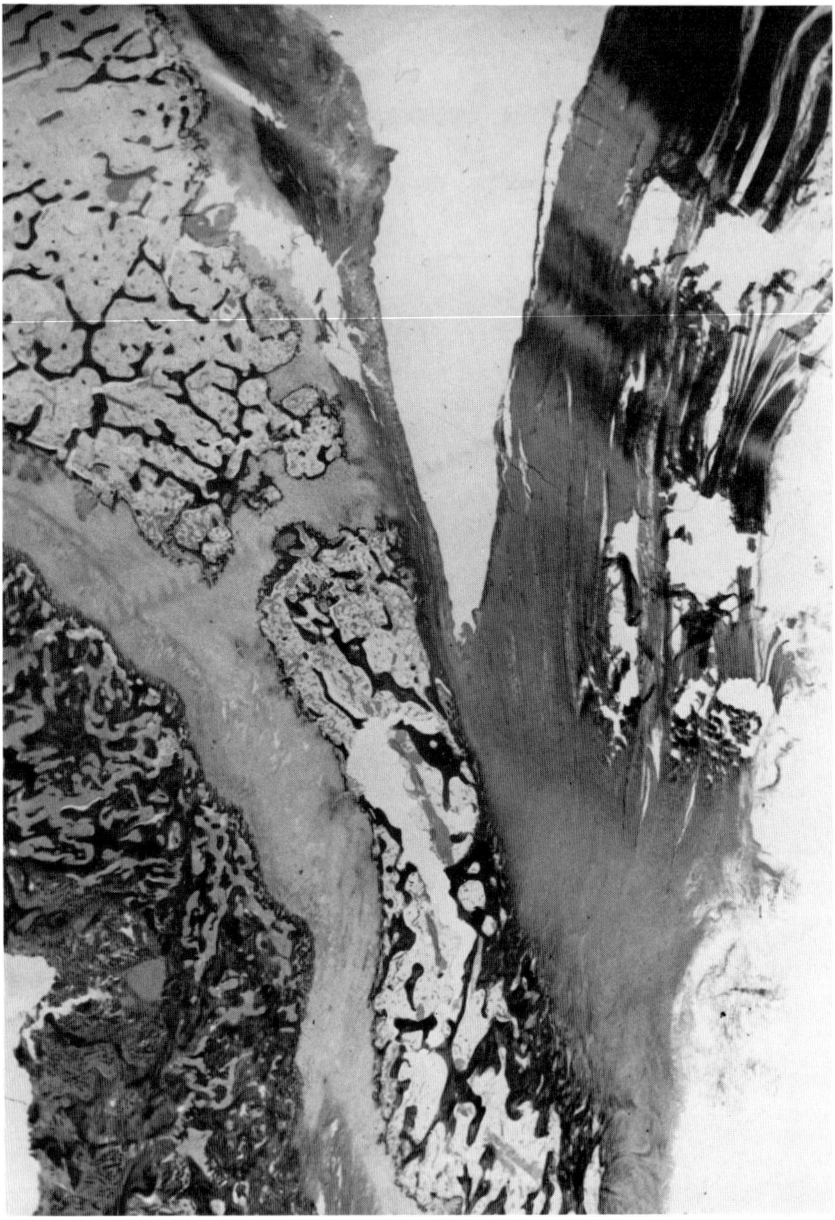

FIGURE 1.21 Histologic section of tibial tuberosity showing attachment of the patella tendon.

FIGURE 1.22 Progressive ossification of the distal tibia and fibula at 6 **(A)**, 9 **(B,C)**, and 13 **(D,E)** years.

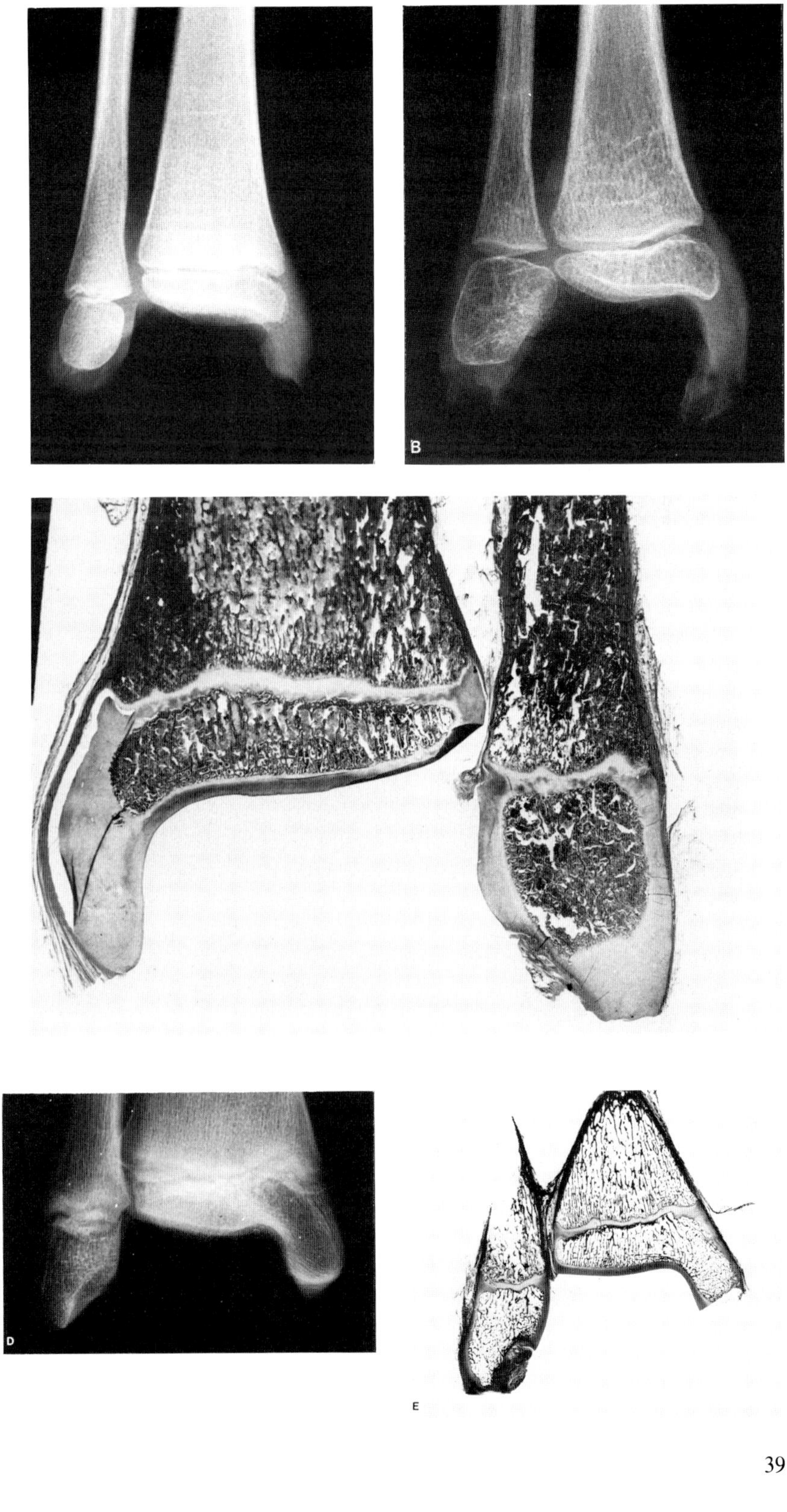
B
D
E

associated with the tibial tuberosity is histologically modified in a proximal to distal gradation of columnar adaption to specific biomechanical demands in this region. Closure of the tuberosity physis occurs in a proximal to distal direction.[41]

Distal Tibia and Fibula

Initially the distal tibial physis is a relatively transverse structure. As the epiphysis matures, undulations develop within the physis and lappet formation occurs peripherally.[32] Within the first 2 years, a significant physeal undulation develops anteriorly above the medial malleolus. This undulation must not be misinterpreted as premature epiphysiodesis following distal tibial fracture. Secondary ossification in the distal tibia begins centrally and initially expands to fill the area over the tibial plafond. At the lateral side of the tibial epiphysis the ossification center may be wedge-shaped. The medial margin adjacent to the medial malleolus is often irregular and may show small peripheral foci of ossification. (Fig. 1.22).

By 7 to 8 years the secondary center expands into the medial malleolus, with complete distal extension often not occurring until adolescence

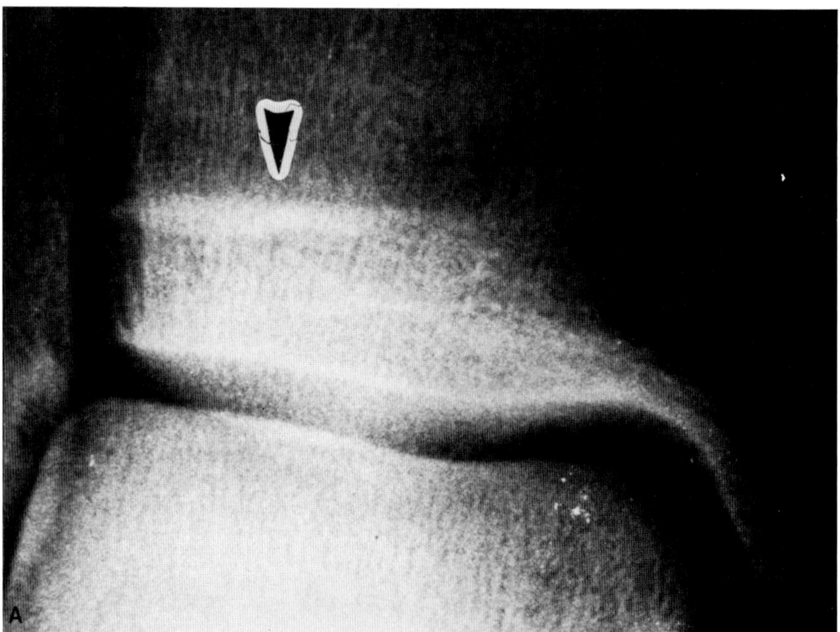

FIGURE 1.23 **A:** Pattern of closure of distal tibia, with more medial side closing and remodeling slightly ahead of the lateral side (*arrow*). **B:** Histologic Section.

(although usually complete by 10 to 11 years). The malleolar tip may exhibit an accessory ossification center. Physiologic epiphysiodesis begins over the medial malleolus and subsequently extends laterally (Fig. 1.23). This pattern of closure appears to predispose to fracture of the lateral portion of the distal tibial epiphysis (fracture of Tillaux), as well as to triplane fractures. The articular surface curves onto the lateral side of the distal tibia to form an articulation with the lateral malleolus (distal tibiofibular joint). A similar extension occurs along the medial side of the fibula. These surfaces extend proximally as a recess to the level of the distal tibial physis, at which point the interosseous ligament begins. This type of minimally mobile joint is termed a syndesmosis.

The initially transverse distal fibular physis becomes a convoluted

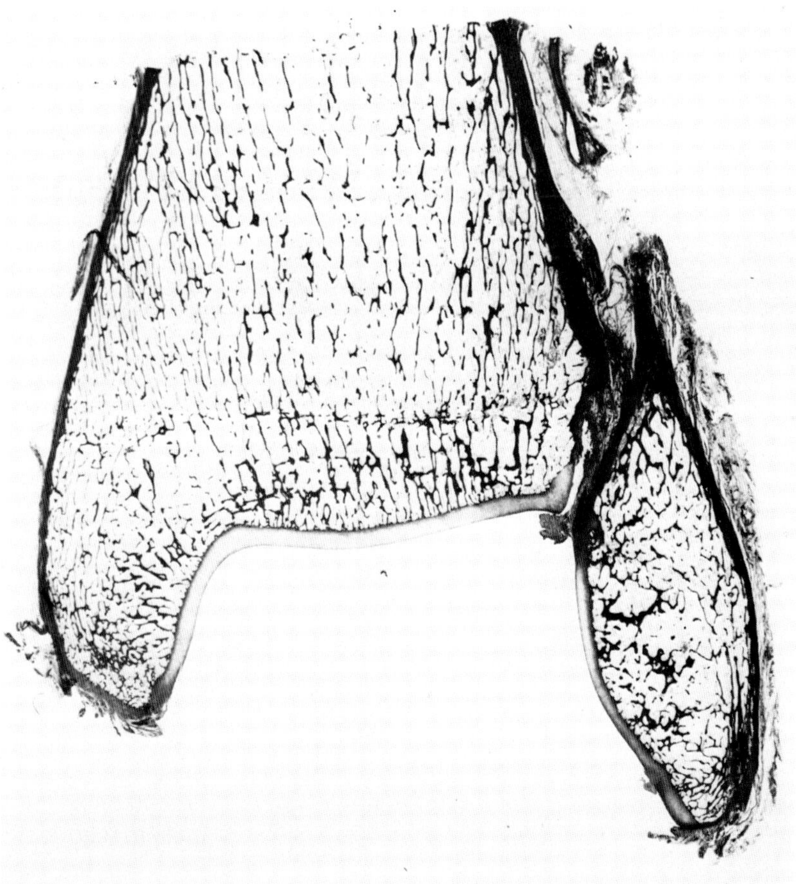

B

FIGURE 1.23 (*Continued*)

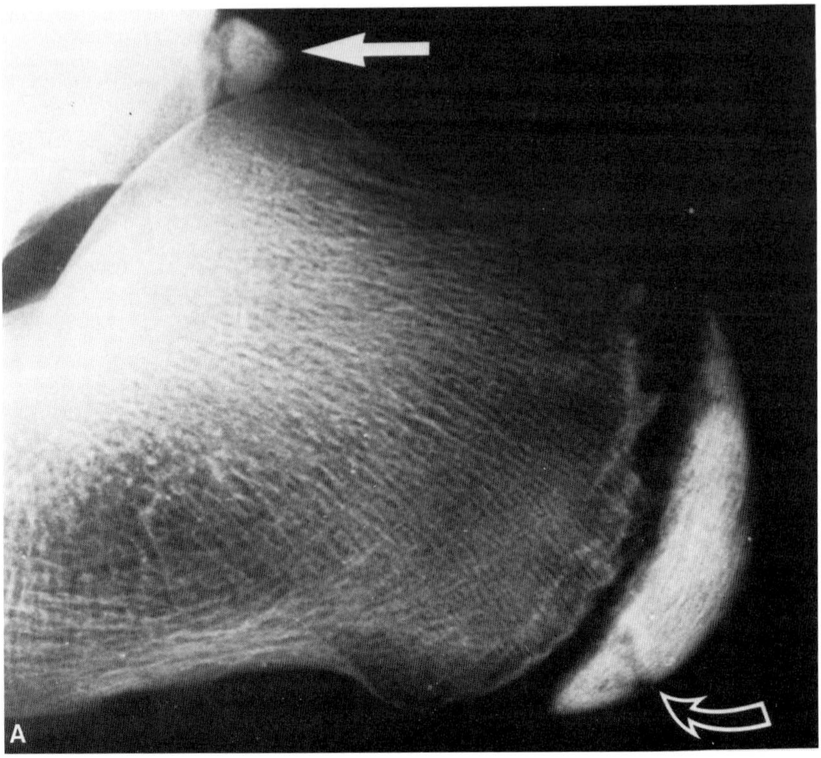

FIGURE 1.24 **A,B:** Variations in the radiographic appearance of the calcaneal apophysis (*open arrows*) and posterior talus (*solid arrow*).

structure with extensive peripheral lappet formation.[32] Within these regions of physeal overlap there may be small areas of accessory ossification (both medially and laterally) that should not be misinterpreted as fractures. This overlapping also minimizes specific physeal separation and displacement (especially when compared with the incidence of distal tibial physeal injuries). The fibular physis normally is level with the tibial articular surface of the distal extent of the tibial ossification center, especially after the second year of life (however, it may be more proximal in infants). As in the medial malleolus, there may be accessory ossification at the tip of the fibula. While this usually is a normal variant of secondary ossification, occasionally it also may result from trauma. Extensive porosity of the distal fibular metaphysis predisposes to buckling or torus injuries that may have severe, multiangular deformation.

Ankle and Foot

Postnatal development of the ankle and foot is probably the most variable of all the elements of the leg. Multiple accessory ossicles exist, many of

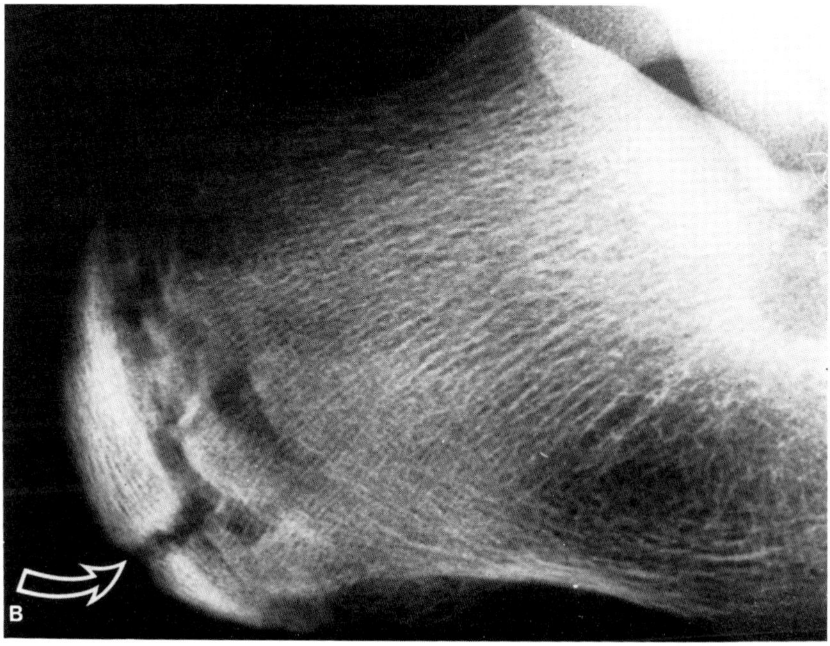

FIGURE 1.24 (*Continued*)

which are not really separate bones but rather secondary ossification within cartilaginous extensions of a principal bone such as the talus (Fig. 1.24) or tarsal navicular.[21,29,30] The calcaneus is the only tarsal bone to regularly develop a secondary ossification center. This calcaneal apophysis has irregular patterns of ossification that are often difficult to interpret when the child has painful heels (Fig. 1.24). The phalanges vary considerably; often the lateral toes lack middle phalanges.

References

1. Bardeen CR, Lewis WH: Development of the limbs, body-wall and back in man. Am J Anat 1:1, 1901.
2. Burkus JK, Ogden JA: Bipartite primary ossification in the developing human femur. J Pediatr Orthop 2:63, 1982.
3. Burkus JK, Ogden JA: Development of the distal femoral epiphysis. A microscopic morphological investigation of the zone of Ranvier. J Pediatr Orthop 4:661, 1984.
4. Caplan AI: The molecular basis for limb morphogenesis, in Littlefield JW, de Groucy J (eds): *Birth Defects*. Proceedings of the Fifth International Conferences. Amsterdam, Excerpta Medica, 1978.
5. Carter DR, Spengler DM: Mechanical properties and composition of cortical bone. Clin Orthop 135:192, 1978.
6. Cauna N: Concerning the nature and evolution of limbs. J Anat 97:23, 1963.

7. Cihak R: Ontogenesis of the skeleton and intrinsic muscles of the human hand and foot. Ergeb Anat Entwicklungsgesch 46:1, 1972.
8. Clark CR, Ogden JA: Development of the menisci of the human knee joint. J Bone Joint Surg Am 65-A:538, 1983.
9. Enlow DH: The functional significance of the secondary osteon. Anat Rec 142:230, 1962.
10. Felts WJL: The prenatal development of the human femur. J Anat 94:1, 1954.
11. Gardner E: Osteogenesis in the human embryo and fetus, in Bourne GH (ed): *The Biochemistry and Physiology of Bone,* ed 2, New York, Academic Press, 1971, pp 77–118.
12. Gardner E, Gray DJ: The prenatal development of the human femur. Am J Anat 129:121, 1970.
13. Gardner E, Gray DJ, O'Rahilly R: The prenatal development of the skeleton and joints of the human foot. J Bone Joint Surg 41-A:847–876, 1959.
14. Gardner E, O'Rahilly R: The early development of the knee joint in staged human embryos. J Anat 102:289, 1968.
15. Gardner E, O'Rahilly R: The early development of the hip joint in staged human embryos. Anat Rec 172:451, 1972.
16. Hert J, Kucera P, Vavra M, et al: Comparison of mechanical properties of both primary and haversian bone tissue. Acta Anat (Basel) 61:412, 1965.
17. Keats TE: Atlas of Normal Roentgen Variants, ed 3. Chicago, Year Book Medical Publishers, 1979.
18. Keats TE, Joyce JM: Metaphyseal cortical irregularities in children: a new perspective on a multifocal growth variant. Skeletal Radiol 12:112, 1984.
19. Laurenson RD: The chondrification of the human ilium. Anat Rec 748:197, 1964.
20. Laurenson RD: The primary ossification of the human ilium. Anat Rec 148:209, 1964.
21. Lawson J, Ogden J, Sella E, et al: The painful accessory navicular. Skeletal Radiol 12:250, 1984.
22. Light TR, McKinstry MP, Schnitzer J, et al: Bone blood flow: regional variation with skeletal maturation, in Arlet J Ficat RP, Hungerford DS (eds): *Bone Circulation*. Baltimore, Williams & Wilkins Co, 1984.
23. McKinstry R, Schnitzer JE, Light TR, et al: Relationship of 99mTc-MDP uptake to regional osseous circulation in immature and mature dogs. Skeletal Radiol 8:115, 1982.
24. Ogden JA: Changing patterns of proximal femoral vascularity. J Bone Joint Surg. 56-A:941, 1974.
25. Ogden JA: Proximal fibular growth deformities. Skeletal Radiol 3:223, 1979.
26. Ogden JA: Development and growth of the musculoskeletal system, in Albright JA, Brand RA (eds): *Scientific Basis of Orthopaedics*. (2nd ed.). New York, Appleton and Lange, 1987.
27. Ogden JA: Chondro-osseous development and growth, in Urist M (ed): *Fundamental and Clinical Bone Physiology,* Philadelphia, JB Lippincott & Co, 1981.
28. Ogden JA: Congenital dysplasia of the hip, in Resnick D,Niwayama G (eds): *Diagnosis of Bone and Joint Disorders*. Philadelphia, WB Saunders Co, 1981.
29. Ogden JA: *Skeletal Injury in the Child*. Philadelphia, Lea & Febiger, 1982.
30. Ogden JA: Anomalous multifocal ossification of the os calcis. Clin Orthop 162:112, 1982.

31. Ogden JA: Development and growth of the hip, in Katz JF, Siffert RS (eds): *Management of Hip Disorders in Children.* Philadelphia, JB Lippincott Co, 1983.
32. Ogden JA: Radiology of postnatal skeletal development VIII. Distal tibia and fibula. Skeletal Radiol 10:209, 1983.
33. Ogden, JA: The uniqueness of growing bones, in Rockwood CA, Wilkins KE, King RE (eds): *Fractures,* vol 3—Children. Philadelphia, JB Lippincott Co, 1984.
34. Ogden JA: Growth slowdown and arrest lines. J Pediatr Orthop 4:409, 1984.
35. Ogden JA: Radiology of postnatal skeletal development IX. Proximal tibia and fibula. Skeletal Radiol 11:169, 1984.
36. Ogden JA: Radiology of postnatal skeletal development X. Patella and tibial tuberosity. Skeletal Radiol 11:246, 1984.
37. Ogden JA, Grogan DP: Prenatal development and growth of the musculoskeletal system, in Albright JA, Brand R (eds): *The Scientific Basis of Orthopaedics,* ed 2. New York, Appleton and Lange, 1987.
38. Ogden JA, Grogan DP, Light TR: Postnatal development and growth of the musculoskeletal system, in Albright JA, Brand RA (eds): *The Scientific Basis of Orthopaedics,* ed 2. New York, Appleton and Lange, 1987.
39. Ogden JA, McCarthy SM, Jokl P: The painful bipartite patella J Pediatr Orthop 2:263, 1982.
40. Ogden JA, Moss HL: Pathological anatomy of congenital hip disease, in *Progress in Orthopaedic Surgery.* New York, Springer-Verlag, 1978.
41. Ogden JA, Tross RB, Murphy MJ: Fractures of tibial tuberosity in adolescents. J Bone Joint Surg 62-A:205, 1980.
42. O'Rahilly R, Gray DJ, Gardner E: Chondrification in the hands and feet of staged human embryos. Contr Embryol Carneg Inst 36:183, 1957.
43. O'Rahilly R, Gardner E: The initial appearance of ossification in staged human embroys. Am J Anat 134:291, 1972.
44. O'Rahilly R, Gardner E: The timing and sequence of events in the development of the limbs in the human embryo. Anat Embryol 148:1, 1975.
45. Resnick D, Greenway G: Distal femoral cortical defects, irregularities and excavations. Radiology 143:345, 1982.
46. Schnitzer JE, McKinstry P, Light TR, et al: Quantitation of regional chondro-osseous circulation in the maturing canine tibia and femur. Am J Physiol 242:H365, 1982.
47. Senior HD: The development of the arteries of the human lower extremity. J Anat 25:55, 1919.
48. Windle WF: Genesis of somatic motor function in mammalian embryos: A synthesizing article. Physiol Zool 17:247, 1944.
49. Zwilling E: Limb morphogenesis. Adv Morphog 1:301, 1961.

2
Genetic and Familial Aspects of Limb Defects with Emphasis on the Lower Extremities

CHARLES I. SCOTT, JR.

Introduction

Limb malformations in human populations are common, with severe birth defects occurring in about 1 in every 200 (0.5%) newborn infants.[1] Environmental agents such as teratogens are often invoked as a cause whenever a child presents with limb deficiencies or malformations. Although it is certainly true that it may be very difficult at times to determine whether or not a defect is hereditary, it is important to realize that genetic factors increasingly are being recognized in this group of conditions. As parents become more knowledgeable about genetics and environmental agents, they want to know the cause of their child's problems and if there is risk of recurrence in subsequent pregnancies.

It is not possible in this brief review to catalog every literature-cited disorder in which there are limb deficiencies of familial or genetic origin. Selected entities are used to illustrate points in recurrence risk counseling.

Congenital deformities may be initiated very early in embryonic life or may develop at various times later in gestational development. Generally, the more severe the deformity, the earlier in fetal life the defect arose. *Malformations* result from defective formation of tissues. *Deformation* is the result of altered mechanical forces on normal tissues. Disruptions are due to breakdown of previously normal tissue.

In a recent review, Brent[2] noted that for 60% to 70% of all human malformations, the etiology is as yet unknown. Environmental causes have been identified in approximately 10% of malformations, with the following breakdown: maternal infections, 3%; maternal disease states, 4%; uterine constraint, 2%; and exposure of the fetus to recognized drugs, chemicals, irradiation, or hyperthermia, 1%. Approximately 5% of malformations have a cytogenetic origin, and about 15% are due to single-gene mutations transmitted in Mendelian patterns.

In this regard, a few words are in order concerning basic principles in genetics. Man has approximately 100,000 genes, which are distributed among 46 chromosomes. The term *congenital* means that a particular disease or somatic abnormality is present at birth. Such conditions may be the result of environmental factors, genetic factors, or a combination of both. Genetic diseases may be recognized at birth or much later in life. The term *familial* indicates that certain disorders occur more frequently in a given family than chance alone would predict. The etiology can be environmental or it can be associated with genetic factors and have significant recurrence risks. The term *hereditary* is generally used in referring to those disorders that are related to traits determined largely by genes or chromosomes.

Autosomal dominant traits are notoriously variable in their clinical presentation. Failure to recognize this characteristic can result in erroneous counseling. *Penetrance* refers to whether the trait is expressed at all, that is, the percentage of patients with the gene who show some manifestation of it. When an individual has the gene and fails to express it, the trait is said to exhibit reduced penetrance. Clinically, this can be the basis for a skipped generation. Many autosomal dominant traits are the result of *new point mutations*. In such instances, entirely normal parents have a child affected by an autosomal dominant trait. These parents have virtually no risk of having another child with the same disorder because a rare mutation occurred in the affected person by chance only and is extremely unlikely to recur. The affected child has an autosomal dominant trait and therefore has a 50% chance of transmitting the trait to any offspring he or she might one day produce. These new autosomal dominant mutations are sometimes associated with a "paternal age" effect, that is, the father is generally older (37 years or more) at the time of conception of the affected person.

Autosomal recessive traits are often associated with a high degree of *consanguinity* of the parents, which is relationship by descent from a common ancestor, such as cousin marriages. Generally, one counsels parents of a child with an autosomal recessive trait that they have one chance in four, or a 25% risk, of having another affected child who will be homozygous for this particular gene. It is quite obvious that there is also a 75% chance that the child will not be affected.

A trait transmitted as an X-linked disorder is expressed by all males who carry the gene because males have only one X chromosome. Females have two X chromosomes, and when one of them carries the mutant X-linked gene, she is said to be a *carrier*. Half of her sons are at risk to receive the X chromosome bearing the trait and would be affected. Half of the carrier's daughters are at risk to be carriers, just like their mother. Half of her sons and daughters may not be affected. If they do not receive the mutant gene, they have no risk of transmitting the X-linked trait to their offspring. The affected male will have all carrier daughters because he can transmit only a mutant X. The sons receive their father's

Y chromosome and, therefore, will be neither affected nor carriers—they cannot transmit the trait.

Multifactorial conditions are not associated with discrete defects of genes or chromosomes; rather, they are attributed to the interaction of two or more genes of small effect that, in themselves, are not deleterious. These disorders are said to be *polygenic*. Because the genes are contributed by both parents and are thought to interact with a variety of environmental agents, the disorders can be considered *multifactorial* in etiology. Commonly these traits are familial. Precise genetic analysis is difficult because of the problems in evaluating the many obvious environmental variables. In general, empiric recurrence risks are quoted in the range of 1% to 15%.

Coxa Vara

The familial tendency of coxa vara as an isolated abnormality has long been observed. This disorder has been reported in three generations of a Cypriot family[3] and is compatible with autosomal dominant inheritance. Affected identical twins[4]—as well as the report of coxa vara in a father, daughter, and niece[5]—are also suggestive of a monogenic cause in some kindreds.

Coxa vara can occur as one manifestation of a number of generalized disorders, including cleidocranial dysplasia, Schmid-type metaphyseal chondrodysplasia, pseudoachondroplastic dysplasia, Schwachman's syndrome, Schwartz-Jampel syndrome, spondyloepiphyseal dysplasia congenita, and spondyloepiphyseal dysplasia tarda. Although this is only a partial listing of the entities in which coxa vara may occur, it illustrates an important general principle in genetics. Before attempting to provide a family with genetic counseling, a specific and accurate diagnosis first must be established. It must be decided if a given condition represents an isolated problem or if it is a part of a more generalized disorder, perhaps affecting a number of organ systems. If counseling were provided on the basis of presumed isolated coxa vara, the patient would be poorly served if, in fact, he or she had an entirely different condition such as Schwartz-Jampel syndrome. Familial isolated coxa vara is an autosomal dominant trait, whereas Schwartz-Jampel syndrome is an autosomal recessive entity. A thorough medical and family history as well as a physical examination can allow differential diagnosis and recognition of specific conditions.

Absence Defects of the Lower Extremities

Cases of complete absence of all four extremities are exceptionally rare, with no evidence to suggest a genetic etiology. Absence defects are usually partial and are likely to be part of a more widespread multiple malformation complex.

Acheiropodia, total absence of the hands and feet, has been reported[6] in multiple members of inbred Brazilian families of Portuguese background in an autosomal recessive mode. The hands and feet are absent, and the extremities end as stumps.

Localized absence defects in the lower extremities are uncommon in comparison with those affecting the upper extremities.

Proximal Focal Femoral Deficiency

Proximal focal femoral hypoplasia (Fig. 2.1) is a rare but well-recognized malformation. It is usually classified by anatomical distribution of the abnormalities, and bilateral changes are much less common than unilateral femoral involvement. The majority of cases are of uncertain cause and until recently have been sporadic. Daentl and associates[7] describe the femoral hypoplasia-unusual facies syndrome in which affected individuals have bilateral femoral hypoplasia/aplasia, variable hypoplasia of the humerus and/or radiohumeral synostosis. They may have a distinctive facial appearance: up-slanting palpebral fissures, short nose, broad nasal tip, long philtrum, thin upper lip, micrognathia, and cleft palate. Maternal

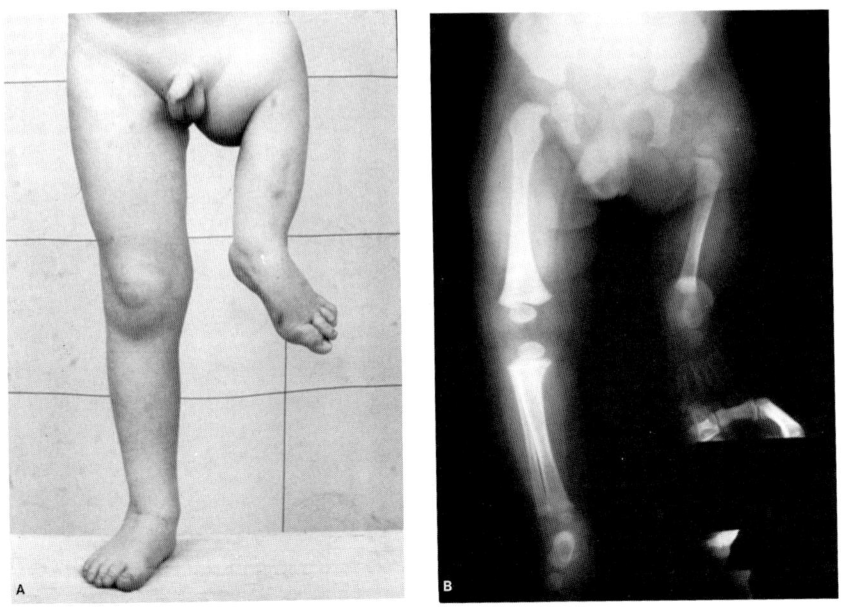

FIGURE 2.1. Clinical photograph (A) and radiograph (B) of a child with proximal focal femoral deficiency.

diabetes has been noted in a few cases. In 1908 Lampert[8] reported the case of an affected father and daughter, suggesting autosomal dominant inheritance. *The author has recently seen a family with three generations affected; only the youngest had the distinctive facial appearance. Clearly the disorder can be inherited as an autosomal dominant trait.* In 1984 Gupta and Gupta[9] reported finding four affected males in a family in two generations, raising the possibility of X-linked transmission of the defect. Hamanishi reviewed a large series of patients with simple congenital short femurs and concluded that there may be a polygenic/multi-factorial basis for these disorders. Thalidomide embryopathy is more often associated with more severe femoral defects, as well as involvement of other long bones, such as the tibia and radius. It is of great importance to obtain a detailed family history of similar skeletal anomalies and deficiencies, to seek prenatal factors such as real or potential teratogen exposures, and to perform a careful physical examination. When these findings are negative, one should counsel families with isolated proximal femoral focal deficiency with caution. Although recurrence risk is unlikely (probably on the order on 1% or less), more studies will be necessary to settle the matter *and resolve the clinical heterogeneity.*

Fibular Defects

Total and partial defects of the fibula usually are sporadic and of unknown etiology. Associated defects involving the upper extremities do occur, such as in the autosomal recessive trait of Robert's syndrome, also called pseudothalidomide syndrome.[11] In this condition, hypomelia varies from phocomelia to lesser degrees of limb reduction, and there are a variety of other abnormalities, including midface defects, cleft iip and palate, prominent external genitalia, and various anomalies of the kidney and heart. Typically, the fibula is absent, and tibiofemoral fusion may be present. An unusual chromosomal abnormality, puffing and splitting of centromeres, is also found. The chromosomal abnormality is considered to be an associated defect, not a cause.

One of the more frequent abnormalities involving the lower extremities is absence or hypoplasia of the fibula. This may occur as an isolated defect or can be found in association with other local aberrations, such as absent fourth and fifth rays, tarsal coalitions, hypoplastic lateral femoral condyles, and proximal femoral deficiency. As part of a widespread skeletal disorder or multisystem entity, fibular deficiency is found in a variety of conditions (Table 2.1). Knowledge of single-gene transmission in these fibular deficiencies allows recognition and delineation of specific conditions as well as proper genetic counseling.

Of interest is the fact that X-linked inheritance seems to be strikingly

TABLE 2.1. Selected genetic disorders of the fibula.

Disorder	Mode of Inheritance	McKusick Catalog Number[a]
Fibular and ulnar hypoplasia	AD	19140
Langer-type mesomelic dysplasia	AR	24970
Fibular aplasia and complex brachydactyly	AR	22890
Fibular aplasia/hypoplasia, femoral bowing, and poly-, syn-, and oligodactyly	AR	22893
Neonatal osseous dysplasia, type I	AR	25605
Fibular aplasia with craniosynostosis	AR	21855
Larsen syndrome	AD	15025
Larsen syndrome	AR	24560

AD = autosomal dominant
AR = autosomal recessive
[a] Phenotype number from McKusick VA: *Mendelian Inheritance in Man*, ed 8. Balitmore, The Johns Hopkins University Press, 1988.

absent in limb deficiencies. However, a newly recognized disorder, oto-palato-digital syndrome, type II,[12] is thought to be transmitted as an X-linked lethal skeletal dysplasia featuring midface hypoplasia, cleft palate, down-slanting palpebral fissures, small thorax, bowed limbs, and absent fibula.

De novo interstitial deletion of chromosome 21 has been reported in a patient with fibular deficiency, ulnar defects, clubfeet, and mental retardation.[13] As a practical point in counseling families, when the proband with a limb deficiency additionally has significant developmental delay or frank mental retardation, chromosomal analysis should be performed.

Tibial Deficiency

Tibial absence/hypoplasia, an uncommon abnormality, is sporadic in the majority of instances and is highly variable in severity. Most cases are part of a systemic syndrome, and associated anomalies may be of major significance. Both autosomal dominant and autosomal recessive modes of inheritance are known (Table 2.2). In these families concurrent defects can allow specific conditions to be differentiated. A detailed family history and careful physical examination are crucial to providing appropriate counseling concerning the risk of recurrence. At times, physical examination and radiographs of various family members may be required to identify those who are affected. Caution must be exercised because of wide interfamilial and intrafamilial variability, not only of tibial defects but also of associated anomalies. As with other limb deficiencies, where mental retardation also exists, karyotyping is indicated.

Obviously, there are a very large number of intrinsic bone dysplasias[14]

TABLE 2.2. Selected genetic disorders of the tibia.

Disorder	Mode of Inheritance	McKusick Catalog Number[a]
Tibia, absence, isolated defect	AR	27522
Tibia, absence, with congenital deafness	AR	27523
Tibia, absence, with polydactyly	AD	18874
Tibia, hypoplasia, with polydactyly	AD	18877
Tibia, absence, with duplication of fibula and ulna	AD	13575
Tibia, absence with triphalangeal thumbs and polydactyly	AD	[a]
Tibia, absence, with split and/foot	AD	[b]
Tibia, absence-micromelia-trigonobrachycephaly	AD	[c]
Robert's syndrome	AR	26830
Tibia vara (Blount's disease)	AD	18870
Tibia vara (Blount's disease)	AR	25920
Tibial torsion, bilateral medial	AD	18880
Pseudoarthrosis, tibial with neurofibromatosis	AD	16220

AD = autosomal dominant
AR = autosomal recessive
[a] Phenotype number from McKusick VA: *Mendelian Inheritance in Man,* ed 6. Baltimore, The Johns Hopkins University Press, 1983.
[b] Canlin S, Lomeli RM, Martinez R, et al: Absent tibiae, triphalangeal thumbs, and polydactyly: Description of a family and prenatal diagnosis. Clin Genet 25:182–186, 1984.
[c] Richieri-Costa A, Ferrareto I, Masiero D, et al: Tibial hemimelia: Report on 37 new cases, clinical and genetic considerations. Am J Med Genet 29:867–884, 1987.
[d] Wiedemann H-R, Opitz JM: Unilateral partial tibial defect with preaxial polydactyly, general micromelia and trigonomacrocephaly with a note on "developmental resistance." Am J Med Genet 14:467–472, 1983.

that result in short stature. Many of these conditions are associated with varying degrees of hypoplasia or dysplasia of the long tubular bones. For the most part, these entities are monogenic and will not be discussed here.

Split-Hand/Split-Foot Deformity

Split-hand/split-foot deformity is heterogeneous and may occur as an isolated malformation or as part of the syndrome. The disorder may affect only the hands or the feet, and there is marked variability of manifestations within as well as between families. It generally is regarded as an autosomal dominant trait. The majority of sporadic cases of split-hand/split-foot defect occur without associated anomalies and are presumed to be due to new dominant mutations. Low penetrance with apparent skipping of generations has been observed by the author and is documented in a number of reports in the literature.[15] Problems arise in counseling these families because there may be genocopies, that is, traits genetically different from phenotypically similar ones. There are reports in the literature[16,17] of split-hand/split-foot deformities that are compatible with autosomal recessive inheritance in a minority of families.[18] Although they are rare, these exceptional family reports are important in counseling a family.

Split-hand/split-foot deformities occur as part of a large number of syndromes that are each inherited as monogenic traits. In the Karsch-Neugebauer syndrome,[19] the affected persons have congenital nystagmus with ectrodactyly. Bonafede and Beighton[20] reported that scalp defects and circumscribed skull defects were associated features of nine affected members of a four-generation kindred with ectrodactyly. Ectrodactyly associated with ectodermal dysplasia and macular dystrophy (EEM syndrome)[21] is an autosomal recessive trait. Ectrodactyly, ectodermal dysplasia, clefting (EEC syndrome), and variable lacrimal duct obstruction[22] is an autosomal dominant trait. Also autosomal dominant is the trait manifested by split-hand/split-foot deformity with triphalangeal thumbs and brachydactyly affecting the index fingers and the third toes, which Carnevale and co-workers[23] reported in two Mexican families.

Ichthyosiform erythroderma, an autosomal recessive trait,[24] is a rare but important malformation syndrome in which lobster-claw deformity may be a manifestation of hemidysplasia. Amelia, transverse defects, hypoplasia of the long bones, or aplasia of fingers or toes is observed on the side affected by unilateral ichthyosiform erythroderma.

A chromosomal abnormality has been reported in one patient with split-hand/split-foot deformity.[25] This child had microcephaly, odd facies, congenital heart disease, and cleft palate and was severely retarded. Karyotyping showed a partial monosomy for the long arm of chromosome 7.

In the clinical setting in which a patient presents for evaluation of a split-hand/split-foot deformity, it is crucial to observe the proband and other family members carefully for all abnormalities. When widespread defects or anomalies are noted, syndrome identification should be attempted. When mental retardation is also present, chromosomal analysis should be performed before final genetic counseling is provided.

Duplication Defects

Duplication of hands and feet is unusual, even when involving one limb. Only three references in the medical literature report duplication of all four limbs.[26–28] There was associated ulnar and fibular dimelia and absence of the radius and tibia as well as peculiar clefting of the nares. Autosomal dominant inheritance was suggested with parent-offspring affectation. Absence of the corpus callosum and hypsarrhythmia were present in one family.

Developmental Morphogenesis

Progress in understanding the pathophysiology of limb morphogenesis has come from a variety of studies. Hootnick and associates,[29] using arteriography and postamputation dissection of human limbs with tibial or fibular absence, found abnormal arterial patterns. They noted persistence of embryonic vascular patterns, absence of certain normal arteries, and failure of formation of the plantar arch vessels. They proposed that these changes predisposed the limb to bony malformations by interfering with the vascular supply during differentiation and development. Similar studies in radial aplasia led Van Allen and colleagues[30] to similar conclusions. Additional research has extended and supported these concepts.[31]

Vascular occlusions during embryonic development have been postulated as the common pathogenetic mechanism whereby a number of congenital abnormalities arise. Robinow and co-workers[32] hypothesized this mechanism to explain a case of peromelia, ipsilateral subclavian atresia, coarctation, and aneurysm of the aorta. This theory is invoked in asymmetric defects that result in destruction or dysgenesis of body parts that had been formed normally.

The role of nervous system involvement in limb development has helped further our understanding of these complex interrelationships.[33] Early rupture of the amnion may cause dysmorphogenesis by compression of the early embryo, resulting in molded deformation and positional abnormalities.[34] Compression can result in polydactyly or syndactyly by interfering with development of normal structures. Similarly, hip dislocation can result. This process has been referred to as the "early amnion rupture spectrum"[35] and offers insight into several congenital abnormalities. In utero constraint of the developing fetus due to the presence of a twin, uterine tumor, uterine malformation, or oligohydramnios may result in deformity by similar mechanisms.[36]

With the advent of recombinant deoxyribonucleic acid (DNA) technology, gene characterization specific to limb development expressed during myogenesis and chondrogenesis can be expected to expand the frontier of developmental genetics. Monoclonal antibodies likewise will offer another technique for studying relationships in the developing limbs. It is anticipated that the molecular biologists working with the developmental biologists will combine their efforts, leading to rapid progress in this exciting field of research.

At present, there is no universally accepted classification or catalog of all limb deficiencies. Dysmorphologists, syndromologists, and geneticists have much to do in lumping and splitting these heterogeneous conditions. In addition to current scientific literature, there are a number of excellent texts available for those who wish to pursue an interest in specific limb defects.[37–45]

Summary

Although the majority of lower limb deficiencies are of sporadic occurrence and of unknown etiology, genetic factors are involved in a significant number. A better informed public is demanding advice concerning cause and recurrence. Careful scrutiny of the medical history and family tree and attention to phenotypic details, can delineate entities. At times, specific laboratory tests are important; for example, when limb deficiencies are associated with mental retardation, with or without other organ system involvement, chromosomal analysis is indicated. We live in a highly litigious age, and it is of great practical value to communicate effectively, especially when giving advice about the cause and recurrence risk of these deficiency states.

References

1. Rogala, E.J., Wynne-Davies, R., Littlejohn, A., Gormley, J.: Congenital limb anomalies: Frequency and aetiological factors. Date from the Edinburgh Register of the Newborn (1964–1968). J. Med. Genet. 11:221–233, 1974.
2. Brent, R.L.: Prevention of physical and mental congenital defects. Part A: The scope of the problem. *In* Marois, M. (ed.): Progress in Clinical and Biological Research. New York, Alan R. Liss. Inc., 1985, Vol. 163A, pp. 55–68.
3. Say, B., Tuncbilik, E., Pirnar, T.: Hereditary congenital coxa vara with dominant inheritance? Humangenetik 11:266–268, 1971.
4. Martin, H.: Coxa vara congenita bei eineugen Zwillingen. Arch. Orthop. 42:230–240, 1942.
5. Almond, H.G.: Familial infantile coxa vara. J. Bone Joint Surg. 38B:534–544, 1956.
6. Freire-Maia, A.: The extraordinary handless and footless families of Brazil—50 years of acheiropodia. Am. J. Med. Genet. 9:31–41, 1981.
7. Daentl, D.L., Smith, D.W., Scott, C.I., Jr., Hall, B.D., Gooding, C.A.: Femoral hypoplasia—Unusual facies syndrome. J. Pediatr. 86:107–111, 1975.
8. Lampert, R.P.: Dominant inheritance of femoral hypoplasia—Unusual facies syndrome. Clin. Genet. 17:255–258, 1980.
9. Gupta, D.K.S., Gupta, S.K.: Familial bilateral proximal femoral focal deficiency. J. Bone Joint Surg. 66A:1470–1472, 1984.
10. Hamanishi, C.: Congenital short femur. Clinical, genetic, and epidemiological comparison of the naturally occurring condition with that caused by thalidomide. J. Bone Joint Surg. 62B:307–320, 1980.
11. Waldenmaier, C., Aldenhoff, P., Klemm, T.: The Robert's syndrome. Hum. Genet. 40:345–349, 1978.
12. Brewster, T.G., Lachman, R.S., Kushner, D.C., Holmes, L.B., Isler, R.J., Rimoin, D.L.: Oto-palato-digital syndrome, type II—An X-linked skeletal dysplasia. Am. J. Med. Genet. 20:249–254, 1985.
13. Reynolds, J.F., Wyandt, H.E., Kelly, T.E.: De novo 21q interstitial deletion

in a retarded boy with ulno-fibular dysostosis. Am. J. Med. Genet. 20:173–180, 1985.
14. Scott, C.I., Jr.: Heritable skeletal dysplasias. *In* Jackson, L.G., and Schimke, R.N. (eds.): Clinical Genetics: A Sourcebook for Physicians. New York, John Wiley and Sons, Inc., 1979.
15. Mackenzie, H.J., Penrose, L.S.: Two pedigrees of ectrodactyly. Ann. Eugen. 16:88–96, 1951.
16. Ray, A.K.: Another case of split-foot mutation in two sibs. J. Hered. 61:169–170, 1960.
17. Freire-Maia, A.: A recessive form of ectrodactyly and its implications in genetic counseling. J. Hered. 62:53, 1971.
18. Verma, I.C., Joseph R., Bhargava, S., Mehta, S.: Split-hand and split-foot deformity inherited as an autosomal recessive trait. Clin. Genet. 9:8–14, 1976.
19. Pilarski, R.T., Pauli, R.M., Bresnick, G.H., Lebovitz, R.M.: Karsch-Neugebauer syndrome: Split-foot/split-hand and congenital nystagmus. Clin. Genet. 27:97–101, 1985.
20. Bonafede, R.P., Beighton, P.: Autosomal dominant inheritance of scalp defects with ectrodactyly. Am. J. Med. Genet. 3:35–41, 1979.
21. Ohdo, S., Hiryama, K., Terawaki, T.: Association of ectodermal dysplasia, ectrodactyly and macular dystrophy: The EEM syndrome. J. Med. Genet. 20:52–57, 1983.
22. Bixler, P., Spivack, J., Bennett, J., Christian, J.C.: The ectrodactyly-ectodermal dysplasia clefting (EEC) syndrome. Clin. Genet. 3:43–51, 1972.
23. Carnevale, A., Hernandez, M., Castillo, V., Torres, P.: A new syndrome of triphalangeal thumbs and brachy-ectrodactyly. Clin. Genet. 18:244–252, 1980.
24. Happle, R., Koch, H., Lenz, W.: The CHILD syndrome: congenital hemidysplasia with ichthyosiform erythroderma and limb defects. Eur.J. Pediatr. 134:27–33, 1980.
25. Pfeiffer, R.A.: Interstitial deletion of a chromsome 7 (q11.2 q22.1) in a child with split-hand/split-foot malformation. Ann. Genet. 27:45–48, 1984.
26. Laurin, C.A., Favreau, J.C., Labelli, P.: Bilateral absence of the radii and tibia with bilateral reduplication of the ulna and fibula. A case report. J. Bone Joint Surg. 46A:137–142, 1964.
27. Sandrow, R.E., Sullivan, P.D., Steel, H.H.: Hereditary ulnar and fibular dimelia with peculiar facies. A case report. J. Bone Joint Surg. 52A:367–370, 1970.
28. Sanchis, A., Cervero, L., Martinez, A., Valverde, C.: Duplication of hands and feet, multiple joint dislocations, absence of corpus callosum, and hypsarrhythmia: Acrocallosal syndrome? Am. J. Med. Genet. 20:123–130, 1985.
29. Hootnick, D.R., Levinsohn, E.M., Randall, P.A., Packard, D.S., Jr.: Vascular dysgenesis associated with skeletal dysplasia of the lower limb. J. Bone Joint Surg. 62A:1123–1129, 1980.
30. Van Allen, M.I., Hoyme, H.E., Jones, K.L.: Vascular pathogenesis of limb defects. I. Radial artery anatomy in radial aplasia. J. Pediatr. 101:832–838, 1982.
31. Hootnick, D.R., Packard, D.S., Jr., Levinsohn, E.M., Lebowitz, M.R., Lubicky, I.P.: The anatomy of a congenitally short limb with clubfoot and ectrodactyly. Teratology 29:155–164, 1984.
32. Robinow, M., Schatzman, E.R., Oberheu, K.: Peromelia, ipsilateral subcla-

vian atresia, coarctation and aneurysm of the aorta resulting from intrauterine vascular occlusion. J. Pediatr. 101:84–87, 1982.
33. Stephens, T.D., Siebert, J.R., Graham, J.M., Beckwith, J.B.: Parasitic conjoined twins, two cases and their relation to limb morphogenesis. Teratology 26:115–121, 1982.
34. Graham, J.M., Miller, M.E., Stephan, M.J., Smith, D.W.: Limb reduction anomalies and early in-utero limb compression. J. Pediatr. 96:1052–1056, 1980.
35. Higgenbottom, M.C., Jones, K.L., Hall, B.D., Smith, D.W.: The amniotic band disruption complex: Timing of amniotic rupture and variable spectra of consequent defects. J. Pediatr. 95:544–549, 1979.
36. Thomas, I.T., Smith, D.W.: Oligohydramnios, cause of the non-renal features of Potter's syndrome, including pulmonary hypoplasia. J. Pediatr. 84:811–814, 1974.
37. McKusick, V.A.: Mendelian Inheritance in Man. 6th Ed. Baltimore, The Johns Hopkins University Press, 1983.
38. Salmon, M.A.: Developmental Defects and Syndromes. Aylesbury, H.M. and M. Publishers, 1978.
39. Gorlin, R.J., Pindborg, J.J., Cohne, M.M., Jr.: Syndromes of the Head and Neck. 2nd Ed. New York, McGraw-Hill Book Co., 1976.
40. Bergsma, D., Lenz, W. (eds.): Morphogenesis and Malformation of the Limb. New York, Alan R. Liss, Inc., 1977.
41. Werthemann, A.: Kie Entwicklungsstorungen der Extremitien. *In* Lubarsch, O., Henke, R., and Rossle, R. (eds.): Handbuch der Speziellen Pathologischen Anatomie und Histologie. Vol. 9, Part 6. Berlin, Springer-Verlag, 1952.
42. Bergsma, D. (ed.): Birth Defects Compendium. 2nd Ed. New York, Alan R. Liss, Inc., 1979.
43. Smith, D.W., Jones, K.L.: Recognizable Patterns of Human Malformations. 3rd Ed. Vol. VII in the Series Major Problems in Clinical Pediatrics. Philadelphia, W.B. Saunders Company, 1982.
44. Birch-Jensen, A.: Congenital Deformities of the Upper Extremities, Copenhagen, Munksgaard, 1949.
45. Temtamy, S., McKusick, V.: The genetics of hand malformations. *In* Birth Defects, Original Article Series. Vol. XIV, No. 3. New York, Alan R. Liss, Inc., 1978.

3
Pediatric Screening and Evaluation

MORRIS S. DIXON, JR.

In the general population the incidence of major congenital deficiencies of the lower limb has not yet been reported. These deficiencies appear to be less common than those in the upper extremity. In one study of a population of 825 children attending child amputee clinics, 359 children (43%) had one or more deficiencies of the lower limb. Of this group, 239 had unilateral involvement and 120 had anomalies of more than one extremity (Table 3.1).[1]

Swanson has published an excellent manual on congenital limb defects, with emphasis on classification.[2] It includes many illustrations of various abnormalities, which can be helpful in understanding and describing each abnormality.

Evaluation of the Newborn

The newborn period of an infant with a significant birth defect is critical, especially for a child with limb deficiency. Statements made and impressions created at this time are remembered by the patients for years, and misconceptions are difficult to change. Blakeslee notes:

> "The first twenty-four hours after the birth of a child or the loss of a limb may be more important to the success of the prosthetic program than any other single factor. Occurrences during these crucial twenty-four hours, and the attitudes and advice of medical personnel (especially if this advice is confusing or contradictory) are most important. The attitudes and advice of other members of the family or even friends also may have an important effect."[3]

It is essential for the pediatrician, usually the first professional to examine the infant thoroughly, to assess the newborn correctly and, in particular, not to give false information about the etiology and prognosis. Parents need to know the answers to five basic questions:

1. What are the problems and what is the diagnosis?
2. What caused the problems and why did it happen to me?

3. What needs to be done now and in the future?
4. What is the prognosis for function and for life?
5. Can it happen again in a subsequent pregnancy?

A careful prenatal and family history may disclose information helpful to the diagnosis; equally important, it will give the mother and father an opportunity to verbalize their concerns about the etiology. Information regarding maternal illness, exposure to drugs and other possible teratogens, plus a complete family history should be recorded for future use in epidemiologic studies. Because the limb bud is formed by the eighth week of gestation, events subsequent to that are unlikely to be responsible for the defect, except with intrauterine cramping or the amniotic band syndrome. Drugs—including oral contraceptives, antidepressants, antiemetics, antimetabolites, anticoagulants, and anticonvulsants—have been reported as possible etiologic agents but the data are still not widely accepted. There are syndromes that are autosomal dominant (i.e., Holt-Oram and ectrodacytyly, ectodermal dysplasia, clefting [EEC]) and autosomal recessive (i.e., Robert's, Miller) in inheritance in which the family history will be important. Table 3.2 gives a useful summary of possible causes of limb deficiencies.

TABLE 3.1 Congenital limb reduction level of amputation.

Unilateral Upper Limb			
Below elbow	=	224	54%
Partial hand	=	85	20%
Above elbow	=	31	7%
Wrist disarticulation	=	30	7%
Elbow disarticulation	=	8	2%
Miscellaneous	=	33	10%
Total	=	411	
Unilateral Lower Limb			
Below knee	=	64	27%
Ankle disarticulation	=	40	17%
Above knee	=	39	16%
Partial foot	=	33	14%
Miscellaneous	=	63	26%
Total	=	239	
Bilateral Upper Limb	=	55	31%
Bilateral Lower Limb	=	39	22%
Double - 1 Upper and 1 Lower	=	11	6%
Triple	=	23	13%
Quadruple	=	47	28%
Total	=	175	

Adapted from Patient Census at Child Amputee Clinics (new cases reported in 1972 and 1980 combined).[1]

TABLE 3.2 Etiology of limb deficiencies.

I. Acquired
- A. Trauma
- B. Malignancy
- C. Other surgical

II. Congenital
- A. *Environmental*
  - 1. Intrauterine infection
    - a. syphilis
  - 2. Drugs
    - a. Proven: thalidomide
    - b. Possible: (no convincing evidence)
      - oral contraceptives
      - synthetic female hormones
      - antidepressents
      - antiemetics (Bendectin®)
      - antimetabolies (Aminopterin)
      - anticoagulants (Warfarin)
      - anticonvulsants (Dilantin®)
      - quinine
      - alcohol
      - etc.
  - 3. Irradiation
  - 4. Maternal health factors
    - a. diabetes mellitus
  - 5. Mechanical factors
    - a. intrauterine cramping
    - b. amniotic band syndrome (Streeter)
  - 6. Other possible risk factors (no good evidence)
    - a. occupational exposure (hydrocarbons)
    - b. pesticide (agent orange)
    - c. pollutants
  - 7. Paternal risk factors (no evidence)
    - a. age
    - b. diabetes mellitus
    - c. environmental exposure
- B. *Genetic*
  - 1. Chromosomal
    - a. Trisomy 13
    - b. Trisomy 18
  - 2. Single gene
    - a. Autosomal dominant
      - Holt Oram
      - ECC (ectrodactyly, ectodermal dysplasia, cleft palate)
      - Fibula agenesis—complex brachydactyly
    - b. Autosomal recessive
      - TAR (thrombocytopenia absent radius)
      - Coney syndrome
      - Fanconi syndrome
      - Baller-Geroid syndrome
      - Hanhart syndrome
      - Robert's pseudothalidomide
      - etc.
- C. *Unknown*
  - 1. Syndromes
    - a. aglossia-adactylia
    - b. Cornelia deLange
    - c. amniotic band syndrome (Streeter)
  - 2. Multiple congenital anomalies (no specific syndrome)
  - 3. Isolated limb deficiency
    - a. single limb
    - b. multiple limb
    - c. PFFD
    - d. fibula agenesis
    - e. tibia agenesis

From Goldberg MJ: Table 2. Orthop Rev, No. 10, p. 50, 1981, with permission.

A meticulous physical examination of the infant is essential to determine overall health, the extent of the lower-limb defect(s), and other abnormalities. In general, a unilateral transverse reduction defect is not associated with other abnormalities. Bilateral lower-limb deficiencies are frequently associated with other anomalies of the skeletal system and other organ systems.[4,5] Syndrome identification will guide the pediatrician in the search for associated anomalies that are not obvious. A useful text for identification of syndromes is Smith's *Recognizable Patterns of Human Malformation*.[6]

Further investigation, including x-rays and consultations, will depend on the type and extent of the malformation and on the experience of the examiners. In the initial interview the pediatrician will need to outline the steps to be taken and continue to update the parents on the results.

Prognosis for life is usually good unless there are associated life-threatening defects. These children usually have normal intelligence, and their future functioning ability depends on the extent of the malformation, whether it is unilateral or bilateral, and whether the upper extremities are involved.

It is extremely important for the pediatrician, and all professionals involved, to be as optimistic as is realistically possible.[7] Patients with a unilateral lower-limb deficiency can usually lead essentially normal lives, including participation in sports such as swimming, skiing, tennis, and horseback riding. Contact sports such as football and hockey are generally not possible.

Bilateral lower-limb deficiencies are more limiting, but with proper guidance and prosthetics, good mobility can almost always be achieved. Having the parents meet and talk to a well-adjusted individual with a similar malformation can be extremely helpful in their acceptance of the child's problem.

A knowledge of the stages that parents go through after the birth of a handicapped child will help the pediatrician understand parental anxieties. Drotar et al[8] described these stages as: 1) initial shock, followed quickly by denial and 2) protracted period of sadness, anger, and anxiety extending perhaps for several months. Drotar et al go on to describe a stage of reorganization characterized by a gradual, positive, long-term acceptance of the child and reinforced by parents' mutual support. Gradually most parents will adapt to their child's handicap and deal with it constructively.

Generally speaking, it is unwise to discuss amputation of the deformed limb during the newborn period (first few months). This is an emotionally charged subject and is better addressed later when the parents and physician have a stronger relationship. It also is important to have the several professionals involved in the care of the child agree on the proposed plan of management, especially in the case of amputation, before presenting it to the parents.

Evaluation of the Infant and Young Child

Assessment of the child beyond the neonatal period requires the same careful history taking and physical examination. There are some differences that commonly occur and should be addressed by the pediatrician.

The history should elicit information given to the parents by previous examiners, particularly with reference to etiology and prognosis. Guilt for having produced a deformed child is an almost universal feeling. It is important to correct misinformation. This will often require repeated explanation and reassurance in subsequent visits.

Misconceptions about prognosis are frequent. An explanation of management and expected result must be offered. As in the newborn, a realistically optimistic outcome should be forecast. There are usually many questions about management because the parents by now have some information along with their own deductions. The subject of possible amputation may have to be addressed, and this requires a sensitive approach.

The degree of parental acceptance of the child and deformity is sometimes difficult to assess in the initial contact, but the medical history should provide the pediatrician with this information. An empathetic pediatrician can ask open-ended questions to determine the fears and attitudes of the parents. More concerns frequently are expressed in subsequent visits.[9]

Most children with lower-limb deficiencies will be able to attend a regular school. However, when multiple limbs are involved, the amputee may be better served in a special class for the orthopedically handicapped.

A booklet such as *Don't Feel Sorry for Paul*[10] can be useful to parents and children, not only in helping them understand the therapy program but also in demonstrating how children can adapt to their disability.

Evaluation of the Older Child and Adolescent

Initial contact with the older child or adolescent also requires the same careful history taking and physical examination as described previously, but the concerns of the child have to be addressed in addition to those of the family. The visit is usually prompted by either questions of management or of adjustment or both. Specific questions about a prosthesis are common and usually require the assistance of an orthopedic surgeon and prosthetist in answering them.

Separate interviews with the parents and the child are very useful in bringing concerns to the surface. Frequently the concerns differ substantially. Teenagers may be more interested in peer relationships and sexual issues, while parents may be more concerned about future employability and the economics of future care.

Once the child has reached adolescence, parental attitudes toward him or her are difficult to change. If parents have been overprotective because of earlier misconceptions or lack of acceptance, this by now has influenced the child's adaptation and behavior. Children may be submissive and overly dependent. They may take the opposite tack and develop an "acting-out" type of aggressive behavior. These problems can be prevented by optimal management earlier by addressing the parental concerns during the newborn period and infancy.

Follow-Up Care

As mentioned above, professionals caring for a child with a limb deficiency will repeatedly be asked the same five questions listed earlier, particularly during the first few months of life. Visits should be frequent during this period to help parents understand the deformity and accept the child.

Other stressful times for parents come at major milestones in their child's life. At about 1 year of age, the normal child is learning to walk, and so parents ask more questions about ambulation. At age 4 to 5 years, concerns are expressed about school adjustment. In the early teenage years, parents worry about peer acceptance, particularly by the opposite sex, and about increasing independence, including driving a car and future employment. Anticipatory guidance by the pediatrician and other professionals can assist in allaying parental and patient anxieties by addressing these issues at the appropriate times, even though the questions may not be asked directly.

The Team Approach

The pediatrician alone is seldom able to provide total care and his or her usefulness is dwarfed by the ongoing, ever-changing challenges and problems of management of these children. Most lower-limb deficiencies will require a team approach that includes the pediatrician, orthopedic surgeon, physical and/or occupational therapist, and a prosthetist. Occasionally, the help of a psychologist and social worker is needed. One individual on the team should serve as medical director so that the parents and child can be given a coordinated treatment plan. A knowledgeable pediatrician can serve in this role effectively.

Limb deficiency clinics provide an additional benefit, allowing children and their parents to meet others with similar deformities. Sharing experiences of adaptation and function can be extremely therapeutic and beneficial and may also provide an ongoing social support system for the parents and for the children.

References

1. Patient census at child amputee clinics. Child Prosthetic-Orthotic Studies, New York University Post-Graduate Medical School, August 1973, April 1982.
2. Swanson, AB: Congenital Limb Defects. Ciba Clin Symp 33: 1981.
3. Blakeslee B: The Limb-Deficient Child. Berkeley, University of California Press, 1963, p 2.
4. Goldberg MJ, Bartoshesky LE, O'Toole D: The pediatric amputee: An epidemiologic survey. Orthop Rev October 1981.

5. Lenz W, Feldman U: Unilateral and asymmetric limb defects in man: Delineation of the femur-fistula-ulna complex. Birth Defects 13:269, 1977.
6. Jones KL: *Smith's Recognizable Patterns of Human Malformation*. Philadelphia, WB Saunders Co, 1988.
7. Marguardt EG: A holistic approach to rehabilitation for the limb deficient child. Arch Phys Med Rehab 64:237, 1983.
8. Drotar D, Baskiewicz A, Irvin V, et al: The adaptation of parents to the birth of an infant with a congenital malformation. Pediatrics 56:710, 1975.
9. Trout MD: Birth of a sick or handicapped infant: Impact on the family. Child Welfare 62:337, 1982.
10. Wolf B: Don't Feel Sorry for Paul. Philadelphia, JB Lippincott Co, 1974.

Section II—Congenital Deficiency of the Lower Limbs

4
Developmental Coxa Vara

THOMAS L. SCHMIDT

Introduction

Developmental coxa vara is a distinct disease process of the proximal femur occurring in the perinatal period of life and involving the inferior portion of the capital femoral physis and adjacent metaphysis. During growth, a decreased neck-shaft angle usually results and subsequent degenerative dysfunction of the hip joint may occur. The behavior of this disease process is unlike other forms of coxa vara because of the nature of its distinctive osteocartilaginous femoral neck defect. Despite its infrequent occurrence, clinical characteristics, natural history, and treatment have been well defined. Treatment for developmental coxa vara has improved but the etiology and successful reliable resolution by treatment of the osteocartilaginous defect remain unsolved.

The earliest descriptions of varus deformity of the proximal femur to include developmental coxa vara first appeared toward the end of the 19th century prior to the availability of roentgenography by Fiorani,[13] Muller,[44] Hofmeister,[21] and Kredel.[34] Various surgical and nonsurgical treatments were introduced by the turn of the century, but the first surgical specimens for histological examination were made available by Hoffa[20] in 1905 and Helbing[19] in 1906, who carried out treatment by excising the entire femoral head and neck and placing the remaining shaft in the acetabulum. Histological evaluation was advanced by Pylkkanen's study[53] in 1960 of 25 biopsy specimens that documented the pathological changes of developmental coxa vara. Proximal femoral valgus osteotomy, the current mainstay of treatment, was first attempted by Keetley[30] in 1888 (reported in 1900 for adolescent coxa vara, thought to be the residual of a rachitic process) and has become recognized as the best form of treatment in the last 50 years.

The incidence of developmental coxa vara is infrequent; Johanning[26] reported one per 25,000 live births in a Scandinavian population. A predilection for sex or race has not been reported. Evidence does exist in some instances for a hereditary factor.[1,10,14,26,40,54] Left and right hip involvement occur in equal numbers. Unilateral involvement is more common than bilateral by two to three times as much.*

Etiology and Pathogenesis

Many proposals have been offered regarding the etiology of developmental coxa vara, including perinatal trauma, metabolic disease, congenital defect, abnormal blood supply, and hereditary tendency. No single factor has, however, been demonstrated to be the cause of the condition. Certainly, some investigators[1,10,14,26,40,54] have identified, in isolated instances, a hereditary tendency but this cannot be shown consistently in all cases. The etiology remains unknown to the present.

Histopathological examination of developmental coxa vara by early investigators and subsequently by others[5,19,20,47] had shown a defect in the endochondral ossification. Pylkkanen[53] studied the histology of 25 specimens taken from the roentgenographically apparent zone of rarefaction in the femoral neck while performing intertrochanteric osteotomies. He confirmed the previous concept of an endochondral ossification defect and added the findings of atrophic metaphyseal bone in the region and the presence of islets of cartilage, leading to a general impression of disturbed cellular architecture. The process of ossification was disorganized and lacking. Significant amounts of connective tissue were interspersed among the cartilage islets and atrophic bone.

Chung and Riser[8] studied the histology of coxa vara following the death (from unrelated causes) in a 5-year-old boy whose height was reported below the third percentile. Their description includes diffuse abnormal findings in the proximal femur as well as growth plates of the iliac crest and ischial tuberosity from the opposite normal side. Histological findings in the region of the osteocartilaginous defect were similar to those described by Pylkkanen, with certain additions. Cartilage cells adjacent to the metaphysis were not hypertrophied as expected nor was the usual calcification of the matrix present, which would initiate development of bony trabeculae. Additionally they found deficient intra- and extraosseous vascular supply to the metaphyseal side of the growth plate. The sum of the histological findings is a deficient production of bone in the metaphysis in the region of the osteocartilaginous femoral neck defect. Deficient growth in this region of the capital femoral physis results in varus deformity of the femoral head on the femoral neck.

Hoyt and Greenberg[24] reported the association, by roentgenographic analysis, of the size of the triangular fragment in the inferior metaphysis of the femoral neck adjacent the capital physis to the degree of varus

---

* References 2–5, 15, 25, 26, 42, 53, 56, 58.

deformity. In general, the smaller the triangular fragment, the greater the amount of varus deformity (Fig. 4.1). It may be difficult to discern the extent of the triangular fragment, or multiple fragments may be present, providing an unclear picture of involvement (Fig. 4.2). The extent of the triangular fragment in concert with the zone of rarefaction and physeal involvement seen on the roentgenogram may be a better indication of the total involvement of the capital femoral physis and therefore of the severity of the disease process and varus deformity.

The extent of the osteocartilaginous defect is an indication of the amount of involvement of the growing process of the capital femoral physis. In animal studies by Hoyt et al[23] and Compere et al[9] it was shown that excision of the inferior capital femoral physis interfered with growth in this region of the physis and led to production of a varus deformity. Relative growth of the superior aspect of the physis to lack of growth inferiorly led to a more vertical orientation of the capital femoral physis and coxa vara. If the osteocartilaginous defect of developmental coxa vara were minimal, the greater degree of normal physeal activity might allow for recovery of a more normal neck-shaft angle with growth. If, however, the defect were greater, recovery to the normal neck-shaft angle might not be possible, with the result of progressive decreasing neck-shaft angle. The more vertically oriented defect would be vulnerable to shearing stress from weight-bearing and lead eventually to a pseudarth-

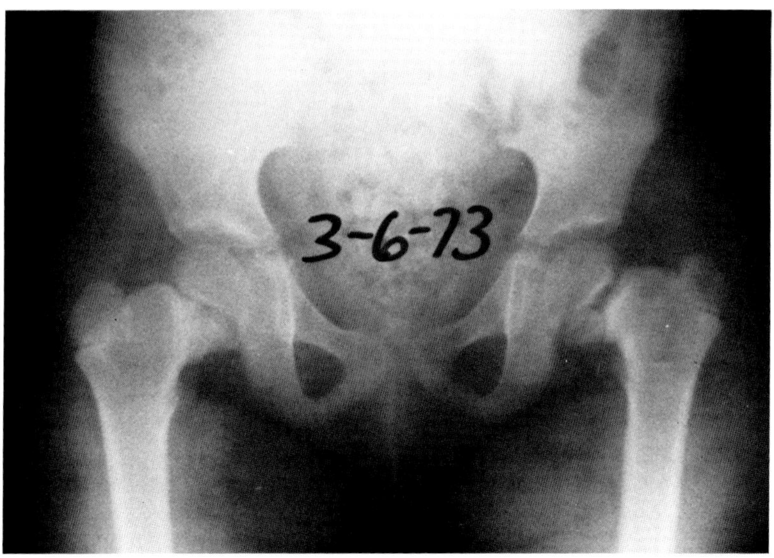

FIGURE 4.1. The triangular fragment in the patient's left femoral neck is small and varus deformity is greater than present in the right hip, which has a larger triangular fragment.

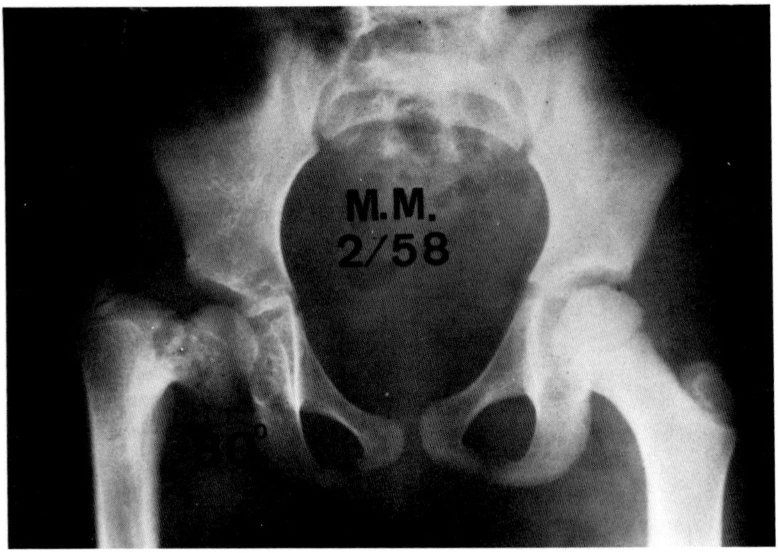

FIGURE 4.2. The triangular fragment is not discernible and multiple fragments are apparent, but the entire femoral neck is involved by irregular ossification, and severe varus deformity is present.

rosis, reflecting a fibrous union of the femoral head to the femoral shaft, as seen in severe untreated coxa vara.

The defect of endochondral ossification is unique to the etiology of developmental coxa vara. If this condition were a reflection of trauma in early childhood, as has been suggested,[8] the osteocartilaginous defect would heal. Varus deformity can result following trauma to the proximal femur, but the healing of an epiphysiolysis or crush injury to the physis does not leave an osteocartilaginous defect similar to that which persists in developmental coxa vara. The defect weakens the femoral neck, which responds to the forces of weight-bearing with progression into varus deformity.[50]

Acetabular development is affected by the osteocartilaginous defect and the resultant varus deformity of the proximal femur. A normally located and formed femoral head is necessary to stimulate acetabular development (Fig. 4.3). In addition, premature closure of the capital femoral physis, which often occurs with or without treatment in coxa vara, leads to abnormal acetabular development.[24,28] Schmidt and Kalamchi[56] noted that if the neck-shaft angle was greater than 110 degrees, the osteocartilaginous defect tended to heal, the neck-shaft angle improved, the physis became more horizontal, assuming a normal attitude and function, and acetabular shape and depth returned to normal. In those hips with less than 110 degrees angle, which tended to progress in varus deformity, physeal position and function deteriorated as well as acetabular shape and depth. Lack of acetabular development reflects the abnormal stress-load conditions of the varus neck-shaft angle, which, in turn, is a reflexion of the severity of the osteocartilaginous lesion.

Clinical Characteristics

Coxa vara is not usually discovered before walking age, although manifestations of its presence—shortening of the lower extremity and limited abduction or asymmetrical range of hip rotation—may make it apparent, particularly in a unilateral occurrence. These are physical signs that should alert any physician who routinely examines infant hips for congenital hip dysplasia. Manifestations that may come to the parent's attention otherwise may include a short, fat thigh and asymmetrical hip rotation. When involvement is bilateral, they may note only stiffness of the hips in diapering the child, which is due to decreased abduction.

Most cases of coxa vara come to the attention of a physician after the onset of walking, when the family notes the child to have a painless gluteus medius limp in instances of unilateral involvement or a painless waddling gait in bilateral involvement. In a series of 98 children, Hoyt and

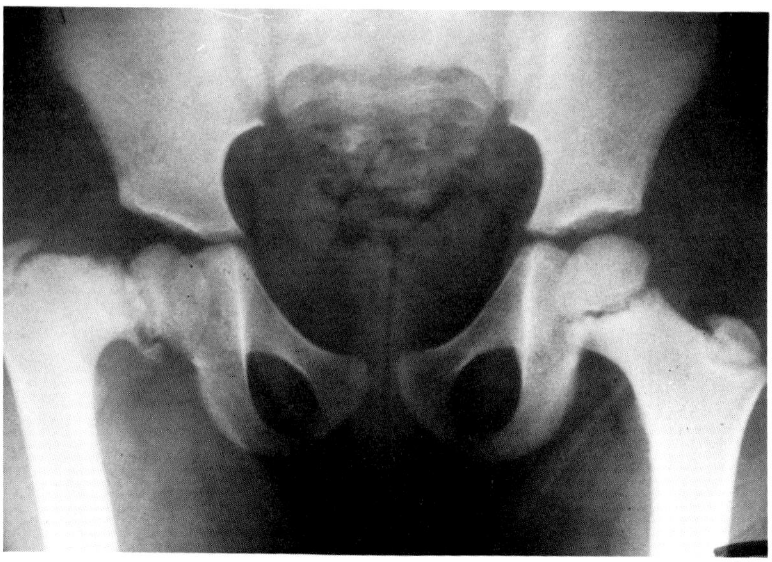

FIGURE 4.3. Acetabular development of the patient's right hip with coxa vara is deficient compared with the normal left hip. Because of varus deformity the femoral head resides more inferior in the acetabulum and does not stimulate normal acetabular growth. The resultant acetabulum is shallow.

Greenberg[24] noted that, in 43%, abnormality was first noticed by the family during the time of early weight-bearing; in 46%, it was noticed between the ages of 3 and 12 years; and in 11% the age of onset was unknown. A consistent age of onset for the disease, however, cannot be deduced from these statistics. Limitation of hip motion can occur in all ranges of motion, but particularly affects abduction and internal rotation. Limitation of hip extension can be masked by the presence of lumbar lordosis, especially with bilateral involvement, but lumbar lordosis is not due solely to hip flexion contracture.[3,4] A leg length discrepancy is apparent in unilateral cases, but obvious telescoping of the hip, as seen in congentially dislocated hips, is absent. Trendelenburg's test is positive in the more severely involved hips but may be equivocal or delayed in mild deformity. A wide perineum may be seen with bilateral coxa vara.

A careful family history is also important since developmental coxa vara has also been reported to be familial in some instances. Other causes such as trauma, infection, bone dysplasias, metabolic disease, and developmental and congenital disorders should be investigated in the history. Subjective complaints from children are improbable but occasionally they may experience fatigue, and later, in the second decade, they may have some discomfort with activity. Symptoms of degenerative arthritis may appear during the third decade.

Roentgenographic Characteristics

When present in infancy, developmental coxa vara may not come to the physician's attention because early clinical examination findings may be normal. Roentgenographic detection may also be difficult. Early roentgenograms taken for suspicion of a hip problem in infancy may deceptively appear normal, especially if the ossific nucleus has not yet appeared. Diagnosis based on roentgenography is made easier if the ossific nucleus is present, at which time it may appear irregular and asymmetrical, with a widened cartilaginous space (inappropriate for the physis alone) occurring between the ossific nucleus and the femoral shaft. Under these circumstances the varus deformity may also be discernible. This appearance may be difficult to distinguish from coxa vara of other causes, but healing response in other conditions will make the diagnosis apparent as the roentgenographic changes in developmental coxa vara persist (Fig. 4.4).

At about 1 year of age, as the femoral neck further ossifies, the triangular fragment representative of the osteocartilaginous defect appears. Other roentgenographic features now become apparent, and the classic findings of coxa vara become distinguishable. Most obvious, varus deformity of the proximal femur will be present, with the physeal plate

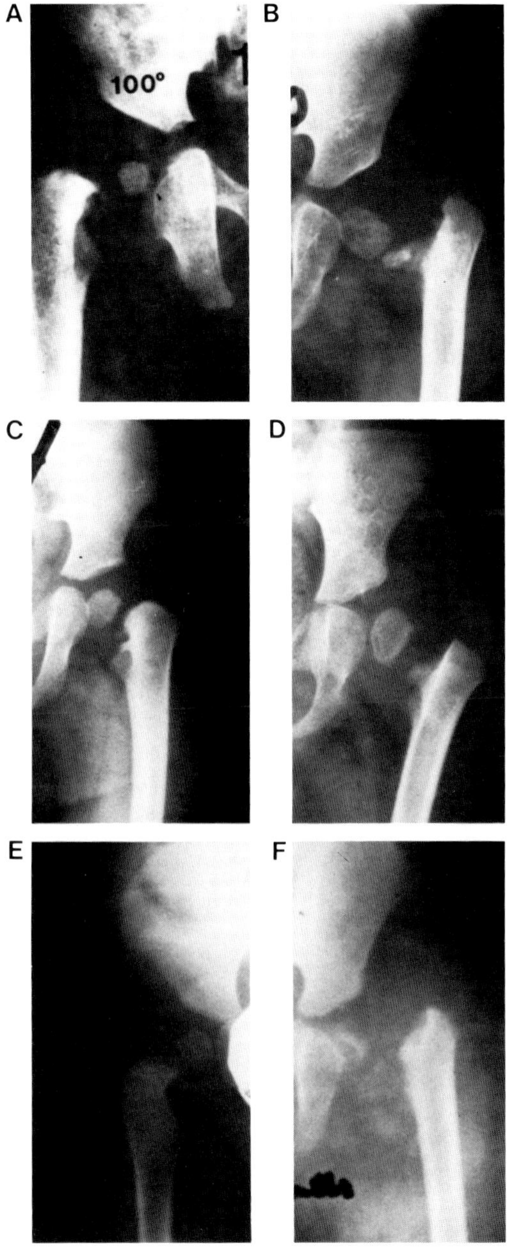

FIGURE 4.4. Conditions that roentgenographically mimic coxa vara early. **A:** Developmental coxa vara at 1 year of age. **B:** Developmental coxa vara in another infant 19 months old. **C:** Boy, 16 months old, with residual varus and femoral neck defect as result of septic arthritis. **D:** Fracture of femoral neck in a boy 3 years and 3 months of age with myelomeningocele. **E:** Fracture, neck of femur in an 18-month-old girl. **F:** Fracture, neck of femur in another girl, 19 months old.

tending toward a vertical attitude and a zone of rarefaction in concert with the physis; this causes the appearance of an inverted Y, delineating the triangular fragment in the inferior femoral neck. The full extent of the femoral head and neck is apparent in the anteroposterior roentgenograph, since the proximal femur is mildly retroverted. The femoral neck is shortened. The femoral shaft appears relatively narrow but may actually be normal in breadth. The shaft is straight without involvement of either varus deformity or bowing and does not have significant increase in cortical thickening of the medial cortex, as seen in congenital coxa vara with bowed femur or short femur. As varus deformity progresses, deformity and osteoporosis of the femoral head occurs. With further growth the acetabulum becomes relatively shallow, with maldevelopment of the medial acetabular wall, as evidenced by deformation of the tear-drop configuration to a V-shaped appearance. The greater trochanter appears enlarged because of overgrowth relative to the femoral head. The femoral head appears to be contained in an inferior position in the shallow acetabulum because of its varus attitude, but if it were placed in more valgus attitude by adduction of the lower extremity, the femoral head would appear to be subluxated due to a shallow acetabular roof. The center-edge angle of Wiberg, therefore, may be misleading in the interpretation of an adequate acetabulum.[56]

Progressive varus deformity becomes severe toward the end of the second decade. The femoral head is deformed, osteoporotic, and lying in the inferior portion of the acetabulum. In some, an apparent lack of continuity exists between the femoral head and remaining portion of the femoral neck, and the acetabulum is significantly malformed (Fig. 4.5). Degenerative changes set in and the greater trochanter, severely overgrown, may readily abut against the ilium with abduction. In cases where the osteocartilaginous defect heals, recovery from the varus deformity occurs early on. The proximal femur assumes a normal neck-shaft angle, and in turn the acetabulum responds by developing normally.

Differential Diagnosis

Generalized musculoskeletal disorders occur in which coxa vara represents one of their characteristic features. Cleidocranial dysostosis and metaphyseal dysostosis can display varus deformity of the hip with an inferior metaphyseal osteocartilaginous defect adjacent to the capital femoral physis. One needs to look for the other differentiating features of these conditions in order not to confuse them with developmental coxa vara. Coxa vara in these situations will usually occur bilaterally. The differentiating features of cleidocranial dysostosis are partial or complete absence of the clavicles and delayed fusion of skull suture lines with the

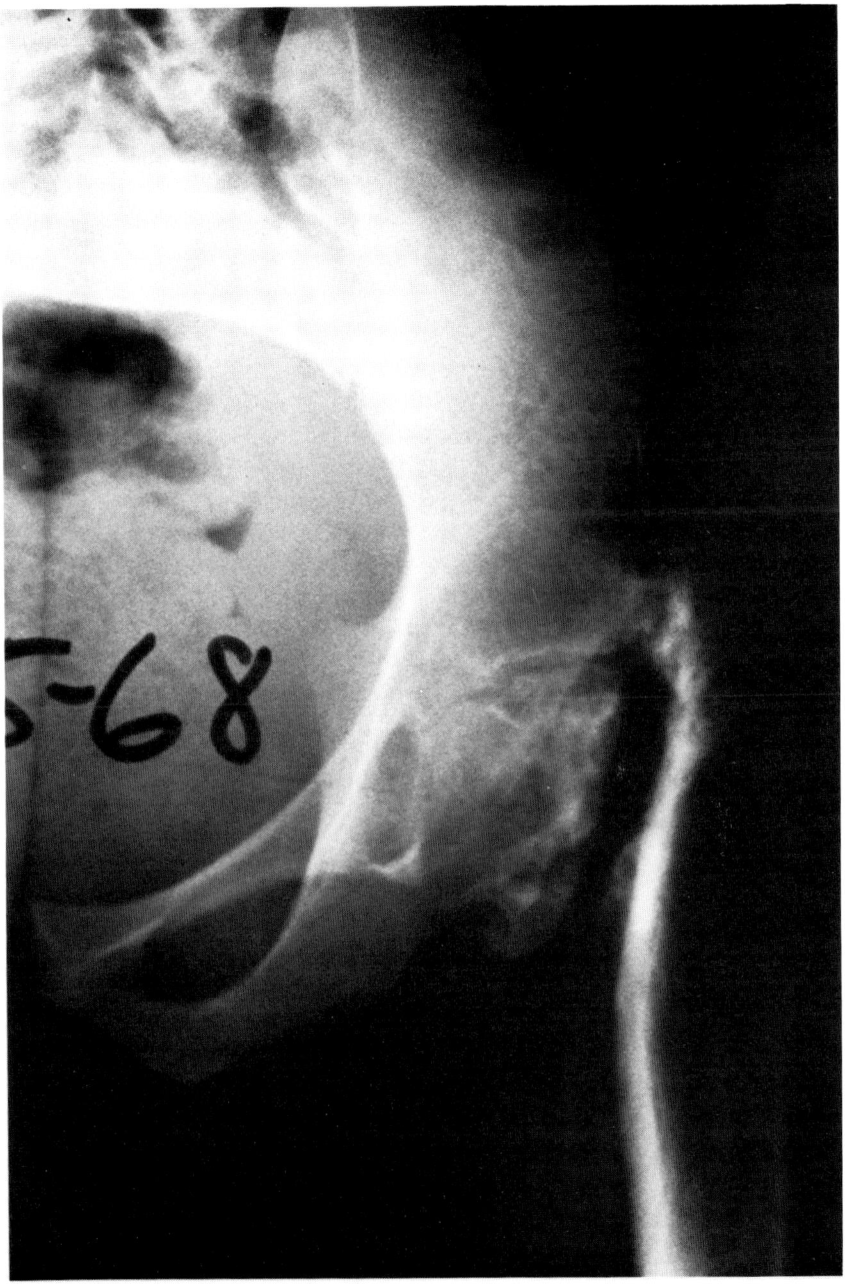

FIGURE 4.5. Severe, untreated coxa vara in an adult male. Note the deformed, osteoporotic femoral head lying in the inferior portion of the malformed acetabulum with discontinuity, pseudarthrosis, between the femoral head and neck.

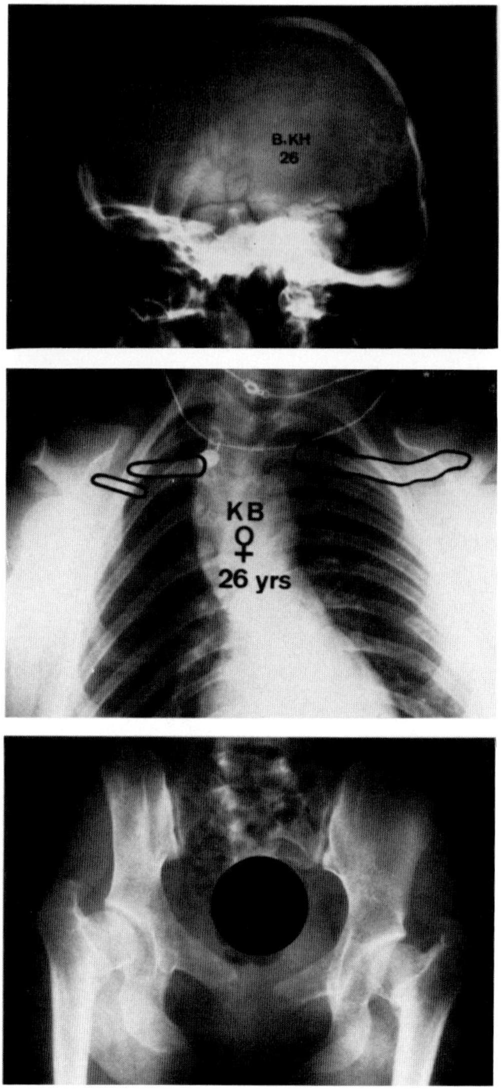

FIGURE 4.6. Woman, 26 years old, with cleidocranial dysostosis. Note cranial defect and Wormian bones, partial absence of clavicles, and lack of development of pubis and ischium at the pubic symphysis. The femoral necks are short with healed defects and premature capital femoral physeal growth arrest. Also note relative overgrowth of greater trochanters and deficient acetabular development. Patient's mother also had cleidocranial dysostosis.

presence of Wormian bones (Fig. 4.6). In metaphyseal dysostosis, particularly of Schmid type, metaphyses elsewhere will appear enlarged and irregular with normal epiphyses and widened physes.[62] Other bone dysplasias, such as osteogenesis imperfecta, pseudoachondroplasia,[62] and osteopetrosis,[31] may have coxa vara as a feature but not the typical roentgenographic picture of developmental coxa vara.

The congenital deformities of short femur and bowed femur can have coxa vara as part of their manifestations. Proximal femoral focal deficiencies also have an associated coxa vara. Special distinction needs to be made regarding the difference between developmental coxa vara and congenital coxa vara. In developmental coxa vara the causal agent of deformity is limited to the femoral neck, the subtrochanteric region being normal. The total length of the femur from the tip of the greater trochanter to the joint surface of the medial condyle of the distal femur is not different from what it would otherwise be in a normal situation, implying no abnormality distal to the osteocartilaginous defect. The osteocartilaginous defect in the inferior metaphysis of the femoral neck and acetabular dysplasia are absent in congenital types of coxa vara. Cases of congenital coxa vara with short or bowed femur are usually apparent at birth with obvious shortening of the limb and have associated skeletal anomalies not limited to the femoral neck. Associated fibular or tibial deficiencies have been noted in 50%.[29] Various foot abnormalities have also been associated with the congenital types. Contribution to varus deformity may occur below the level of the trochanters, with increased thickening of the medial cortex and narrowing of the medullary canal. The acetabulum appears essentially normal. Most obvious, the relative overall length of the femur is shorter than normal, and the thigh may clinically appear externally rotated and flexed.[3,4,17,29,51,55] (Fig. 4.7).

Acquired causes should be excluded before making the diagnosis of developmental coxa vara. The residual effect of trauma to the hip, infection, and metabolic diseases can produce a coxa vara. Epiphysiolysis[48,61] and femoral neck fractures from child abuse can mimic early developmental coxa vara. Later, the residual of femoral neck fractures and slipped capital femoral epiphysis can mimic coxa vara. Infection in early infancy destructive of the metaphysis or of the physis and epiphysis can result in varus deformity. Metabolic conditions having coxa vara are rickets and Gaucher's disease. Additionally, fibrocystic disease of the proximal femur can result in coxa vara deformity.[7] A common acquired cause is avascular necrosis of the proximal femur either as the result of treatment in congenital hip dislocation or as a manifestation of the residuals of Perthes disease or slipped capital femoral epiphysis. Cerebral palsy and myelomeningocele have also been reported to have coxa vara deformity.[16,60]

Natural History

The natural history of untreated developmental coxa vara relates to the severity of the varus neck-shaft angle and is a reflection of the extent of the endochondral ossification defect. Coxa vara with an angle greater than 110 degrees tends to improve with further growth, healing the endochondral defect, improving the neck-shaft angle, deepening the acetabulum, and preserving capital femoral physis function (Fig. 4.8). Deformities less than 100 degrees tend to progress. Deformities that have neck-shaft

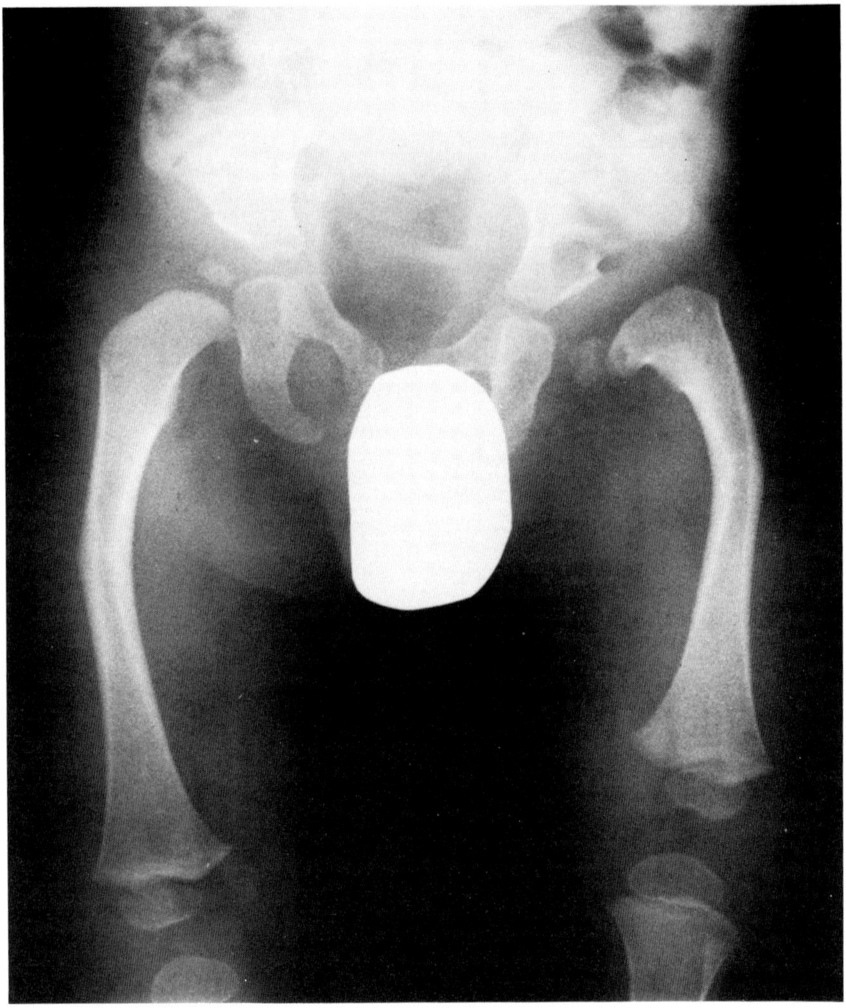

FIGURE 4.7. Boy, 2 years and 2 months old. Congenitally short, bowed femur with coxa vara on the patient's left. The patient's right side represents a congenitally bowed femur with a relative coxa vara.

angles between 100 and 110 degrees are in a gray zone and require observation to determine whether they will resolve or progress (Fig. 4.9).

For those deformities less than 100 degrees, progressive decrease in the neck-shaft angle occurs with resultant vertical orientation of the physis, persistence of the endochondral defect, and defective acetabular development. Early closure of the physeal plate is common. The femoral head becomes deformed and resides in the inferior aspect of the shallow acetabulum. Shearing forces of weight-bearing lead to ossific disconti-

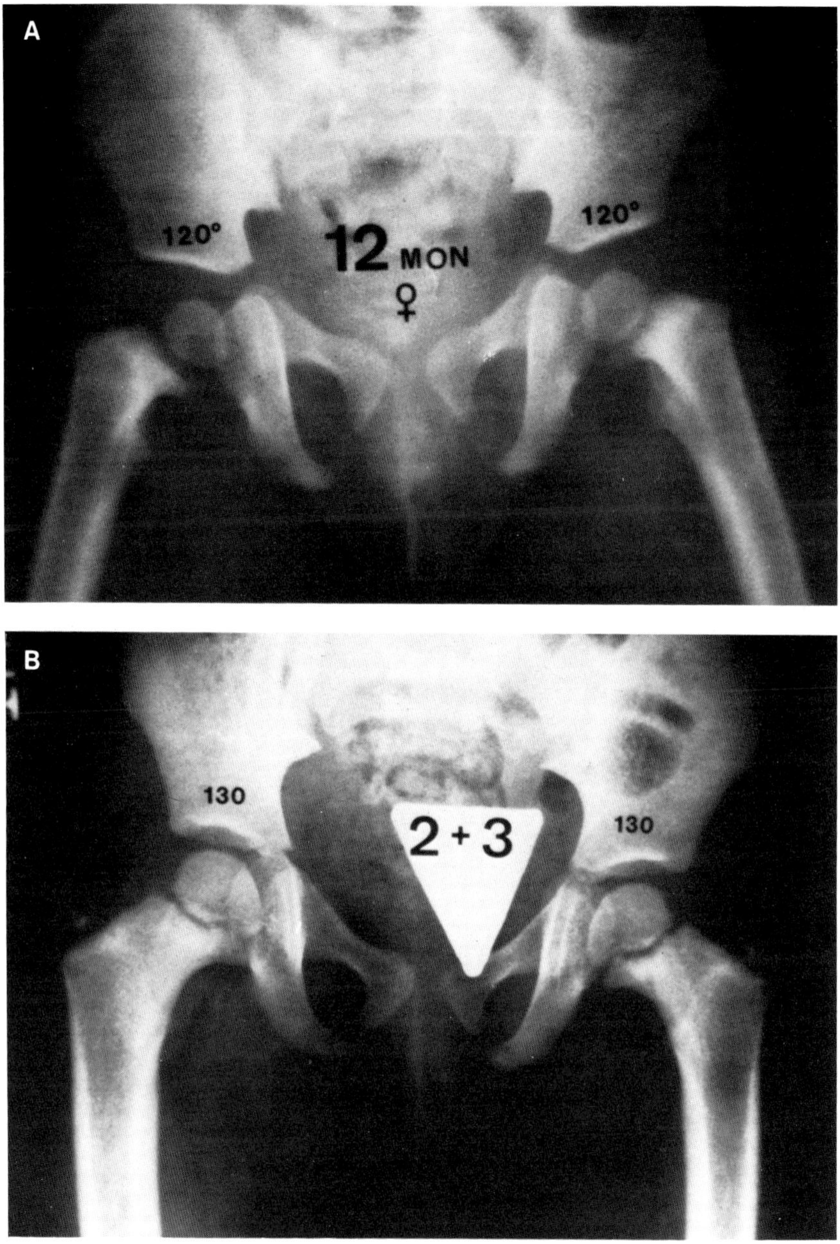

FIGURE 4.8. **A:** Girl, 1 year old, with varus deformity of 120 degrees and small triangular fragments. **B:** At 2 years and 3 months of age, the hips have grown out of varus deformity, the triangular fragments have healed, and the acetabula are developing normally.

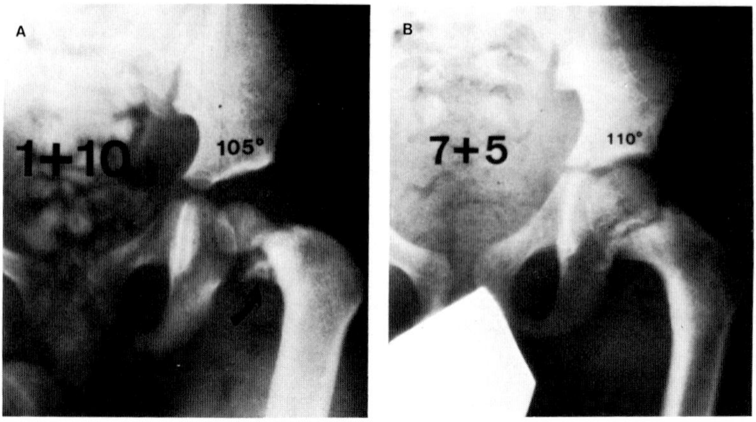

FIGURE 4.9. **A:** Boy, 1 year and 10 months old, with bilateral coxa vara. The right hip had varus deformity of 100 degrees and was treated with valgus osteotomy previously. The left hip, seen here, had varus deformity of 105 degrees and a triangular fragment. **B:** The left hip was observed with no treatment. At 7 years and 5 months of age the triangular fragment has healed. Varus deformity has improved, and acetabular development toward a normal configuration has occurred.

nuity developing, in some, a true pseudarthrosis between the femoral head and neck. Degenerative changes set into the joint. The relative greater trochanteric overgrowth impinges against the ilium in abduction. Degenerative changes, pain, limitation of motion, and abductor weakness lead to gait disturbance and progressive disability (Fig. 4.10).

Treatment

Fiorani[13] is attributed with the first description of coxa vara in 1881[12] and, therefore, was possibly the first to devise treatment. His impression was that the condition resulted from rickets, and he advised antirachitic therapy and relief from weight-bearing.[13,25] Keetley[30] in 1888 performed a corrective osteotomy in the subtrochanteric region. Kraske[33] in 1896 carried his correction out with a wedge osteotomy in the femoral neck, but this was abandoned because of bad results. Hoffa[20] in 1905 and Helbing[19] in 1906 excised the entire femoral head and neck and placed the resultant femoral shaft in the acetabulum. Elmslie[12] in 1907 recommended early splintage of the hip in abduction and internal rotation. Nilsonne[45,46] in 1924 used abduction positioning as did LeMesurier[38] in 1948 who added traction; results, however, did not sustain this as a form of treatment. Nilsonne[46] in 1929 and Lasserre[37] in 1931 endorsed subtrochanteric

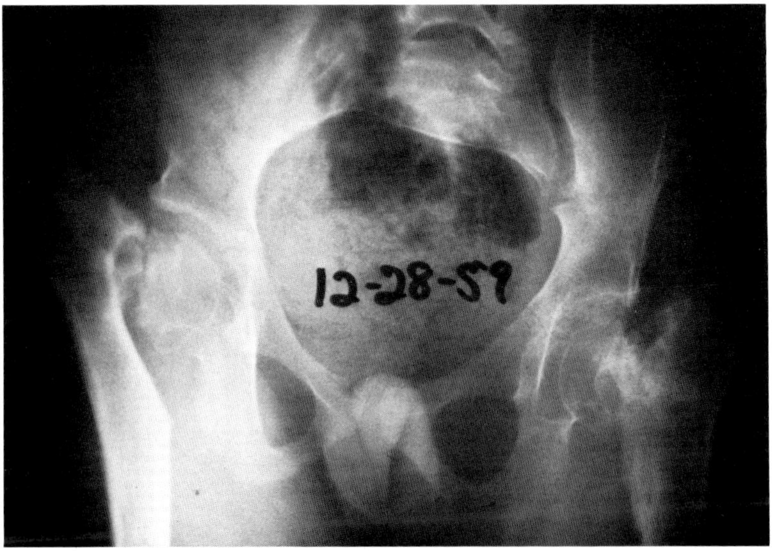

FIGURE 4.10. Bilateral developmental coxa vara with varus deformity less than 100 degrees untreated leading to severe varus deformity and consequent deterioration of the hips.

valgus osteotomy with Lasserre, suggesting the usefulness of adding adductor tenotomy. Zadek[63] in 1935 reported using subcapital drilling to unite bone across the endochondral defect with subtrochanteric osteotomy to correct varus but results varied. Pauwels[49] described an intertrochanteric osteotomy in 1935 that provided good results and paved the way for valgus osteotomy as a popular form of treatment. LeMesurier (1948),[38] Horwitz (1948),[22] and Lian (1950)[41] transfixed the cervical defect with pins, bone graft, or both. Subsequent growth of the femoral neck was prevented and deformity remained uncorrected.[30] Lian suggested adding a subtrochanteric valgus osteotomy as a second stage.[41] Langenskiold and Salenius[36] and Pylkkanen[53] performed greater trochanteric epiphysiodesis in moderate cases but review by Langenskiold and Salenius[36] in 1967 indicated results were unreliable. Following the introduction of Pauwels' osteotomy in 1935, this form of treatment is now the mainstay of therapy, with many forms of the intertrochanteric osteotomy being described. All have the similar goal of correction of varus deformity but techniques have varied, and improvement in both technique and fixation of the osteotomy fragments has progressed.

Present-day approaches to treatment have been well established. Treatment does not always lead to cure but results in modification of the outcome, improving the biomechanics of the involved joint. The goal of treatment is to remove the shearing stress from the area of weakness, the endochondral defect, and, if possible, to convert the forces to compression loading through that area. Currently, restoration of a normal neck-shaft angle by valgus osteotomy most closely accomplishes this goal. In doing so, damage to the capital physis and greater trochanteric apophysis should be avoided. The desired result is a healed endochondral defect, continued growth of the capital physis, and return of normal acetabular development.

Valgus correction should be achieved early in a progressive coxa vara when the growth plate is least affected and the endochondral defect has not had the opportunity to advance across the femoral neck. Early correction will also have the greatest potential of returning the acetabulum to normal. The concern in performing early surgical correction is that physeal arrest might be precipitated, resulting in further shortening of the limb. Delay of treatment to preserve physeal function, however, leaves the proximal femur in its disease state. Further limb shortening results, since any growth in the physis is horizontal rather than vertical. Greater involvement of the physis by the endochondral defect increases the likelihood that it will arrest. Delaying neck-shaft angle correction to an older age does not take advantage of the potential for acetabular remodeling. Late osteotomy and placement of the femoral head in a valgus position results in uncovering of the femoral head in an already shallow, deficient acetabulum (Fig. 4.11).

The role of nonoperative treatment is very limited. Certainly, a varus deformity above 110 degrees can be observed without treatment and will usually resolve with return of normal neck-shaft angle and acetabular configuration.[56] In those hips where deformity lies between 100 and 110 degrees, while observation for progression is being carried out, a shoe lift can be used if significant leg-length discrepancy is present. Abduction exercises can be used if adductor contracture is present. Nonoperative management is contraindicated in varus deformity below 100 degrees unless surgery is contraindicated or has to be delayed for medical reasons. If necessary, the involved hip should be protected against weight-bearing stresses with either bracing or bedrest, and weight reduction is advisable[47] but not confirmed by study.

The most reliable means to achieve correction and encourage healing of the endochondral defect and acetabular development in a progressive coxa vara is a proximal femoral valgus osteotomy. The prime indication for proceeding with an osteotomy is a femoral neck endochondral defect and a neck-shaft angle less than 100 degrees. If the neck-shaft angle is less than 110 degrees and progression is observed, valgus osteotomy should be carried out. Haraldsson[18] and Weinstein et al[59] introduced the Hilgenreiner epiphyseal angle as a method of assessing the need for operative treatment (Fig. 4.12). If this angle was greater than 60 degrees, operative treatment was indicated. Angles between 45 and 60 degrees represented a gray zone in which observation for progression was advised

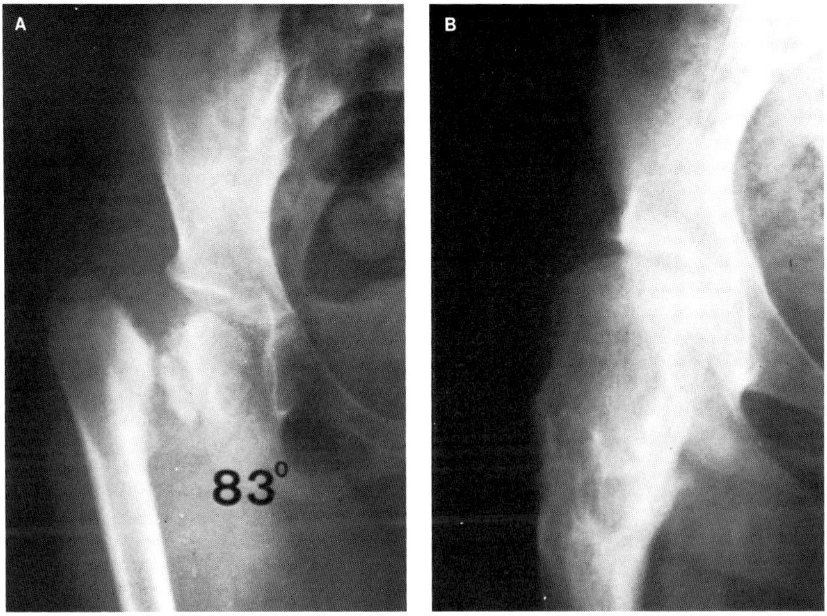

FIGURE 4.11. **A:** Girl, 6 years and 7 months old, with bilateral coxa vara. The acetabulum of her right hip has not been stimulated to develop since the femoral head is in the inferior portion of the acetabulum. Potential for future acetabular development is diminished owing to her age. **B:** Valgus osteotomy was performed at 6 years and 8 months of age with correction of the neck-shaft angle to 145 degrees. Proximal femoral capital physeal closure was noted 4 months later at 7 years of age. This roentgenogram at 13 years and 5 months of age shows no response of acetabular development to the valgus correction.

before proceeding to osteotomy; angles less than 45 degrees were expected to correct spontaneously. The angle measurement was taken from supine, not weight-bearing, roentgenograms. The accuracy and consistency of measurements can be subject to pelvic obliquity and inconsistent lower-limb placement since the measured angle occurs across a joint.

The goal of osteotomy is to restore the neck-shaft angle to 140 degrees, thereby converting shear forces across the physis and endochondral defect to compressive forces. This results in realignment of the capital physis to a normal position. Excessive overcorrection and damage to the capital physis and greater trochanteric apophysis should be avoided. The normal biomechanics of the hip joint should be restored and effective length of the abductor muscles reestablished.

The method of proximal femoral osteotomy is not as important as long as neck-shaft angulation of 140 degrees is reestablished through the intertrochanteric region. Many techniques of osteotomy have been de-

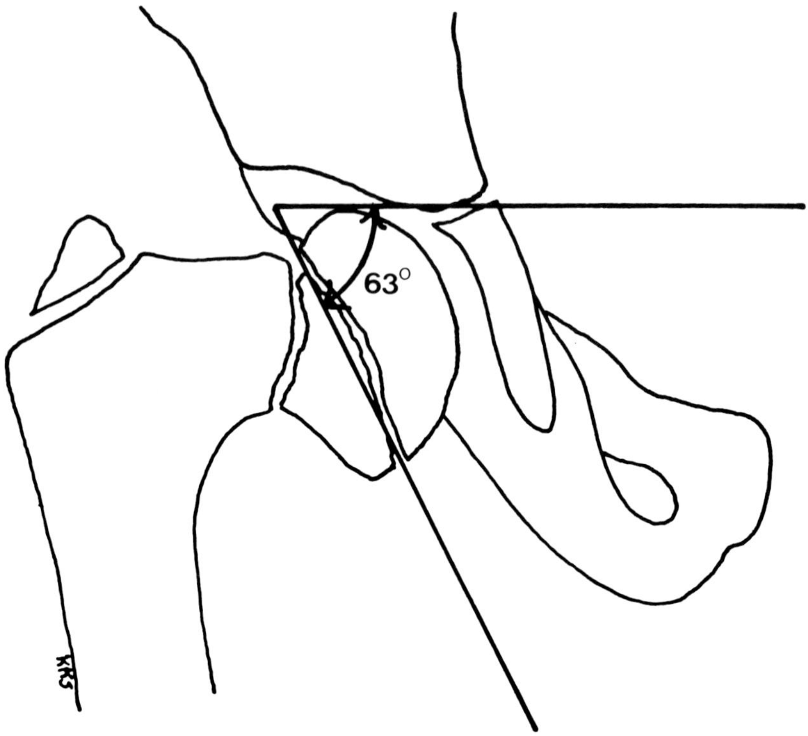

FIGURE 4.12. Hilgenreiner epiphyseal angle measurement used to assess need for operative treatment.

scribed and all can be effective. Simply transecting the bone and securing proper angulation with a children's hip osteotomy device is all that is needed. Weighill,[58] Lasserre,[37] and Johanning[27] point out that adductor tenotomy prior to osteotomy helps in obtaining the amount of neck-shaft angle correction needed by reducing the tension across the osteotomy. Weighill reported that inadequate correction occurred only in instances where adductor tenotomy had been omitted. Flexion at the osteotomy site should be avoided. This can be prevented by release and transposition of the iliopsoas tendon with lesser trochanter.

Postoperative care depends on the type of fixation used but usually involves immobilization in a hip spica cast for 6 weeks or until the osteotomy is healed. Following cast removal, weight-bearing is protected on the affected side until the endochondral defect is observed to have healed, usually within 4 to 12 months.[24] After this, observation should be carried out for possible early closure of the physis and adequate acetabular development.

Results of osteotomy are reported universally as good, but consistency

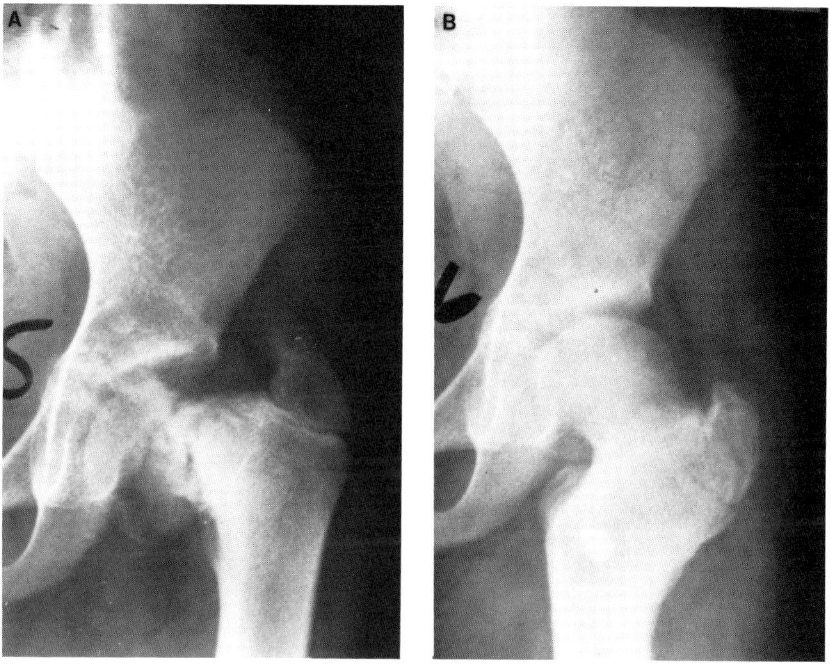

FIGURE 4.13. **A:** Coxa vara of 86 degrees in a girl 7 years and 11 months of age prior to valgus osteotomy. Adductor tenotomy was not done. **B:** Seven months after valgus osteotomy of 140 degrees the triangular defect has healed and the capital physis has closed.

as to what constitutes a good result is lacking. The variables to be assessed are an adequate amount of neck-shaft angle correction, age of patient at time of osteotomy, presence of physeal arrest, and degree of acetabular development, all of which affect the quality of the final outcome. Early neck-shaft angle correction to 140 degrees in a very young child is recommended, with observation for progression and repeat osteotomy if necessary. Extreme valgus is not recommended because the femoral head will not exert an adequate remodeling stimulus for acetabular development. Besides defining an adequate neck-shaft angle correction in evaluating results of osteotomy, the problems of physeal arrest and adequate acetabular development should be assessed.

Many authors† have noted premature physeal arrest following valgus osteotomy for developmental coxa vara. The incidence is not well established, but it would seem to occur in a significant number. Schmidt and Kalamchi[56] reported that premature closure of the capital physis was

† References 2–4, 6, 11, 15, 22, 24, 38, 42, 52, 53, 56–58.

seen in 89% of 16 hips after valgus osteotomy (Fig. 4.13). The endochondral defect healed in all hips having adequate valgus correction. Physeal closure was present 2 to 41 months postoperatively, with 81% of the closures occurring within 18 months of osteotomy. No relationship between closure and age at time of osteotomy or amount of neck-shaft angle correction was noted. Surgical technique could be indicted as the possible cause in only one instance.

Why the physis closes prematurely after osteotomy is as yet unexplained. Changing the posture of the physis and the proximal femur changes the biomechanical forces through the femoral neck region. Muscle tension is increased, particularly in the adductors and iliopsoas. The role that increased tension plays on a possibly precarious vascular supply to the endochondral defect is unknown. A change in this vascular balance may contribute to early closure. More experience with release of these muscles at the time of osteotomy is needed to determine if this treatment modification will have a positive effect in reducing the incidence of capital physeal closure. In many instances the extent of the endochondral defect is too great to overcome the involvement of too much physis for recovery of function, causing early closure regardless of surgery. A change, then, in the position of the capital physis with subsequent change in the biomechanical stresses may either precipitate physeal closure if involvement of the endochondral defect is too great or may allow further growth if the physis is relatively intact.

Acetabular dysplasia associated with developmental coxa vara has been described previously,‡ but little has been said about it in relation to treatment. The center-edge angle of Wiberg has been used to evaluate acetabular dysplasia,[53] but this can be a misleading indicator for assessing the effectiveness of the acetabular containment of the femoral head. The center-edge angle describes the relationship of the acetabular rim to the femoral head. It does not reflect the widening and flattening and consequently the deficient depth of the acetabulum, which becomes even more apparent after osteotomy. We have used an acetabular depth index (Fig. 4.14) to evaluate the effectiveness of acetabular development following osteotomy.[56] The acetabular depth tended to improve following an osteotomy that regained correction to 140 degrees. Valgus correction less than 140 degrees did not result in any significant change in acetabular depth. It seems then that valgus correction needs to be adequate and is more effective when applied early if acetabular depth is to be influenced. Return of a tear-drop configuration to the medial acetabular wall confirms acetabular development and the effectiveness of the valgus correction, particularly when performed at younger ages.[56]

Concern for a sufficient acetabulum arises in the older child when

‡ References 3, 4, 7, 15, 24, 32, 35, 42, 43, 53, 56, 58.

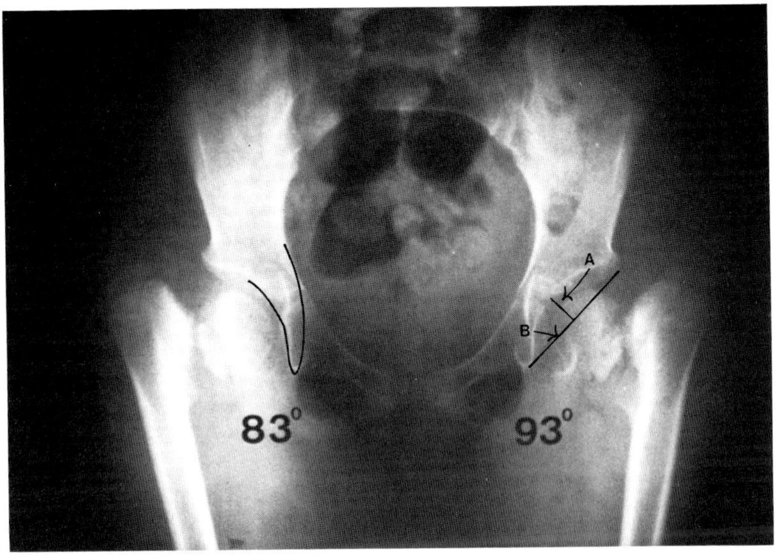

FIGURE 4.14. Measurement of the acetabular depth index is illustrated on the patient's left hip. The index is determined by dividing the depth (A) of the acetabulum by one half the width (B) of the acetabular opening. The point at which the depth is determined is defined by a line bisecting and perpendicular to the line extending from the superior rim to the inferior rim of the acetabulum. The right hip demonstrates lack of development of normal tear-drop configuration of the medial acetabular wall, reflecting acetabular dysplasia. The acetabulum appears flattened with widening of the acetabular opening. It can be seen that the center-edge angle of Wiberg can be a misleading indicator for assessing the acetabulum.

overcorrection beyond 150 to 155 degrees occurs or when valgus correction greater than 140 degrees is performed in the presence of a very shallow acetabulum. The femoral head may become relatively uncovered, causing inadequate transmission of weight-bearing stress to the pelvis with the result that degenerative changes occur (Fig. 4.11). Acetabular development following valgus correction in these circumstances should be observed, and treatment should be considered for the acetabular side of the joint if necessary.

Greater trochanteric overgrowth and leg-length discrepancy are two problems that complicate the occurrence of capital physeal closure. Arrest of the greater trochanteric apophysis or transfer of the greater trochanter may be required to maintain the effectiveness of abductor power. Leg-length discrepancy in unilateral involvement should not exceed 4 cm, even with early closure of the capital physis, and can be effectively dealt with by appropriately timed epiphysiodesis.

Recurrence of varus deformity has been observed, especially if osteotomy has been performed early in childhood, or if valgus correction is inadequate.[24] Repeat valgus osteotomy may be necessary, particularly if the endochondral defect has not healed within a year after surgery. Limitation of range of hip motion may be present following valgus correction.

Complications directly related to the osteotomy itself include malunion or nonunion, failure of internal fixation, avascular necrosis, infection, and greater trochanteric apophysis arrest. The closure of the greater trochanteric apophysis can contribute to further valgus deformity of the proximal femur.[9,23,24]

In a rare instance, a neglected coxa vara with a femoral neck pseudarthrosis in a skeletally mature individual may come to the attention of the orthopedic surgeon. Treatment should be directed to securing the femoral head to the neck with bone graft in addition to valgus osteotomy, as Johanning[27] suggests, with internal fixation extending into the femoral head. Langenskiold has described using the Brackett procedure in which the proximal femoral shaft is inserted into the base of the femoral head with transposition of the greater trochanter.[35] Surgical reconstruction may also be necessary on the acetabular side of the hip joint. Other surgical alternatives for consideration include fusion of the hip joint or total joint replacement. In both treated and untreated cases the sequelae of degenerative arthritis may set in, requiring the orthopedic surgeon to approach this problem as he would any other severe degenerative arthritis.

References

1. Almond HG: Familial infantile coxa vara. J Bone Joint Surg 38B:539–544, 1956.
2. Amstutz HC: Developmental (infantile) coxa vara—a distinct entity. Report of two patients with previously normal roentgenograms. Clin Orthop 72:242–247, 1970.
3. Amstutz HC, Freiberger RH: Coxa vara in children. Clin Orthop 22:73–92, 1962.
4. Amstutz HC, Wilson PD: Dysgenesis of the proximal femur (coxa vara) and its surgical management. J Bone Joint Surg 44A:1–24, 1962.
5. Barr JS: Congenital coxa vara. Arch Surg 18:1909–1919, 1929.
6. Bell M: Surgical management of coxa vara. Orthop Trans 3:344, 1979.
7. Calhoun JD, Pierret G: Infantile coxa vara. Am J Roentgenol Radium Ther Nucl Med 115:561–568, 1972.
8. Chung SMK, Riser WH: The histological characteristics of congenital coxa vara: A case report of a five year old boy. Clin Orthop 132:71–81, 1978.
9. Compere EL, Garrison M, Fahey JJ: Deformities of the femur resulting from arrestment of growth of the capital and greater trochanteric epiphyses. J Bone Joint Surg 22:909–915, 1940.
10. Duncan GA: Congenital coxa vara occurring in identical twins. Am J Surg 37:112, 1937.

11. Duncan GA: Congenital and developmental coxa vara. Surgery 3:741–765, 1938.
12. Elmslie RC: Injury and deformity of the epiphysis of the head of the femur: Coxa vara. Lancet 1:410, 1907.
13. Fiorani G: Sopra una forma speciale di zoppicamento. Gazz Osp 2:717, 1881.
14. Fisher RL, Waskowitz WJ: Familial development coxa vara. Clin Orthop 86:2–5, 1972.
15. Golding JSR: Infantile coxa vara (congenital coxa vara). in Rang M (ed): *The Growth Plate and Its Disorders*. London, Livingstone, 1969, pp 155–161.
16. Gordon SL, Cotler JM: Coxa vara in three patients with concommitant cerebral palsy. Clin Orthop 137:175–180, 1978.
17. Hamanishi C: Congenital short femur. J Bone Joint Surg 62B:307–320, 1980.
18. Haraldsson S: The epiphyseal angle in coxa vara infantum and its relation to results. Acta Orthop Scand 39:76–81, 1968.
19. Helbing C: Die coxa vara. Z Orthop Chir 15:502, 1906.
20. Hoffa A: Die angeborenen coxa vara. Dtsch Med Wochenschz 31:1257, 1905.
21. Hofmeister F: Coxa vara, a typical form of. Beitr Klin Chir 12:245, 1894.
22. Horwitz T: The treatment of congenital (or developmental) coxa vara. Surg Gynecol Obstet 87:71–75, 1948.
23. Hoyt WA Jr, Troyer ML, Reef T, et al: The proximal femoral epiphyses: experimental and correlated clinical observation of their potential. J Bone Joint Surg 48A:1026, 1966.
24. Hoyt WA Jr, Greenberg BJ: Congenital coxa vara, in Tronzo R (ed): *Surgery of the Hip Joint*. Philadelphia, Lea & Febiger, 1973, pp 157–172.
25. Hoyt WA Jr, Greenberg BJ, Melby A III: Congenital coxa vara, in Tronzo RG (ed): *Surgery of the Hip Joint*. New York, Springer-Verlag, 1984, vol 1, pp 203–223.
26. Johanning K: Coxa Vara Infantum I. Clinical appearance and aetiological problems. Acta Orthop Scand 21:273–297, 1951.
27. Johanning K: Coxa Vara Infantum II. Treatment and results of treatment. Acta Orthop Scand 22:100–125, 1952.
28. Kalamchi A, MacEwen GD: Avascular necrosis following treatment of congenital dislocation of the hip. J Bone Joint Surg 62A:876–888, 1980.
29. Kalamchi A, Cowell HR, Kim KI: Congenital deficiency of the femur. J Pediatr Orthop 5:129–134, 1985.
30. Keetley CB: Coxa vara. Lancet 1:1115–1118, 1900.
31. King RE, Lovejoy JF Jr: Familial osteopetrosis with coxa vara, a case report. J Bone Joint Surg 55A: 381–385, 1973.
32. Knowles KG: Congenital coxa vara, presentation of a case. RI Med J, 46:594–596, 1963.
33. Kraske P: Uber die operative Behandlung der statischen Schenkelhalsverbiegung Zentralbl Chir 6:121, 1896.
34. Kredel L: Coxa vara congenita. Contralb Chir 23:969, 1896.
35. Langenskiold F: On pseudarthrosis of the femoral neck in congenital coxa vara. Acta Chir Scand 98:568–575, 1949.
36. Langenskiold A, Salenius P: Epiphyseodesis of the greater trochanter. Acta Orthop Scand 38:199–219, 1967.
37. Lasserre C: Subtrochanteric oblique osteotomy in coxa vara, with temporary external fixation of the fragments. J Bone Joint Surg 13:296–298, 1931.

38. LeMesurier AB: Developmental coxa vara. J Bone Joint Surg 30B:595–605, 1948.
39. LeMesurier AB: Developmental coxa vara. J Bone Joint Surg 33B:478–482, 1951.
40. Letts RM, Shokier MHK: Mirror-image coxa vara in identical twins. J Bone Joint Surg 57A:117–118, 1975.
41. Lian C: Congenital coxa vara and Perthes' disease. Acta Orthop Scand 19:527–535, 1950.
42. Magnusson R: Coxa vara infantum. Acta Orthop Scand 23:284–308, 1954.
43. Michelsson JE, Langenskiold A: Coxa vara following immobilization of the knee in extension in young rabbits. Acta Orthop Scand 45:399–411, 1974.
44. Muller E: Torsion of the femoral neck during the growth period, A new disease picture. Beitr Chir 4:137, 1889.
45. Nilsonne H: Beitrag zur kenntnis der kongenitalen form der coxa vara. Acta Radiol 3:383–408, 1924.
46. Nilsonne H: On congenital coxa vara. Acta Chir Scand 64:217–219, 1929.
47. Noble TP, Hauser ED: Coxa vara. Arch Surg 12:501–538, 1926.
48. Ogden JA, Lee KE, Rudical SA, et al: Proximal femoral epiphysiolysis in the neonate. J Pediatr Orthop 4:285–292, 1984.
49. Pauwels F: Zur Therapie der kindlichen Coxa vara. Verh Dtsch Orthop Ges 30:372–387, 1935.
50. Pauwels F: Congenital coxa vara, in *Biomechanics of the Normal and Diseased Hip*. New York, Springer-Verlag, 1976, pp 42–80.
51. Pavlov H, Goldman AB, Freiberger RH: Infantile coxa vara. Radiology, 135:631–640, 1980.
52. Peabody CW: Subtrochanteric osteotomy in coxa vara. Arch Surg 46:743–749, 1943.
53. Pylkkanen PV: Coxa vara infantum. Acta Orthop Scand 48:1–120, 1960.
54. Say B, Taysi K, Pirnar T, et al: Dominant congenital coxa vara. J Bone Joint Surg 56B:78–85, 1974.
55. Schatz SL, Kopits SE: Proximal femoral focal deficiency. Am J Roentgenol 131:289–295, 1978.
56. Schmidt TL, Kalamchi A: The fate of the capital femoral physis and acetabular development in developmental coxa vara. J Pediatr Orthop 2:534–538, 1982.
57. Trueta J: *Studies of the Development and Decay of the Human Frame*. Philadelphia, WB Saunders Co, 1968, pp 274–278.
58. Weighill FJ: The treatment of developmental coxa vara by abduction subtrochanteric and intertrochanteric femoral osteotomy with special reference to the role of adductor tenotomy. Clin Orthop 116:116–124, 1976.
59. Weinstein JN, Kuo KN, Millar EA: Congenital coxa vara. A retrospective review. J Pediatr Orthop 4:70–77, 1984.
60. Weisl H: Coxa vara in spina bifida. J Bone Surg 65B:128–133, 1983.
61. Wojowycz M, Starshak RJ, Sty JR: Neonatal proximal femoral epiphysiolysis. Radiology 136:647–648, 1980.
62. Wynne-Davies R, Fairbank TJ: *Fairbank's Atlas of General Affections of the Skeleton*. Second edition. New York, Churchill Livingstone, 1976.
63. Zadek I: Congenital coxa vara. Arch Surg 30:62–102, 1935.

5
Congenital Short Femur

ROBERT EILERT

Congenital short femur refers to the type of femoral deficiency wherein all the components of the femur are present, but where there is significant shortening, i.e., greater than 4 cm.

This chapter is concerned with congenital short femur in its variations. Analysis of each patient must be customized to formulate a logical treatment plan, but experience with the variety and combination of problems seen can provide a guide to this evaluation and planning.

Peter Ring[31,32] popularized application of the term "congenital short femur" to the presentation of a child with a proportionally shortened femur. Typically, the clinical presentation is of a shortened femoral segment that is more bulky than the normal side with an external rotation deformity (Fig. 5.1). The greater trochanter may be high riding if there is associated coxa vara. The amount of shortening varies between 10% and 35% of the normal limb. In more than 75% of the cases there is some associated anomaly of the lower leg, such as fibular hemimelia or shortened tibia (Table 5.1). Frequently there is anterior-posterior instability of the knee joint because of absence of the anterior cruciate ligament. Muscular power and movement are normal other than the restriction of internal rotation of the hip. The defect is recognizable at birth, although it may go undetected if the percentage of shortening is small.

The x-ray appearance is of a complete femur that is hypoplastic, i.e., shortened in its length although all the elements of the upper and lower end of the femur are present (Fig. 5.2). The diaphysis may be bowed laterally with some thickening of the lateral cortex. There may be a coxa vara of the femoral neck, although the triangular fragment seen in the femoral neck in cases of isolated congenital coxa vara is not present.[26]

Classification

Various systems of classification have been proposed in the literature,[29,34] including those of Aitken,[2] Hamanishi,[18] Amstutz,[4] and Kalamchi et al.[21]

There has been a fascination in creating classifications of femoral

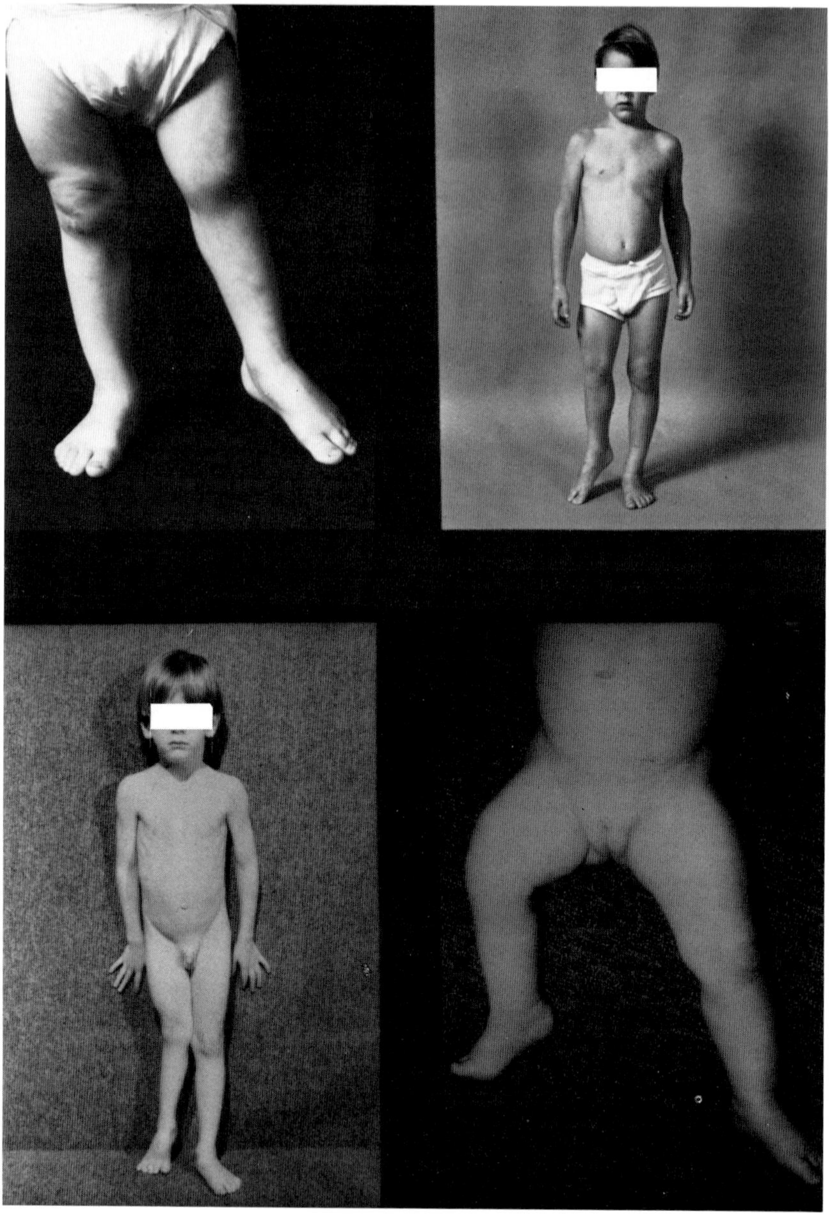

FIGURE 5.1. Four different patients with congenital short femur demonstrating consistency of clinical presentation.

TABLE 5.1. Associated anomalies (in order of occurence).

Knee Deficiency
Absent anterior cruciate ligament
Meniscal anomalies (ring meniscus)
Fibular Deficiency
Everted foot, absent rays
Genu valgum
Ball-and-socket ankle
Tarsal coalition
Tibial Deficiency
Short angulated tibia
Absent tibia

deficiency based on radiologic appearance of the deformity. A spectrum of progressively more severe deficiency has been outlined by numerous authors. None of these classifications has gained wide acceptance, as they are complicated and unwieldy. In trying to place a specific case into one of the proposed categories, one finds that it does not quite fit, and, indeed, it has been suggested that there may be as many categories and subcategories as there are number of cases.

Functionally, severe limb-length discrepancy is the outstanding problem of the femoral-deficient patient such that prosthetic management for ambulation becomes the cornerstone of treatment, with surgery mainly employed to improve alignment or to aid in prosthetic fitting.

The advent of the Wagner technique as a safe, reliable method of limb lengthening has served to separate femoral deficiency into two broad therapeutic groups.[13] One group presents the possibility of limb-length equalization by surgical technique. The second group is associated with such severe shortening and joint deficiency that equalization is possible only by prosthetic devices.

The first group can be collected under the term of congenital short femur, and the second group is designated proximal focal femoral deficiency.[27]

Differential Diagnosis

Differential diagnosis includes congenital dislocation of the hip, congenital coxa vara, proximal focal femoral deficiency, and hemihypertrophy. The hip is located in cases of congenital short femur, but the most common cause of apparent femoral shortening in the newborn is congenital dislocation of the hip. The absence of Ortolani or Barlow's sign and the normal alignment of the hip on x-ray rule out the diagnosis of congenital dislocated hip. Congenital coxa vara in its isolated form is associated with

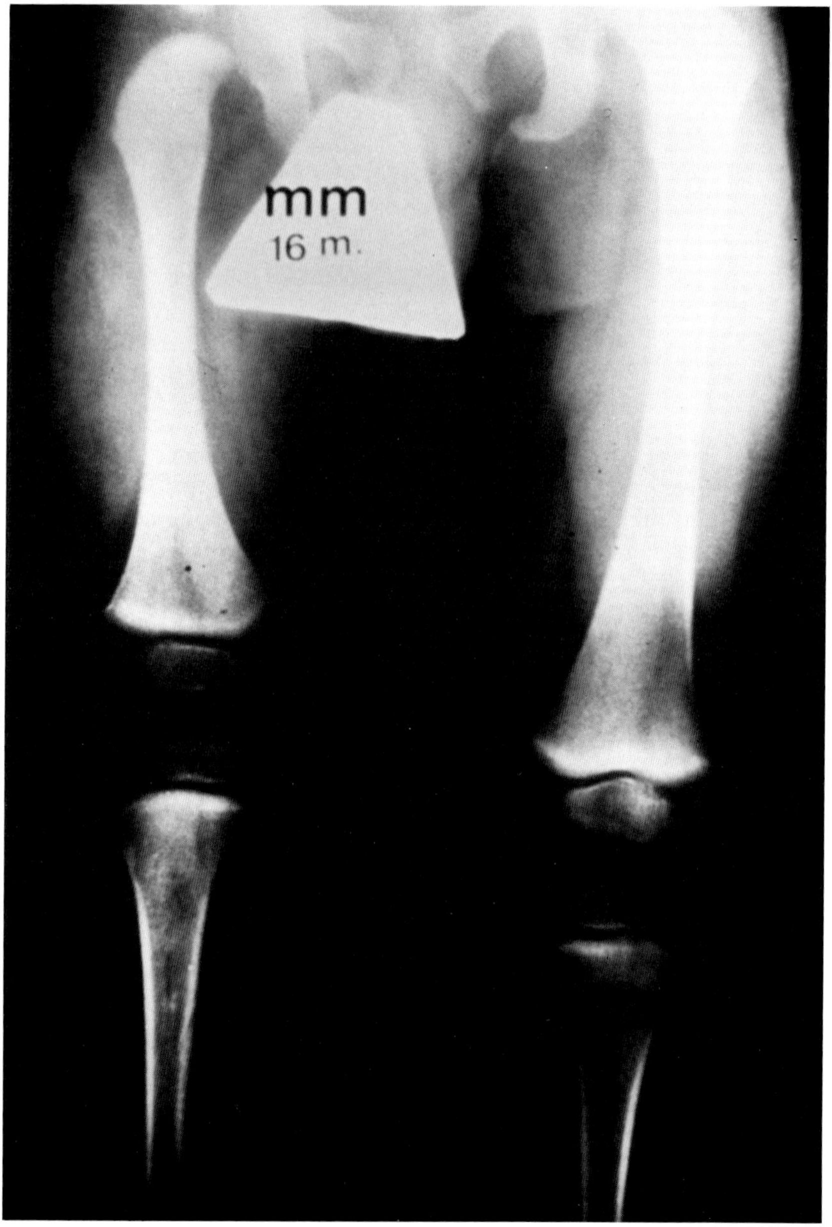

FIGURE 5.2. Radiograph of congenital short femur in patient 16 months old.

a femur of nearly normal length.[3,14] The x-ray appearance of the decreased neck-shaft angle and triangular fragment in the lower portion of the femoral neck is diagnostic of congenital coxa vara and not present in this syndrome.[15] Proximal focal femoral deficiency produces a more severe shortening with obvious severe deformity and complete or partial absence of the femoral head and neck resulting in an absence of acetabular development, which is evident from birth. Congenital hemihypertrophy produces a bulky leg on the involved side, but can be differentiated by the enlargement of soft tissues of the thigh, leg, and foot on the involved side. X-ray examination reveals generalized hypertrophy of the femur with no bowing or cortical thickening and the shorter side appears proportional.

Associated Anomalies

A variety of associated anomalies have been described with congenital short femur. The most common is genu valgum in that there is lateral angulation of the leg. Frequently, the anterior cruciate ligament is deficient such that there is a positive pivot shift present on examination and laxity on both Lachman's test and drawer sign. There may be anomalies of the meniscus, with a ring meniscus being documented in some cases, indicating that the embryologic material for the anterior cruciate ligament has been included in the meniscus (Fig. 5.3). The tibia is shortened frequently and may be angulated anteriorly, particularly if there is fibular deficiency. Fibular deficiency may vary in its presentation from the fibula being hypoplastic with shortening of the leg segment to complete absence of the fibula. If there is fibular deficiency of lesser degree, it may be associated with a ball-and-socket ankle plus or minus fusion of some of the tarsal bones. If there is severe fibular deficiency, frequently the lateral rays of the foot will be absent as well. Less commonly, absence of the tibia occurs in association with congenital short femur.

These associated anomalies are important considerations in planning and implementing treatment for these children. Generally, the greater the number of associated anomalies, the fewer the therapeutic options.

Natural History

Progressive limb length discrepancy is the major clinical problem in congenital short femur. The amount of shortening tends to be proportional, so that the femur that is 10% short at birth will be 10% short at maturity. This geometric progression of shortening was described by Amstutz[5] and can be mathematically expressed as the difference in femoral length divided by the length of the normal femur. This observation has been confirmed by numerous authors,[12,18] including the present. The only major disagreement in the literature is from Shapiro, but it is unlikely that he limited the diagnosis of congenital short femur to the type described in this chapter. If there are severe associated anomalies, the growth pattern is not as predictable.

If the neck-shaft angle is decreased, thereby presenting as a coxa vara deformity, this angulation may be progressive such that the neck-shaft angle decreases with growth. Therefore, a progressive coxa vara deformity may be part of the natural history.

Pain is not generally a feature of the natural history, although progressive coxa vara may produce arthritic changes if left untreated.

Treatment Principles

The preeminent problem for treatment in these children is management of the significant limb length discrepancy, which may be severe in the most hypoplastic femur. The goals of treatment are: (1) to anticipate the

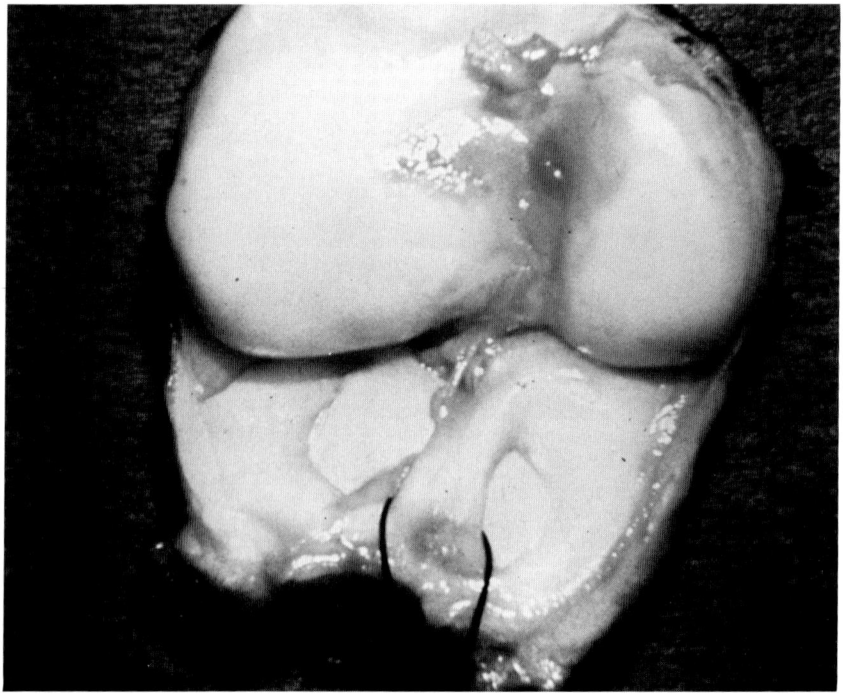

FIGURE 5.3. Resected knee joint in instance where knee fusion was performed for severe femoral deficiency. The suture is looped under the ring meniscus. The anterior cruciate ligament was absent.

ultimate discrepancy; (2) to maximize function even if it means the wearing of some type of prosthesis; (3) to deal effectively with the associated anomalies; (4) to consider the appearance of the limb and minimize psychological negative impact; and (5) to minimize the number of operations and hospitalizations.

The author's approach to management is based on a problem list for each patient. Obviously, the problems increase with the increasing amount of shortening and associated anomalies.

The frequency of follow-up depends on the amount of shortening and on the psychological support necessary for the family. In early infancy I usually see these patients every 3 or 4 months, mainly to help the parents adjust to the deformity and to educate them about the prognosis. The parents are concerned about the impact of the abnormality on their child's life. These children generally have normal mental capabilities since mental retardation is not associated. The parents are greatly encouraged by meeting children similar to their own who are succeeding in school, in sports, and in life. Therefore, an effort is made to get these families together for mutual support and edification.

During childhood a scanogram for limb length and wrist film for bone age are obtained on at least a yearly basis to plot the relative growth and development of the limb. This allows the therapeutic program to be established with some security as to the pattern of growth and percentage of discrepancy present (Table 5.2).

Treatment Recommendations

Valgus Osteotomy of the Proximal Femur

In cases of congenital short femur coxa vara may be present. Persistent severe coxa vara produces deformity of the femoral head and arthrosis[18,30] (Fig. 5.4). The femoral head becomes bullet-shaped rather than round, and degenerative arthritis can occur in the young adult. The coxa vara seen with congenital short femur is not the same as isolated congenital coxa vara.[6] In the isolated form, the femur is only slightly shortened and the x-ray appearance is different, with a triangular fragment in the lower part of the femoral neck. These radiographic findings

TABLE 5.2. Scale for treatment of limb-length discrepancy[a]: shortening vs lengthening.

0–2.5 cm	Shoe lift
2.5–4 cm	Epiphysiodesis
4–18 cm	Limb lengthening
> 18 cm	Prosthetic fitting with or without amputation

[a] Based on Stephens & Wagner.[39] (Stephens DC: Femoral and Tibial Lengthening. J Pediatr Orthop, 3:424–430, 1983.)

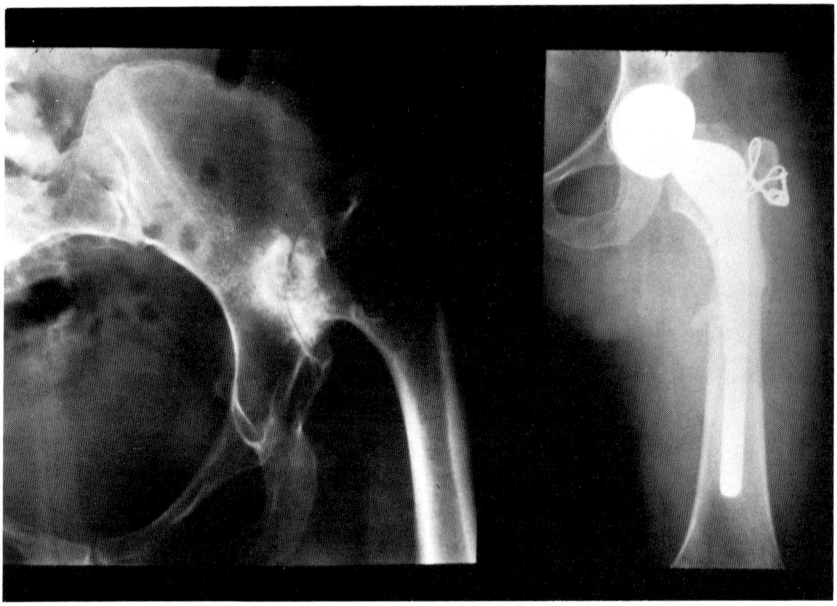

FIGURE 5.4. Degenerative arthritis secondary to coxa vara associated with congenital short femur. This adult was treated with a customized hip prosthesis. (Courtesy D. Messner, M.D.)

are not present in the congenital short femur cases, and there is greater shortening of the femur, with the changes of bowing and cortical sclerosis as previously described.

The coxa vara deformity mechanically weakens the force of the abductor muscles, and the angulation contributes to the shortening of the femur. The indications for operation are: (1) severe coxa vara with a 90-degree neck-shaft angle or less, and (2) progressive coxa vara such that the neck-shaft angle diminishes with growth. Hamanishi has documented that the progressive type of coxa vara may be predicted by measuring the growth-plate angle. If the growth-plate angle is 60 degrees or more, there is high likelihood that the coxa vara will be progressive[18] (Fig 5.5).

The coxa vara deformity can be corrected by valgus osteotomy of the proximal femur, bringing the femur to an angle of at least 150 degrees.[20] If the deformity is progressive, repeat operation may be necessary. Kalamchi showed that in cases of isolated coxa vara, arrest of the growth plate may follow osteotomy, but this has not been the experience in cases of congenital short femur associated with coxa vara.

Various techniques of osteotomy have been employed, but the author's preferred technique is that of Pauwel's,[30] where a lateral closing wedge permits correction of the angulation. It is appropriate at the same time to gain rotational correction if the usual external rotation deformity is

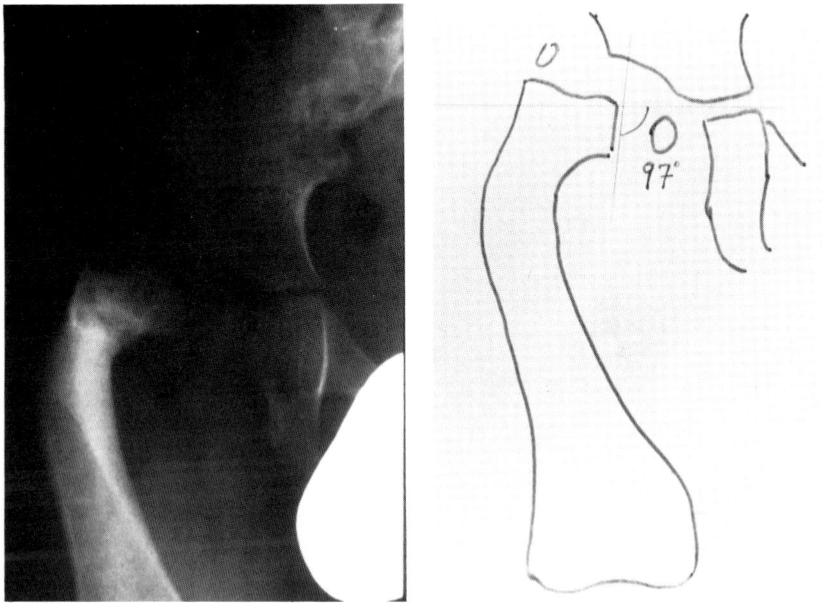

FIGURE 5.5. Growth-plate angle measured by method of Hamanishi[18] is 97 degrees and the coxa vara will be progressive.

present. Fixation in younger children has been effectively maintained with the use of a tension band wire suture as advocated by Pauwel (Fig. 5.6).

The timing for valgus osteotomy of the femur depends on whether the deformity is progressive. Early or severe progression would mandate early operative procedure. Usually the operation is performed about age 5 years.

Van Nes Rotation-Plasty

In cases of severe shortening, the femoral length approaches 50%. In these cases, femoral lengthening for equalization is not a reasonable or possible option. In these instances, the ankle joint may be rotated to function as a knee joint. The patient can be fitted with a below-knee prosthesis using the ankle for the pivot at the knee level as opposed to using an above-knee prosthesis with a mechanical knee joint. The van Nes procedure was originally described by Borggreve[9] and popularized by van Nes[37] and more recently by Kritter[25] and Kostuik et al[24] (Fig. 5.7).

The advantages of the van Nes procedure are that the prosthesis can be simpler and, in successful cases, the gait is more rhythmic and smooth than that of a similar patient fitted with an above-knee prosthesis.

Drawbacks to the operation are the objectionable appearance of the

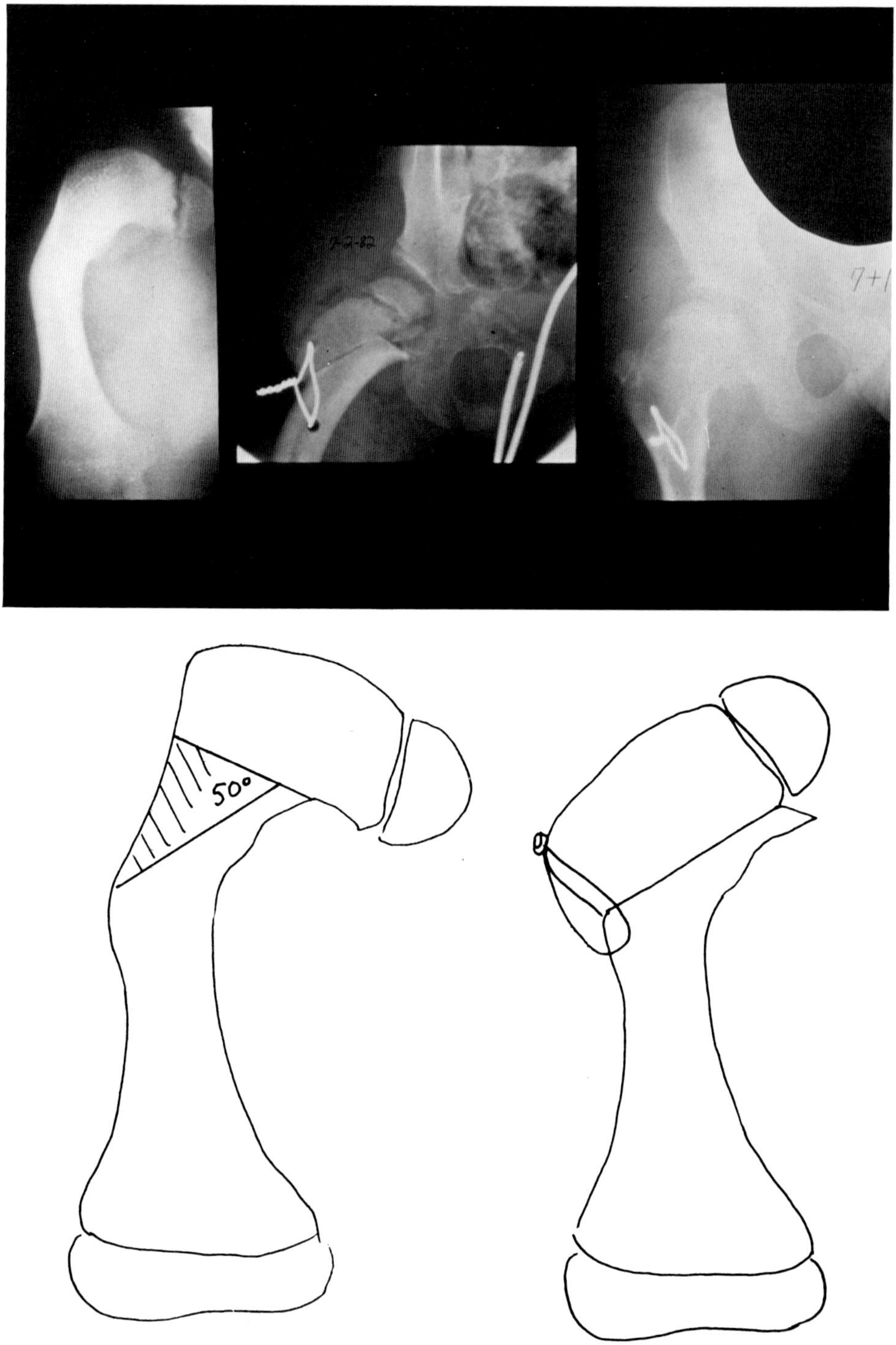

FIGURE 5.6. **A:** Congenital short femur with severe coxa vara. **B:** Immediately following valgus osteotomy by Pauwel's technique. **C:** Three-year follow-up. **D:** Planning diagram for Pauwel's valgus osteotomy. **E:** Drawing of final plan for osteotomy.

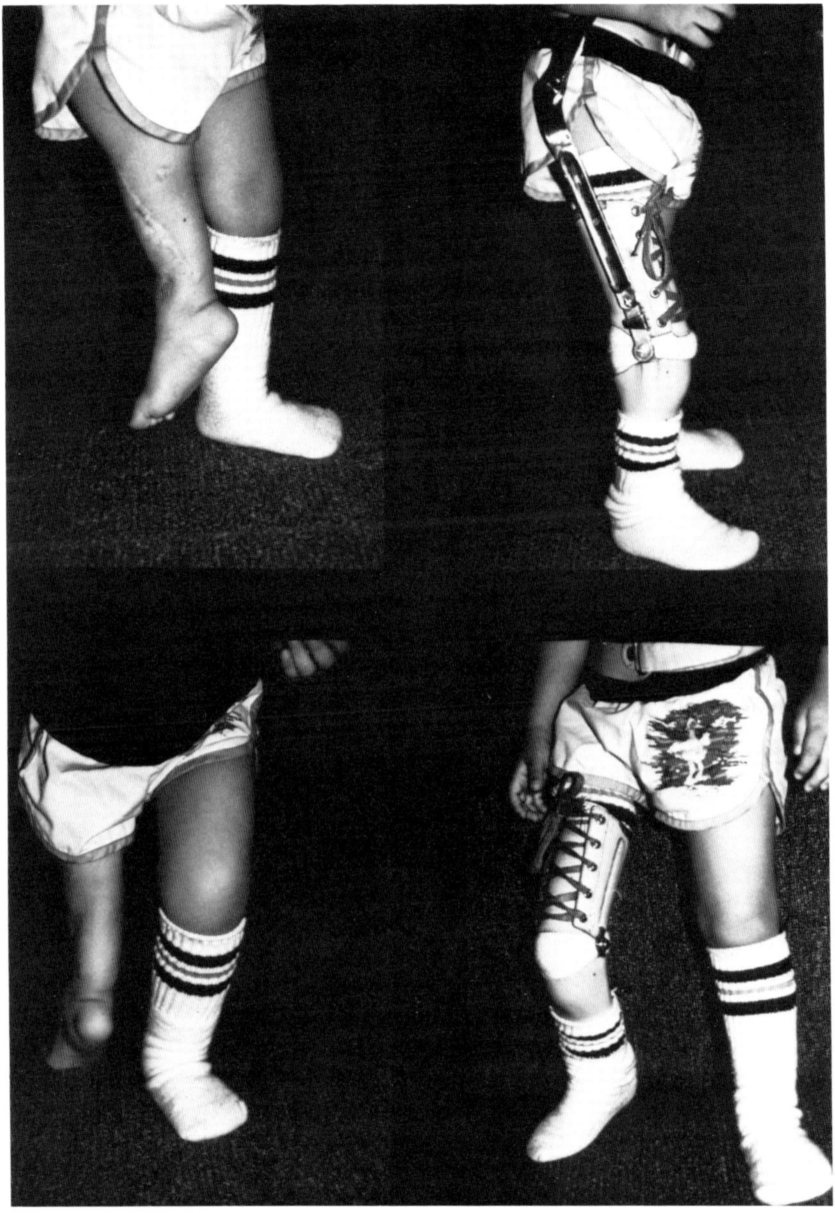

FIGURE 5.7. **A:** Patient following van Nes turnaround procedure showing ankle joint functioning as a knee. **C,D:** Prosthetic fitting.

reversed foot, which generally is not acceptable to females, including the mothers of male patients. The operation is, for the most part, more applicable to proximal focal femoral deficiency where severe shortening of 50% or greater is a feature.

The operation is usually combined with arthrodesis of the knee to stabilize the proximal segment. In cases of fibular hemimelia, which is frequently an associated problem, the ankle joint is not fully formed and does not function well after a van Nes procedure.

Another problem with the rotation-plasty is the tendency for the limb to derotate as the child grows, necessitating multiple operative procedures to maintain the position of the foot with the heel facing forward. The advantage of operating early is that flexibility and the ability to train the patient are greater. On the other hand, the older patient has less problems with derotation and the operation does not have to be repeated. Gillespie[24] originally suggested that the operation should be postponed until age 12 years, but more recently has resected a longer segment of bone at the time of derotation, thereby providing better relaxation of muscle and avoiding some of the derotation problem.

Knee Arthrodesis

In severe cases, which are those with the highest percentage of shortening, the knee is unstable. This is due to congenital anomalies within the knee joint, such as absence of the anterior cruciate ligament and abnormalities of the meniscus, which at times even produce a ring-shaped meniscus. The range of motion of these knee joints is limited, as is the muscle power. The knee then becomes a point of deformity, either angular or rotatory, rather than functioning as a true hinge joint. In its extremely high position, the knee does not provide for functional gait in most instances. By arthrodesis of the knee, correction of alignment may be obtained, especially flexion deformity. Stabilization of the knee joint by arthrodesis produces better function for the above-knee prosthesis, providing a stronger stump with better control[22,23] (Fig. 5.8). In cases where the van Nes rotation-plasty is done or planned at the ankle level, arthrodesis is an excellent ancillary procedure for alignment and stabilization.

Two basic techniques for arthrodesis have been proposed: the intramedullary or central pin technique and the compression or Charnley-type technique. In both instances the cartilage is debrided from the end of the bone to expose the epiphyseal bony center. Fusion then occurs between the epiphyseal center of the femur and that of the tibia. By this technique the growth plates are preserved on either side of the knee joint, if they are present, and further growth can occur.

The timing of knee arthrodesis has been variously proposed as being between 2 and 4 years of age, but it probably should be done closer to 4 years.

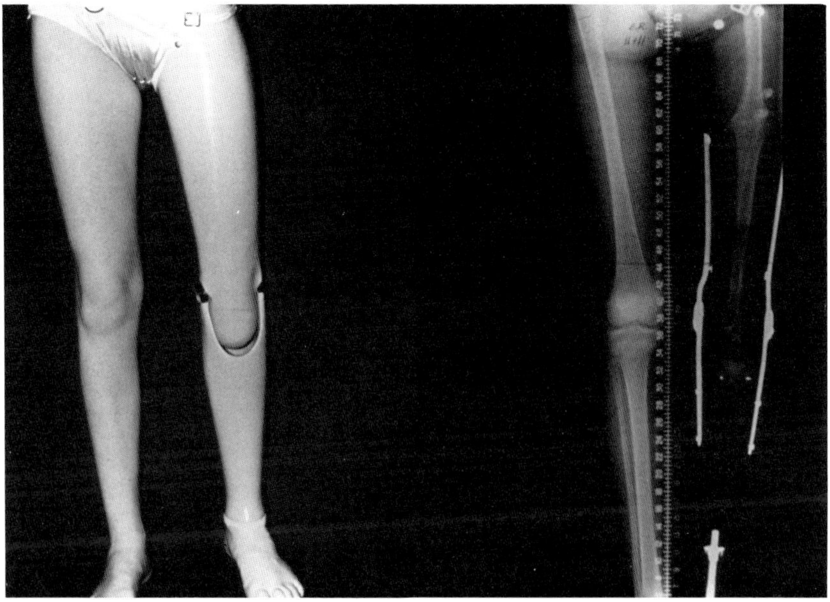

FIGURE 5.8. Severe congenital short femur and absent fibula treated by knee arthrodesis and Syme's amputation; fitted with above-knee prosthesis.

Syme's Amputation

In the patient with shortening beyond 30% of the length of the normal femur, equalization by surgical technique is not practical and prosthetic equalization is necessary. Syme's amputation can be used in these cases of severe shortening to facilitate standard prosthetic fitting.[10,17] Frequently in severe shortening cases, there are associated anomalies that also dictate amputation as a reasonable procedure for converting the limb to an evenly contoured stump.[1,11] These associated anomalies may be fibular hemimelia or tibial hemimelia in which there is severe joint deformity at the ankle or knee level as well as a severely deformed foot.

Syme's amputation provides an end-bearing stump using the heel cushion as a weight-bearing structure. The heel cushion is a specialized anatomic structure in that there are cells within the pad defined by the perpendicular fibrous septae between the skin and the bone. These cells function as hydraulic compression units and are not shifted by shear stress.[11]

The technique for Syme's amputation[36] is well described by Harris,[19] who popularized this procedure after World War II as a good amputation level for function. Its appropriateness for children has been well documented. Major details include maintaining the heel pad intact and carefully centering and attaching the heel pad perpendicular to the shaft of the bone at the time of operation.[11,40]

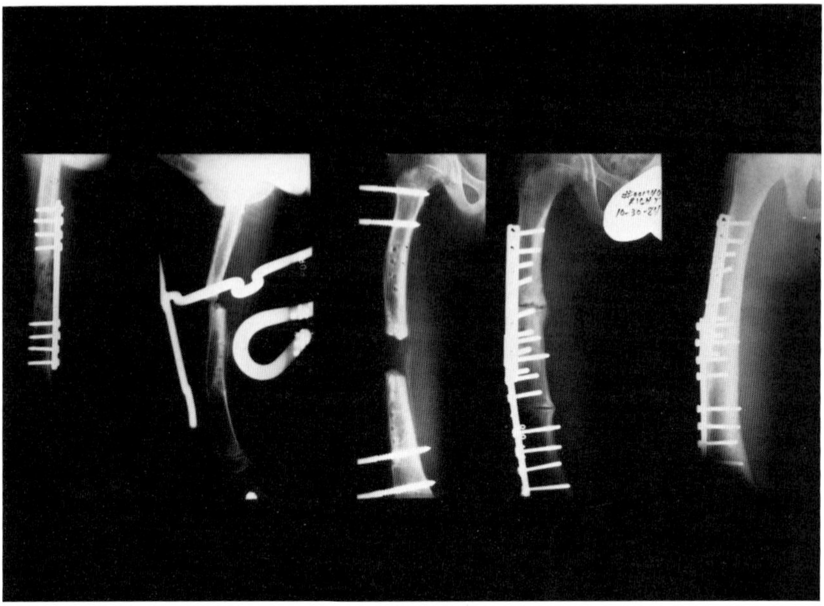

FIGURE 5.9. Two-stage femoral lengthening by Wagner technique. **A:** Postoperative appearance after 6-cm lengthening, grafting, and plating. **B:** Fracture occurring several months after plate removal. **C:** Opportunistic lengthening after fracture with Wagner device and Schantz pins. **D:** Double osteotomy to correct bowing after second lengthening. **E:** Postoperative 2 years with 13-cm total femoral lengthening.

Syme's amputation or the Boyd variant can be performed about the time the child begins to stand and walk in cases where the natural history is well established and the parents are fully oriented. The amputation serves as a salvage or fallback procedure at a later age or in instances where the van Nes rotation-plasty may have failed or not been accepted.

Distal Femoral Epiphysiodesis

Epiphysiodesis is a reasonable procedure for discrepancy of 2.5 to 4 cm. A lesser discrepancy can be equalized easily by shoe lifts, and a larger discrepancy mandates either femoral lengthening or prosthetic management.

Epiphysiodesis of the distal femur may be used on the ipsilateral side to adjust the height of the prosthetic knee in cases where knee arthrodesis is performed. It may be used on the contralateral side more frequently to make up the last bits of discrepancy in cases where surgical lengthening has approximated the normal side.

The prerequisite for performing epiphysiodesis is a good growth study record in which the growth pattern has been documented by repeated scanograms and bone age studies.[7,8,16,28] In congenital short femur the expected growth pattern is a geometric one in that the percentage of shortening present at birth does not change throughout growth. In other words, if the femur is 85% of the length of its normal opposite mate, that proportional relationship will continue throughout growth and in an adult the femur will still be 85% of the normal length.

Femoral Lengthening

The advent of the Wagner technique and device for performing femoral lengthening has provided a reproducible method by which lengthening of 15% to 20% can safely be obtained.[38,39]

There are several requirements for femoral lengthening to be entertained as a possibility: (1) The hip and knee must both be stable. (2) There must be a reasonable expectation of equalization of limb length. (3) A cooperative patient and family are imperative for completion of the lengthy and complicated procedure.

If a patient is of average height, a 20% gain in length would mean approximately 10 cm. In one session of femoral lengthening, 6 to 7 cm is the usual gain. My personal best femoral lengthening is 14 cm in two sessions, which would approximate 28% of normal femoral length. Wagner has related to me that he has lengthened a femur as much as 18 cm in as many as three sessions, which would represent close to a 35% gain in length (Figure 5.9).

It is possible to gain lengthening approaching 30% if one anticipates at least two sessions, but it is certainly difficult to persuade the usual American patient to go more than two sessions, since the process is slow and laborious, gaining about 1 cm per week during the lengthening procedure. Bone grafting is necessary in a high percentage of cases, and ancillary procedures for placing and removing bone plates are also a part of the procedure. In counseling parents, I generally explain that the total time for supervision on a particular lengthening session is about 8 months from inception to the completion of satisfactory healing, i.e., the point that full unprotected weight-bearing is permitted.

Femoral lengthening is complicated and complications are an expected part of the procedure. It is never a question of whether complications will arise, but simply when they will arise; consequently, you expect them and treat them. These complications include pin tract infection, loss of motion, joint subluxation, fracture, osteoporosis, psychosis, and malunion. The procedure, therefore, is not to be undertaken lightly.

A few technical points are important when performing a lengthening for congenital short femur. The soft tissues are "programmed" to be short in these limbs as opposed to shortening by trauma or infection where the soft tissues are "programmed" to normal length and respond better to lengthening. The fascia must be resected, including the lateral intramuscular septum as far as it can safely be reached. This avoids some problem with angulation during lengthening and allows more lengthening to occur. The pins should be placed anterior to the fascia lata to allow flexion of the knee during lengthening so that range of motion can be maintained. A range of motion of at least 70 degrees needs to be maintained by vigorous twice daily physical therapy during the lengthening procedure.

Frequently, preliminary procedures are necessary to stabilize the knee or hip joint, and it is suggested that severe varus angulation or derotation of the femur be corrected prior to the lengthening. Lesser angulatory deformities of 15 or 20 degrees may be corrected simultaneously with lengthening, but greater amounts of angulation are better corrected by preliminary operation.

The timing of operation should be around age 8 in those cases where double or triple sessions will be necessary, but may be postponed until age 10 or 12 in cases where a single lengthening will provide equalization. This would be in instances where 6 or 7 cm is required, representing 15 to 20% of the femoral length. Multiple sessions are spaced at 2 to 3 years apart to allow for bony healing and for removal of hardware prior to the next session.

Varus Osteotomy of the Distal Femur or Proximal Tibia

The valgus deformity at the knee is a frequent feature of congenital short femur. It may be especially prominent in cases where the fibula is deficient or absent. The deformity becomes more obvious as rotation and angulation of the proximal and midfemur are corrected. The choice of the distal femur or proximal tibia is determined by which level will leave the knee joint parallel to the floor. In most of my cases, this has resulted in an osteotomy of the proximal tibia below the tibial tubercle to avoid damage to the growth of the upper tibia.

Timing for the varus osteotomy at the knee level is somewhat later, as it is a good "fine tuning" procedure. Early on, some adjustments and compensation can be made in the prosthesis for those who are prosthetic wearers. It is worthwhile waiting to observe the effect of time in cases of fibular deficiency, as the angular deformity may decrease with growth.

The technique for osteotomy is usually an opening/closing wedge osteotomy so that it is opened part way on the lateral side and closed on the medial side with transfer of a bone wedge. This type of osteotomy tends to pivot the correction in the mid-portion of the bone and give a better appearance to the limb.

Summary

Congenital short femur is a form of femoral deficiency that presents the possibility of surgical equalization of limb length. By observation of growth patterns and careful planning, surgical treatment can enhance the management of this congenital long-bone deficiency.

References

1. Aitken GT: Amputation as a treatment for certain lower-extremity congenital abnormalities. J Bone Joint Surg 41-A: 1267–1285, 1959.
2. Aitken GT: Proximal femoral focal deficiency—Definition, classification, and management, in Aitken GT (ed): *Proximal Femoral Focal Deficiency, A Congenital Anomaly*. National Academy of Sciences, 1969, pp 1–22.
3. Almond HG: Familial infantile coxa vara. J Bone Joint Surg 38-B: 539–544, 1956.
4. Amstutz HC: The morphology, natural history, and treatment of proximal femoral focal deficiencies, in Aitken GT (ed): *Proximal Femoral Focal Deficiency, A Congenital Anomaly*. National Academy of Sciences, 1969, pp 50–76.
5. Amstutz HC: Prognosis for growth and development of congenital anomalies of the lower extremities, abstracted. J Bone Joint Surg 49-A: 1011, 1967.
6. Amstutz HC, Wilson PD Jr: Dysgenesis of the proximal femur (coxa vara) and its surgical management. J Bone Joint Surg 44-A: 1–24, 1962.
7. Anderson M, Green WT, Messner MB: Growth and predictions of growth in the lower extremities. J Bone Joint Surg 45-A: 1–14, 1963.
8. Anderson M, Messner MB, Green WT: Distribution of lengths of the normal femur and tibia in children from one to eighteen years of age. J Bone Joint Surg 46-A: 1197–1202, 1964.
9. Borggreve J: Kniegelenksersatz durch das in der Beinlängsachse um 180° gedrehte Fussgelenk. Arch Orthop Unfallchir 28: 175–178, 1930.
10. Davidson WH, Bohne W: The syme amputation in children. J Bone Joint Surg 57-A: 905–909, 1975.
11. Eilert RE, Jayakumar SS: Boyd and syme ankle amputations in children. J Bone Joint Surg 58-A: 1138–1141, 1976.
12. Fixsen JA, Lloyd-Roberts GC: The natural history and early treatment of proximal femoral dysplasia. J Bone Joint Surg 56-B: 86–95, 1974.
13. Gillespie R, Torode IP: Classification and management of congenital abnormalities of the femur. J Bone Joint Surg 65-B: 557–568, 1983.
14. Golding FC: Congenital coxa vara. J Bone Joint Surg 30-B: 161–163, 1948.
15. Golding C: Congenital coxa vara and the short femur. Proc R Soc Med 32: 641–648, 1938.
16. Green WT, Anderson M: Skeletal age and the control of bone growth, in: *Instructional Course Lectures, The American Academy of Orthopaedic Surgeons*, vol XVIL. St Louis, CV Mosby Co, 1960, pp 199–217.
17. Hall JE, Bochmann D: The surgical and prosthetic management of proximal femoral focal deficiency, in Aitken GT (ed): *Proximal Femoral Focal Defi-*

ciency, A Congenital Anomaly. National Academy of Sciences, 1969, pp 77–99.
18. Hamanishi C: Congenital short femur. Clinical, genetic and epidemiological comparison of the naturally occurring condition with that caused by thalidomide. J Bone Joint Surg 62-B: 307–320, 1980.
19. Harris RI: Syme's amputation. The technical details essential for success. J Bone Joint Surg 38-B: 614–632, 1956.
20. Hoyt WA, Greenberg BJ: Congenital coxa vara, in Tronzo RG (ed): *Surgery of the Hip Joint*. Philadelphia, Lea & Febiger, 1973, pp 157–172.
21. Kalamchi A, Cowell HR, Kim KI: Congenital deficiency of the femur. J Pediatr Orthop 5(2): 129–134, 1985.
22. King RE: Proximal femoral focal deficiencies, in Tronzo RG (ed): *Surgery of the Hip Joint*. Philadelphia, Lea & Febiger, 1973, pp 126–156.
23. King RE: Some concepts of proximal femoral focal deficiency, in Aitken GT (ed): *Proximal Femoral Focal Deficiency, A Congenital Anomaly*. National Academy of Sciences, 1969, pp 23–49.
24. Kostuik JP, Gillespie R, Hall JE, et al: Van Nes rotational osteotomy for treatment of proximal femoral focal deficiency and congenital short femur. J Bone Joint Surg 57-A: 1039–1046, 1975.
25. Kritter AE: Tibial rotation-plasty for proximal femoral focal deficiency. J Bone Joint Surg 59-A: 927–934, 1977.
26. LeMesurier AB: Developmental coxa vara. J Bone Joint Surg 30-B: 595–605, 1948.
27. Lloyd-Roberts GC, Stone KH: Congenital hypoplasia of the upper femur. J Bone Joint Surg 45-B: 557–560, 1963.
28. Moseley CF: A straight-line graph for leg-length discrepancies. J Bone Joint Surg 59-A: 174–179, 1977.
29. Pappas AM: Congenital abnormalities of the femur and related lower extremity malformations: Classification and treatment. J Pediatr Orthop 3(1): 45–60, 1983.
30. Pauwels F: *Biomechanics of the Normal and Diseased Hip. Theoretical Foundation, Technique and Results of Treatment. An Atlas*. New York, Springer-Verlag, 1976.
31. Ring PA: Congenital abnormalities of the femur. Arch Dis Child 36: 410–417, 1961.
32. Ring PA: Congenital short femur—simple femoral hypoplasia. J Bone Joint Surg 41-B: 73–79, 1959.
33. Schmidt TL, and Kalamchi A: The fate of the capital femoral physis and acetabular development in developmental coxa vara. J Pediatr Orthop 2(5): 534–538, 1982.
34. Shands AR Jr, Macewen GD: Congenital abnormalities of the femur. Acta Orthop Scand 32: 307–314, 1962.
35. Shapiro F: Developmental patterns in lower-extremity length discrepancies. J Bone Joint Surg 64-A: 639–651, 1982.
36. Syme J: Surgical cases and observations. Lond Edinb Mon J Med Sci 26: 93–96, 1843.
37. Van Nes CP: Rotation-plasty for congenital defects of the femur. Making use of the ankle of the shortened limb to control the knee joint of a prosthesis. J Bone Joint Surg 32-B: 12–16, 1950.

38. Wagner H: Operative lengthening of the femur. Clin Orthop 136: 125–142, 1978.
39. Wagner H: Surgical lengthening or shortening of femur and tibia. Technique and indications, in Hungerford DS (ed): *Leg Length Discrepancy—The Injured Knee*. New York, Springer-Verlag, 1977, pp 71–94.
40. Westin GW, Sakai DN, Wood WL: Congenital longitudinal deficiency of the fibula. Follow-up of treatment by Syme amputation. J Bone Joint Surg 58-A: 492–496, 1976.

6
Proximal Femoral Focal Deficiency

IVAN KRAJBICH

Introduction

Congenital abnormalities of the femur with or without involvement of the hip joint are numerous and have been widely reported in the literature. Among them is a group of conditions involving primarily the subtrochantric area of the proximal femur. The rest of the femur and iliofemoral articulation are involved to a certain degree as well. These conditions have a rather distinct clinical and radiographic appearance.

It was not until the pioneering work of Aitken, King, Amstutz,[1,2,3,4,5,19,22] and several others[6,7,39,29] in the 1960s that these conditions were recognized as a distinct entity of differing severity and became known under the name of proximal femoral focal deficiency (PFFD). The term describes a rather unique spectrum of congenital femoral deficiency with characteristic clinical and radiographic features. At the same time it excludes other congenital abnormalities of the femur, which were frequently associated with femoral deficiency in the past, such as congenital coxa vara (also called cervical developmental infantile coxa vara), cogenital short femur, and phocomelia. The PFFD varies in severity—from the relatively mild case, with a defect of ossification in the subtrochanteric area and a significantly short femur yet relatively normal iliofemoral articulation—to a condition where the hip joint is completely absent and the only femur present is a small ossicle of the distal femoral epiphysis. The defect may be unilateral or bilateral. Bilateral cases can be symmetrical or asymmetrical, but have a tendency to be of a more severe degree.

Etiology

The etiology of this condition remains unknown; however, some conclusions can be drawn from embryologic studies.[22,32,33] We know that the limb bud starts to develop at approximately 32 days of fetal life.

Thereafter the limb develops rather rapidly from proximal to most distal. The development then progresses gradually through mesenchymal condensation, chondrification and eventually ossification of the bones. The hip joint components—the head, the femoral head, neck, and the acetabulum—develop from a common block of cartilage. The hip joint appears as a cleft between the head of the femur and acetabulum in the common cartilagenous anlage. The cleft gradually propagates, separating the two components until a definite joint cavity is formed. Based on these data and on a review of radiographic examinations of patients with PFFD, King[22] pointed out that the development of the femur and the acetabulum were mutually dependent. The presence of an adequate acetabulum, which can be ascertained on early radiographs, always means that the femoral head is likewise present, although its ossification may be delayed significantly. Similarily, if no acetabular development can be ascertained, no femoral head will develop. As limb bud development and hip joint formation occur in the first 2 to 7 weeks of fetal life, it seems reasonable to assume that this is the time when the ethiologic factors come into play in the development of the PFFD. This corresponds to the clinical finding of significant congenital limb deformities in children of mothers who took thalidomide in the first 4 to 6 weeks of gestation.[16,25] However, no similar agent has been identified as an ethiologic factor in cases of PFFD. Whatever the insult to the developing limb bud may be, it leaves a profound deficit in the formation of the proximal femur, in the muscle development in the proximal thigh, in the knee joint, and, to a variable degree, in the lower leg. The spectrum of severity we encounter clinically and the high incidence of other congenital skeletal abnormalities associated with the PFFD are likely to correspond to the severity of the intrauterine insult and its timing (earlier insult leading to more profound deficit).

Clinical Manifestation

The clinical appearance of the child born with PFFD is very typical. The thigh segment is abnormally short, held in flexion, abduction, and external rotation. Hip and knee flexion contractures are present, and this—together with the abrupt change in diameter of the proximal thigh closely adjacent to the calf—gives the child's leg an appearance of a ship's funnel. Owing to the combination of the short femoral segment and the flexion contracture at the iliofemoral articulation and knee joint, the foot of the affected extremity is frequently at the level of the opposite knee, showing a characteristically severe leg-length discrepancy (Fig. 6.1). There is always significant instability of the knee joint in the anteroposterior (AP) plane, due to deficient or absent cruciate ligaments. The condition itself is frequently associated with some degree of fibular

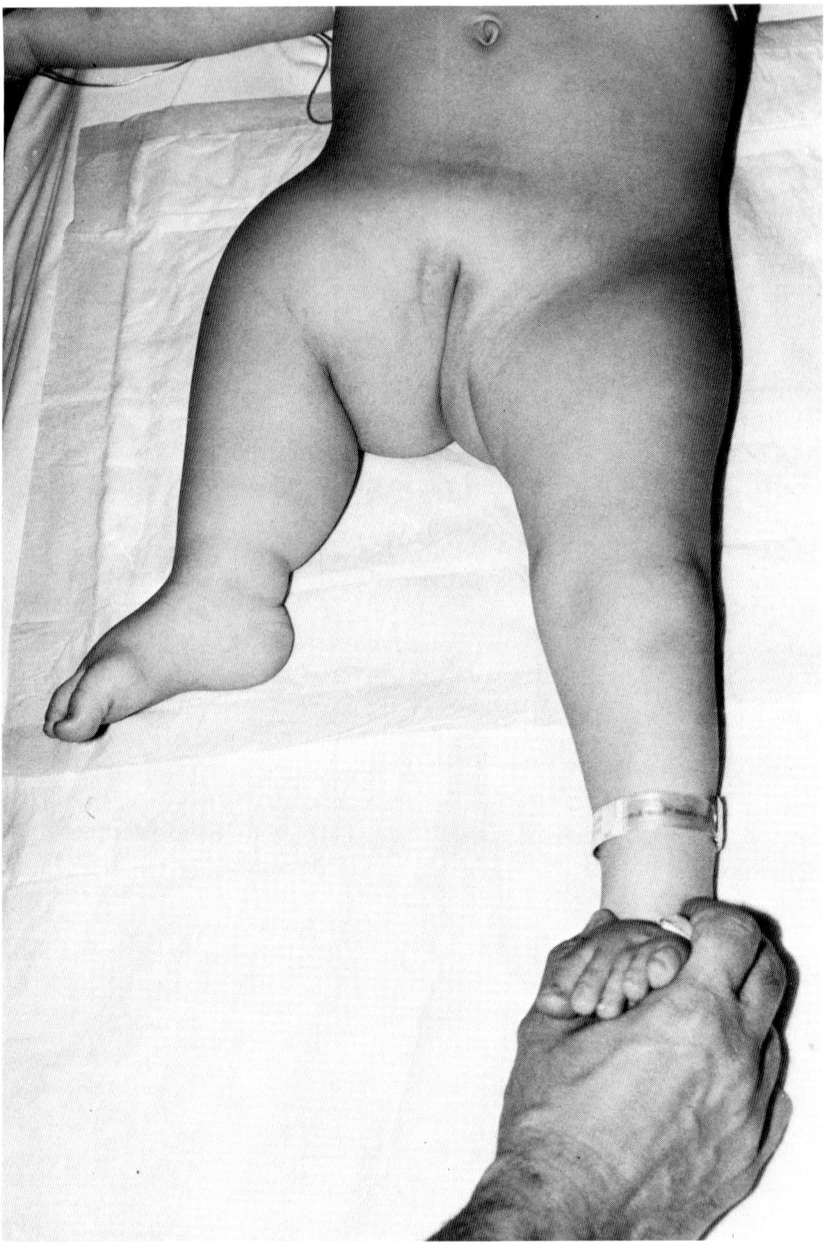

FIGURE 6.1. Clinical appearance of a child with PFFD.

hemimelia, with an incidence of 70 to 80% reported by most authors.[7] The fibular hemimelia can manifest itself as a mildly hypoplastic fibula on one end of the spectrum to a condition where the fibula is completely absent and the foot deformed. Presence or absence of significant foot deformity is of some importance as it has implication for treatment. There is a high incidence of associated congenital abnormalities in the remainder of the skeleton. In the report of Bevan-Thomas,[7] almost 50% of patients had abnormality involving other limbs. The same percentage has been reported by Aitken[3] and observed in our PFFD patient population. These figures, combined with the fact that approximately 15% of PFFD cases are bilateral, make it obvious that many of these children are in the multihandicapped category. Cases of bilateral PFFD frequently have the more severe form of the condition associated with absent fibula and foot abnormalities.

Diagnosis is almost always possible on the first examination. The profound shortening of the extremity, ship-funnel appearance, together with the knee and hip contracture, are quite characteristic. The delay in diagnosis, which sometimes does occur, is almost always due to the examiner's infamilarity with the condition.

Difficulty in interpreting the initial radiographs, which can be misleading to the uninitiated, also contributes to the occasional initial misdiagnosis. Physical examination, however, is of little value in determining the severity of the condition. Assessment can be made with the help of the radiographs, with the newer methods of imaging such as ultrasonography and nuclear magnetic resonance imaging (NMRI) being helpful on occasion. Different degrees of PFFD are then classified according to the radiographic appearance. A physical examination will help to assess the integrity of the rest of the limb (particularly integrity and function of the foot and ankle) and the rest of the peripheral skeleton. This, more than anything else, will determine child's treatment and his or her's ultimate function.

Classification

Several classifications have been proposed for PFFD.[2,3,5,13,16,18] The difficulty in establishing a uniform classification system stems from the attempt to classify a condition that occurs in the continuous spectrum of severity with no clear agreement on end points. Original classification was put forward by Aitken[3] and included only the conditions that would be classified as true PFFD by most authors. Other classifications, such as one by Amstuz,[4,5] have been more inclusive, including a condition known as congenital short femur. More recently, Kalamchi[18] attempted to include PFFD in a broader classification of congenital deficiencies of the femur. However, it was Gillespie and Torode[13] who in their classification pointed out the fundamental difference between the congenital short

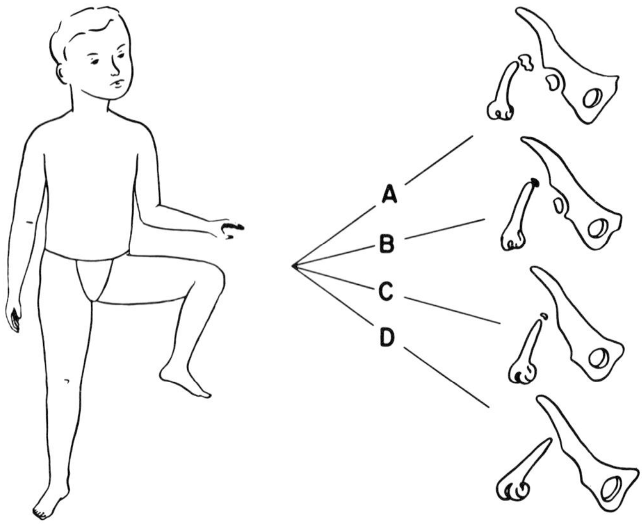

FIGURE 6.2. Four types of PFFD. (Reprinted with permission from Aitken GT: Proximal femoral focal deficiency: definition, classification and management. A Symposium on Proximal Femoral Focal Deficiency—A Congenital Anomaly, National Academy of Sciences, 1969, p. 7.)

femur and a true PFFD. This distinction is important, particularly so with respect to the treatment of the two conditions.

Generally, I believe that the original classification by Aitken[3] still best describes the major stages of severity for this condition despite the inherent problem of trying to categorize into distinct groupings a condition that occurs in a continuous spectrum. The Aitken classification (Fig. 6.2) is used in this text when referring to grading. The classifications based only on radiographic appearance have the drawback of interpreting radiographs of children with various degree of skeletal maturity in a condition that manifests itself not only by the absence of certain skeletal element, but also by delayed ossification in the ones present.

Class A (Figure 6.3 A,B)

Radiographs show an obvious defect in the subtrochanteric area of the proximal femur; however, the head of the femur is present, together with adequate acetabulum. The femoral segment is invariably quite short. Despite radiographic defect, there is a cartilaginous connection that has a tendency to progressively ossify with advancing skeletal maturity. This

FIGURE 6.3. **A:** PFFD Aitken Class A, age 1 year. Note good acetabulum and presence of femoral head. **B:** Same patient at age 8 years. Note surgical knee arthrodesis has been performed.

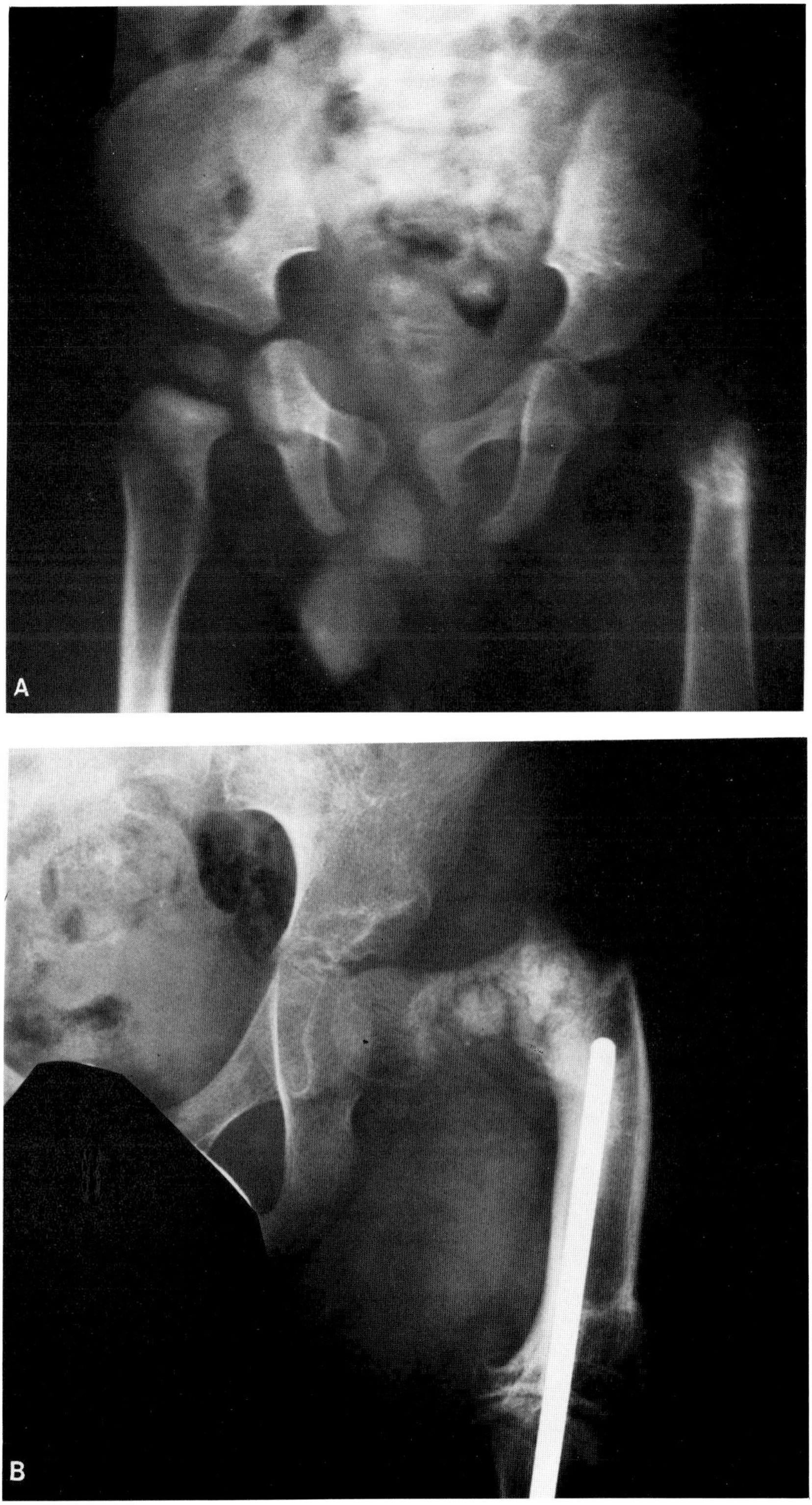
A
B

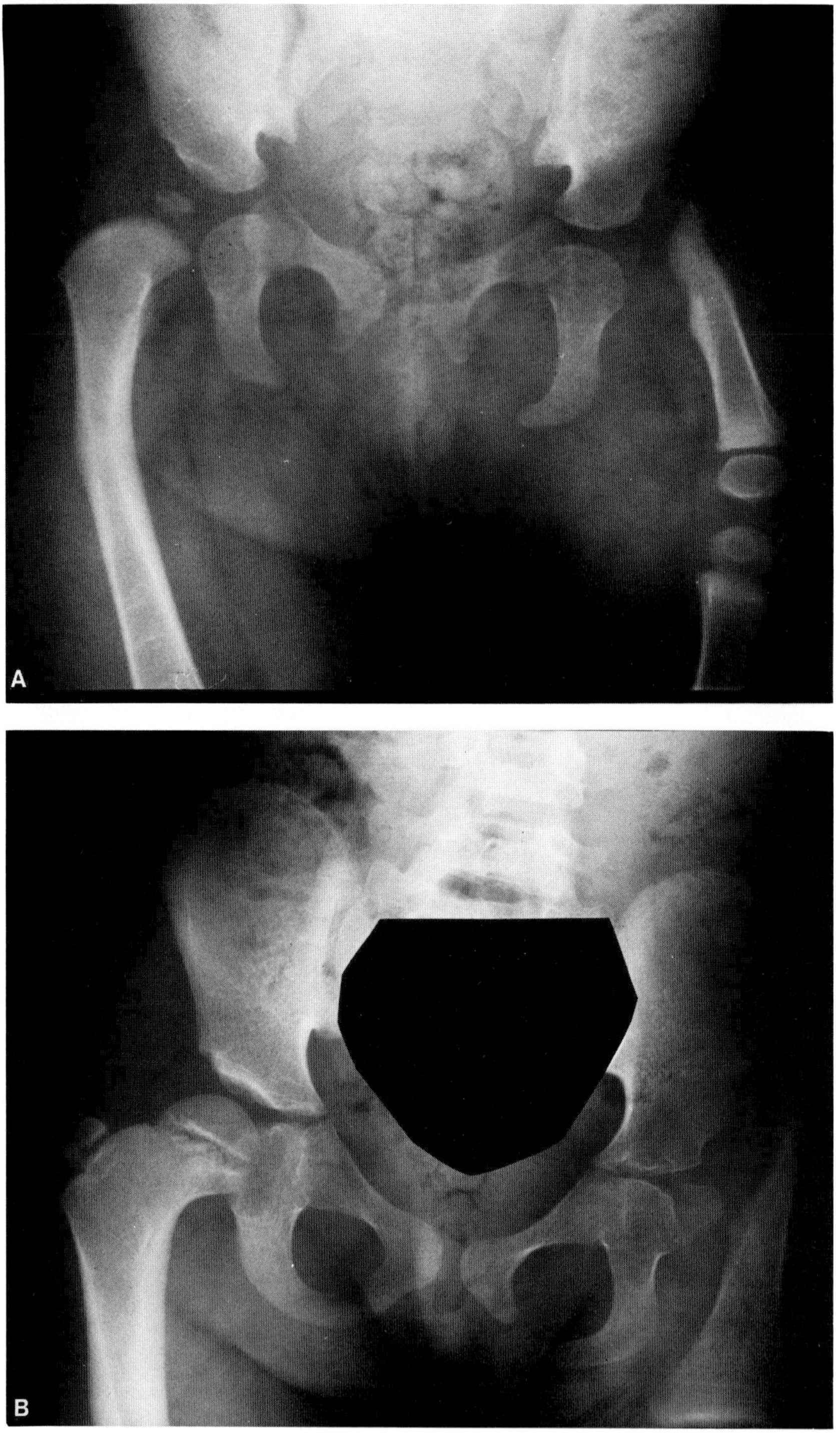

FIGURE 6.4. **A:** PFFD Aitken Class B on the left side at age 1 year. Note abnormal femur on the right as well. **B:** Class B, same patient at age 5 years. Note persistent defect and high-riding proximal femur.

can go on to complete ossification in some cases. The relationship of the trochanteric area, neck and head of the femur, even in cases that ossify by the end of skeletal maturity, is a marked subtrochanteric varus.

Class B (Figure 6.4 A,B)

The radiographic defect of the proximal femur is more extensive. The femoral head and adequate acetabulum are present, although the head is frequently delayed in ossification and its presence can only be deduced from the shape of the ilium, showing an adequate acetabulum. Use of ultrasound or NMR can help to demonstrate the presence of a cartilaginous femoral head. The femoral shaft is always short and deformed. Although some ossification does gradually occur, the defect always persists into skeletal maturity. The proximal end of the femur is proximal to the acetabulum and frequently has a small bony tuft on its end.

Class C (Figure 6.5 A,B)

This group is characterized by severely dysplastic acetabulum and by a femoral head that never ossifies and is most likely absent in most cases. The femoral shaft shows proximal migration and frequently an ossified tuft on its proximal end.

Class D (Figure 6.6 A,B)

The ilium in these patients has a featureless smooth lateral outline with complete absence of the acetabulum. The femoral head and neck and the trochanter area are completely absent. The shaft is extremely short and the proximal end is pointed. In the most severe cases only a small segment of the distal femur is present, with marked knee abnormality. Some of these show complete lack of ossification in the femur on the initial radiographs and can be misdiagnosed as a congenital absence of femur. Only later, when the cartilaginous distal femoral fragment ossifies, does the true nature of abnormality become clear. Again ultrasonography or NMRI can be helpful initially to make the distinction. Interestingly, bilateral cases are commonly Class D.

Treatment

A number of treatment options have been described in the literature over the years.* Even now a uniformity of opinion does not exist. It has frequently been said that each case of PFFD needs to be treated on its

---

* References 1,5,8,10,12–15,17,20,21,24–27,31,35–39.

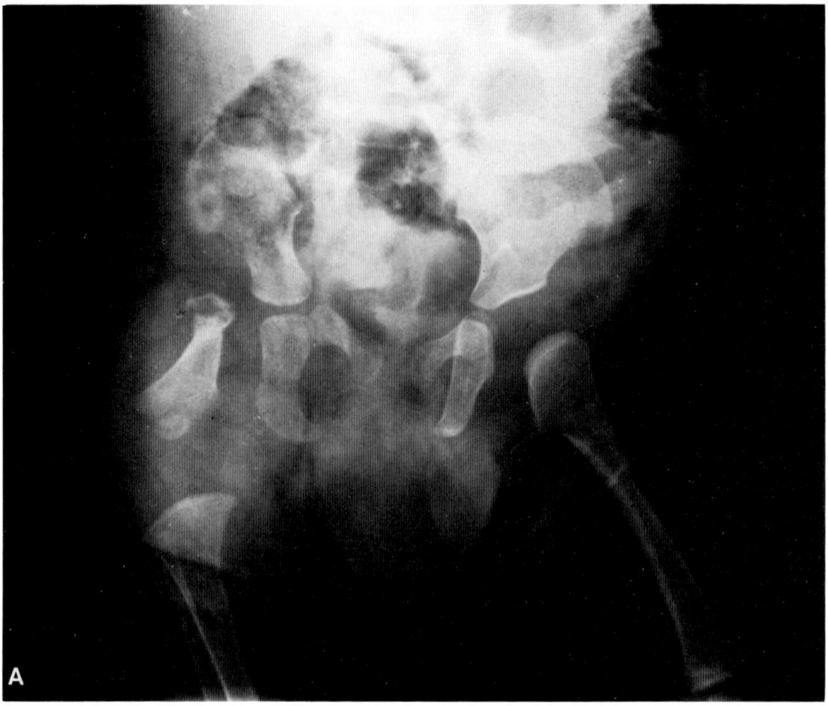

FIGURE 6.5. **A:** PFFD Aitken Class C, age 7 months. Note inadequate acetabulum and short femoral segment. **B:** Same patient with the femur abducted.

own merrit. To a degree this is true, yet some basic principles do apply and help with the decision-making. Both treatment modalities, prosthetics and surgery, play an important role.

The goal of treatment is, of course, optimal improvement in function together with acceptable cosmesis. We base our treatment on several basic parameters: (1) bilaterality or unilaterality of the condition, (2) severity grade (Aitken types A and B verses types C and D), and (3) presence or absence of functional foot and ankle.

Bilateral PFFD

Bilateral PFFD (Fig. 6.7) almost always requires prosthetic treatment only. Many of these children are functional without any treatment, having acceptable gait on the short extremities. Bilateral extension prostheses are provided, allowing the children to function at their peers' height.

Surgery in the bilateral condition is reserved for cases of severe associated foot deformities, which preclude reasonably normal weightbearing. These are usually children with normal upper extremities and

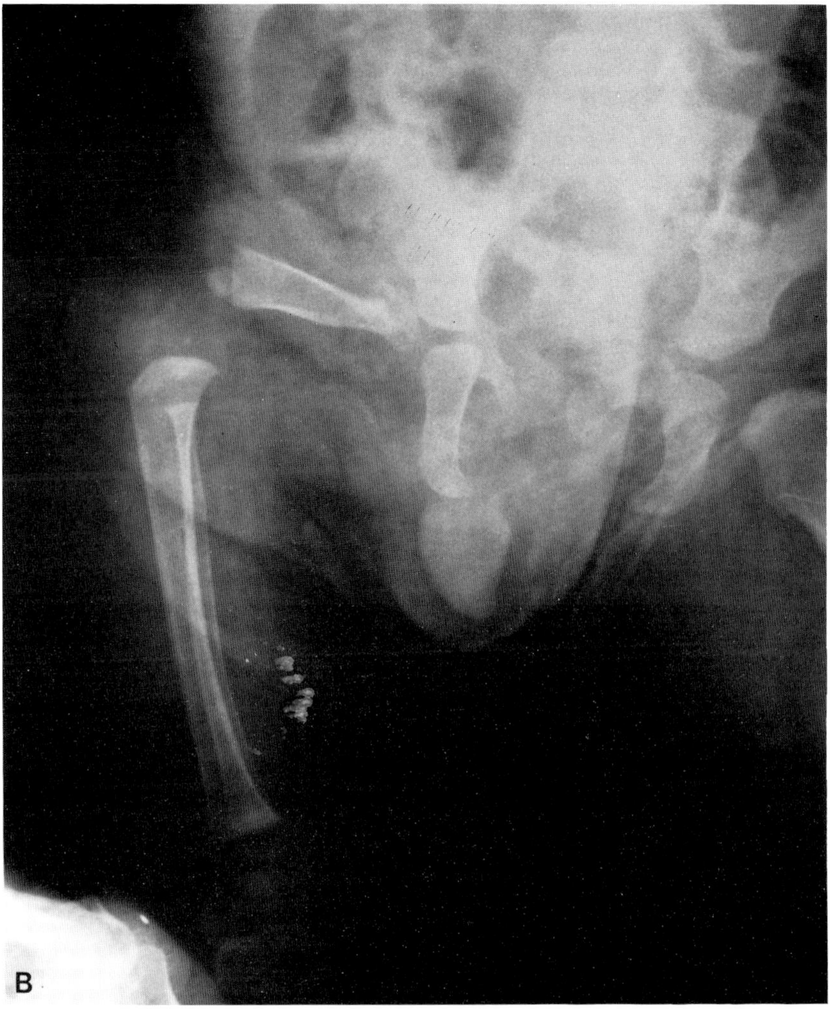

FIGURE 6.5. *Continued*

severe foot deformities who have had bilateral Syme's amputation and prosthetic fitting or surgical foot reconstruction, making the feet plantigrade. A far more complicated problem are the children who have upper extremity abnormalities and who are using their feet as the main prehensile organ. In these children foot amputation or reconstructive surgery, which would diminish suppleness and function in the feet, would be disastrous. Every effort should be made in such cases to accommodate the feet in an orthosis or a prosthesis that can be easily put on or taken off so that the patient can enjoy both the benefit of walking with the help of the appliance and the natural dexterity of the feet, which substitute for the

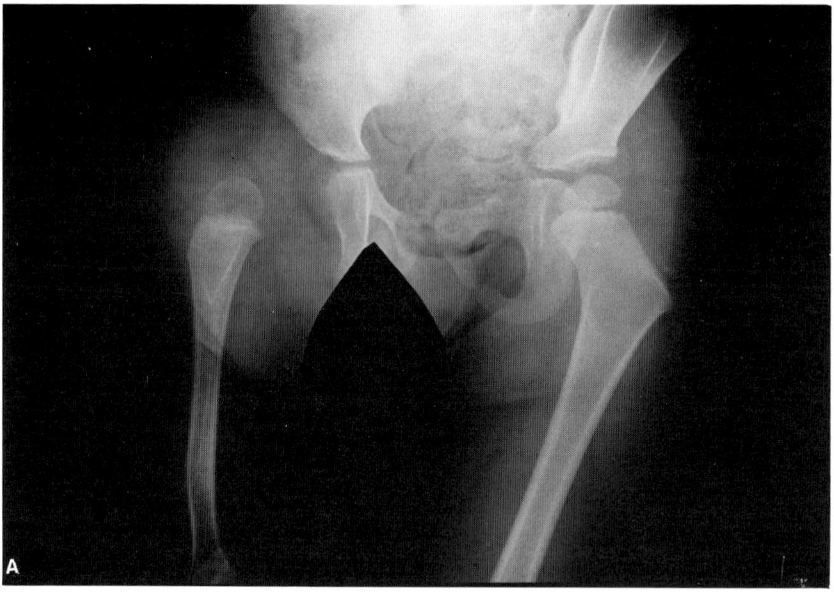

FIGURE 6.6. **A:** PFFD Aitken Class D, age 2 years. Note only cartilaginous fragment of the distal femur is present at this stage. What appears to be the femur is in actual fact tibia. No acetabular development. **B:** PFFD Aitken Class D, age 1 year, different patient. Note short femoral segment and complete absence of acetabular development.

child's hands. The occasional child with a lower-grade (Aitkens type A or B) bilateral PFFD may benefit from a hip stabilization procedure to improve gait. We, as a rule, have been very conservative in our surgical approach to this group of patients and have achieved satisfactory functional results.

Unilateral PFFD

Treatment in this group almost always requires both surgical and prosthetic intervention. The patient is always faced with a large leg-length discrepancy and an unstable hip. The goal of the surgical treatment is to provide a more stable hip whenever possible and to optimize the leg as a stump for a prosthetic fitting. Ultimately, each of these patients will require a prosthesis for bipedal locomotion; thus, providing them with optimal "stump" is of paramount importance. Nevertheless, the opinion regarding the advisability of surgery in this situation differs from center to center. There are some who believe that surgical treatment is not advisable in the majority of cases and that the prosthesis can be fitted around the patient's leg and upper thigh. It is my opinion and that of a number of other treating surgeons that the stump fitting can be signifi-

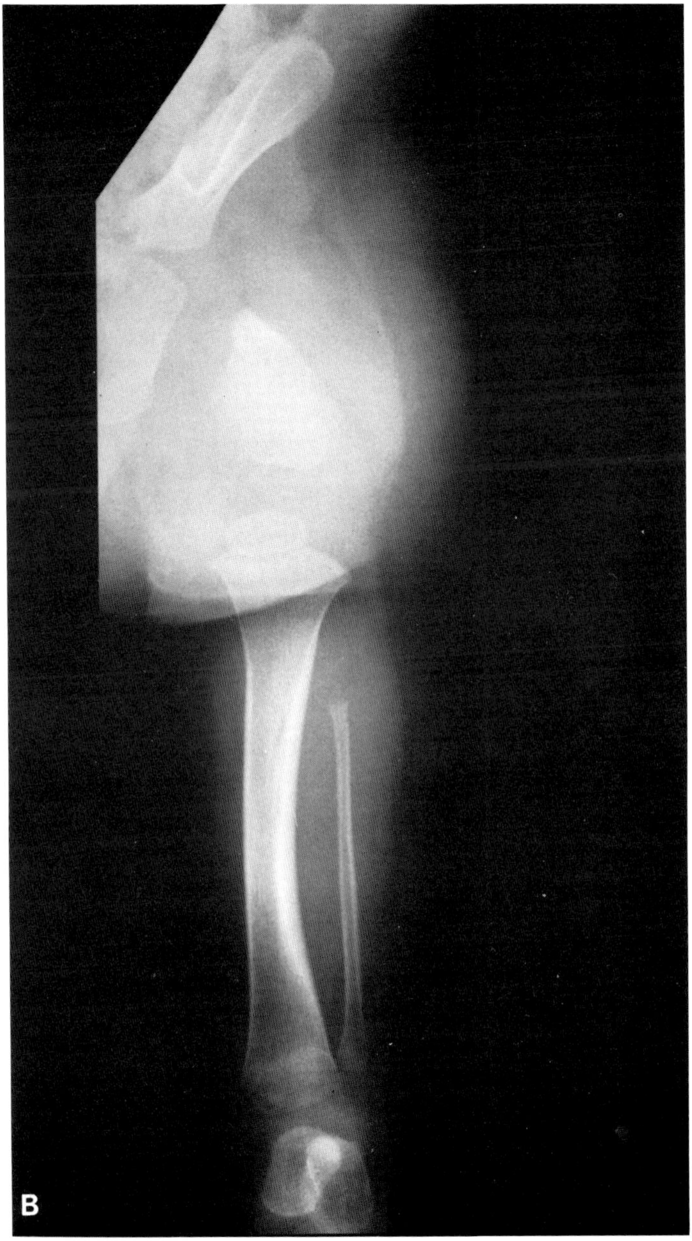

FIGURE 6.6. *Continued*

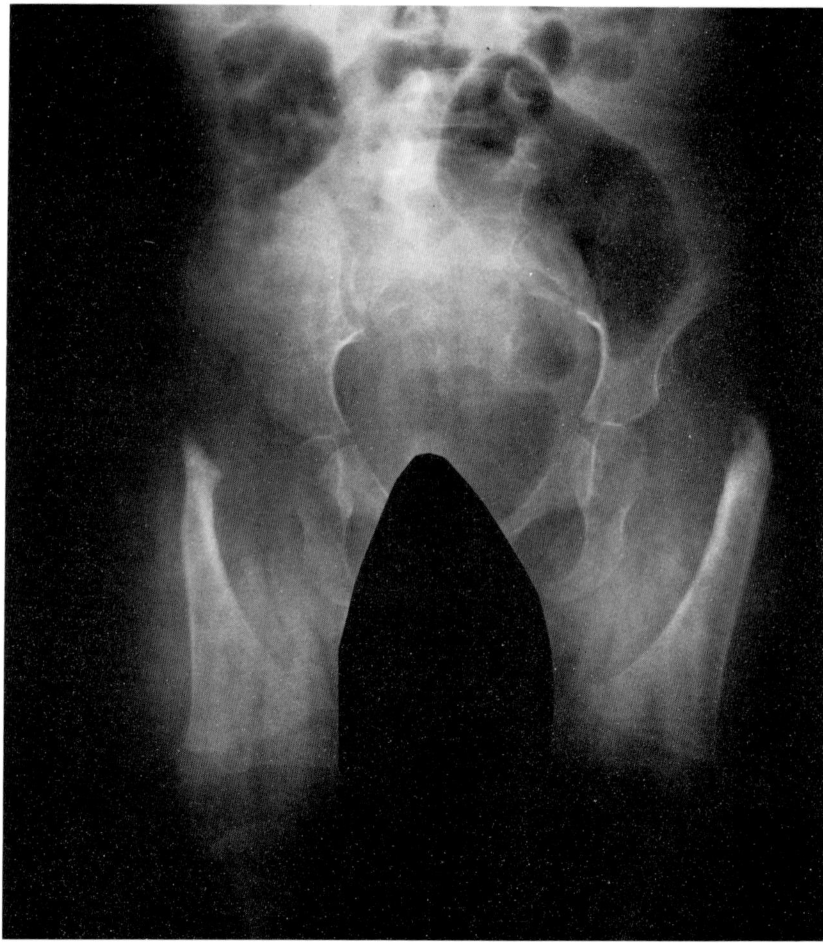

FIGURE 6.7. Bilateral PFFD in a 2-year-old child. Note associated absence of fibulae.

cantly improved by surgery. Two problems can be thus addressed. The first is that of the fixed flexion deformity of the hip and knee, making the prosthetic fitting difficult proximally, where the thigh has a tendency to slide out of the prosthesis and the prosthesis loses contact with its ischial weight-bearing area. The second problem is one of the foot. The foot is forced into equinus to accommodate the cosmetically acceptable prosthesis, making the proximal stump too long, or the prosthesis is fitted around the foot in a more natural plantigrade position, making it cosmetically less acceptable. Our feeling is that both these problems can be adequately addressed by a proper surgical approach. The hip and knee contracture can be significantly improved by performing knee arthrodesis. This produces one bone thigh of approximately normal length, allowing a good lever arm to be fitted inside a prosthesis.[21,24] Extension at the hip joint generated by the momentum of the long lever arm with the standard above-knee prosthesis allows for gradual stretching of the flexion contracture of the hip joint. We find this procedure useful and offer it routinely to our PFFD patients with unilateral deformity. Knee surgery is usually performed at the age of 2 or 2 ½ years, and one of the epiphysis around the knee is preserved to allow for some additional growth of the thigh segment.

The problem of the foot is somewhat more controversial. There are essentially three alternatives. One is to leave the foot alone and fit the prosthesis around it with a standard prosthetic knee joint below the level of the foot. Another option is Syme's amputation, which has gained in popularity and which we use in patients who have a significantly deformed foot or inadequate ankle joint secondary to the associated fibular hemimelia. This procedure provides for a good end-bearing stump, and the child can be fitted quite well as a conventional above-knee amputee with an ischial-bearing socket for the unstable hip joint. The third option is a Van Nes rotation-plasty. This operation was originally described by Borgrave in Germany in the 1930s[9] for severe infection of the knee joint. It was Van Nes who described the operation in the English literature after World War II, applying it to femoral deficiencies.[36] The rotation-plasty has been used extensively in our center in Toronto by Dr. John Hall in the 1960s[14] and Dr. Robert Gillespie[13] in the '70s. We still recommend it for children who have an adequate foot and ankle (Fig. 6.8). The operation is extremely useful to convert what would be a functional above-knee amputee to a functional near below-knee amputee. The drawback to this operation has been said to be its poor cosmesis and hence poor psychological acceptance by the patient. This has not been our experience. The operation is well accepted by patients and their families if one explains the benefits to the family and, in our setting, has a former patient demonstrate the functional benefits as well.

The second objection to rotation-plasty is that it has a tendency to derotate and thus the operation has to be repeated one or two times during the child's growth. This is a valid observation, and many of our patients did, indeed, require a second procedure to correct gradual derotation. In the last few years we have concentrated on accomplishing the rotation completely through the knee joint at the time of knee fusion and with reattachment of all the muscles crossing the knee joint. This achieves a situation where the muscles, namely, the gastrocnemius and hamstrings, together with the quadriceps and anterior compartment of the leg, pull in a straight line so as not to cause bony derotation. Results of patients treated with this approach have so far been satisfactory with not a single patient requiring further derotation. Follow-up, however, is still short term and final evaluation of these patients is not available. Nevertheless, even with

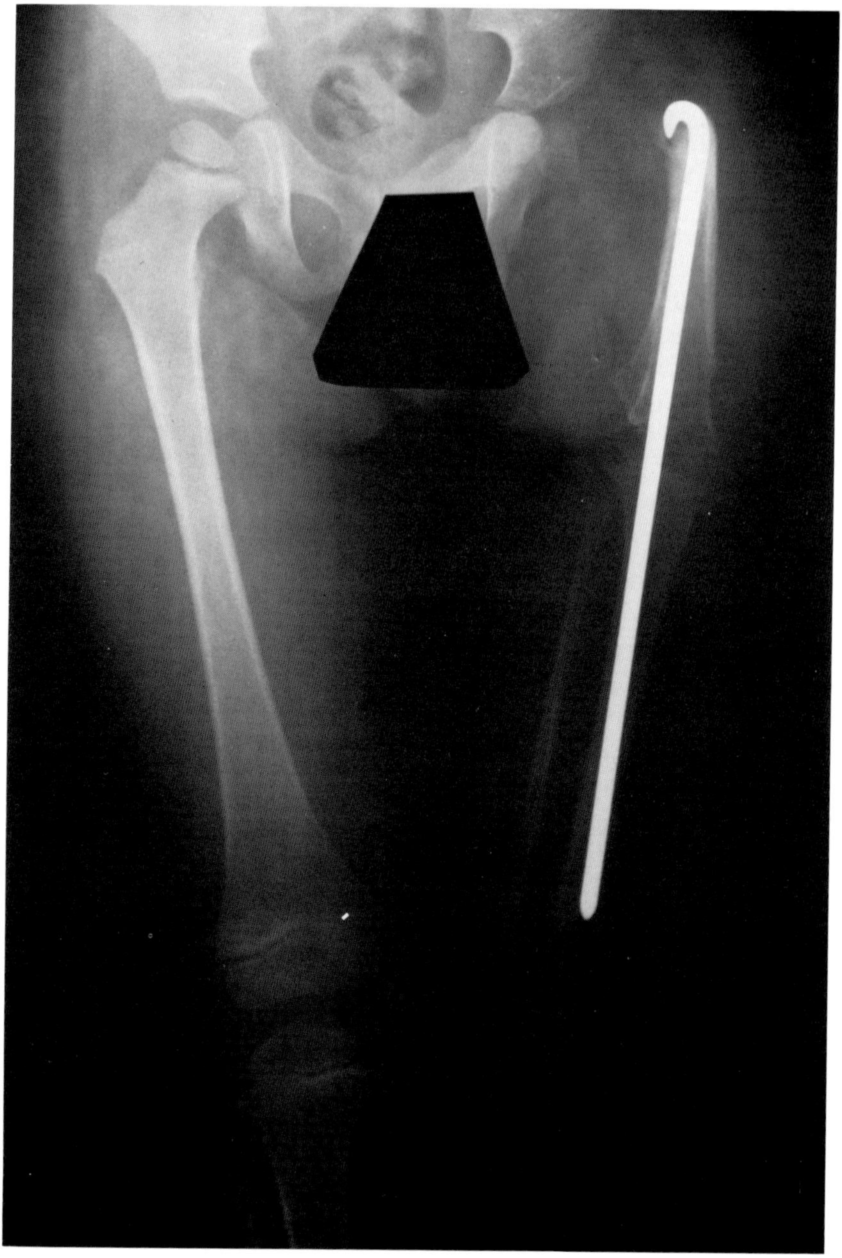

FIGURE 6.8. Knee arthrodesis and van Nes rotation-plasty. Note medial position of the fibula after the rotation.

the prospect of the patient requiring a second derotation operation, the Van Nes rotation-plasty is functionally beneficial to the patient as it gives the child a knee that has active extension and flexion and significantly improves the biomechanics of gait.

In summary, treatment to improve the leg as a prosthetic stump consists of knee fusion and Syme's amputation in a child who has a severe degree of fibular hemimelia with an abnormal foot and ankle. In a child who has a reasonable ankle and foot with a good range of motion at the ankle joint, the treatment is knee fusion accompanied by Van Nes rotation-plasty through the knee fusion. The child with Syme's amputation is fitted with an above-knee prosthesis modified for PFFD, usually with an ischial-bearing socket. The child with a Van Nes rotation-plasty is fitted with a Van Nes rotation-plasty below-knee prosthesis, which in cases of an unstable hip joint requires an ischial-bearing socket.

The second goal of surgery is to improve the stability of the hip joint whenever possible. The current state of art can accomplish this only in patients with lower grade PFFD, that is, Aitken type A or B. Most patients, in this less severe group, can benefit from valgus osteotomy of the hip joint. The osteotomy consists of resection of the pseudarthrosis area proximally to the level of the ossified femoral neck and distally to the ossified femoral shaft. The femoral head and neck are then fixed in maximum valgus (155°–170°) on the femoral shaft. It is important to resect a significant portion of the nonossified cartilaginous enlage or a portion of the ossified proximal femur to allow the extreme valgus to be accomplished (Fig. 6.9 A,B).

We find that, indeed, if a good valgus position is achieved during surgery, the osteotomy heals with improved ossification of the whole proximal femur, including the femoral head. The overall functional improvement, however, does not depend only on bony stability of the hip joint but also on adequate muscle power. The abductors are frequently deficient in this condition and may remain so even in cases of surgically stabilized hip. Such patients will still exhibit a significant Trendelenburg lurch during gait owing to weak abductors. However, if the abductors and their insertion into the proximal femur can be identified during surgery and then reattached to the proximal femur in the area where the greater trochanter would normally be, the functional results can be very good indeed. These patients can significantly improve their preoperative Trendelenburg lurch. The surgery is performed between the ages of 5 and 7 years, when significant portions of the proximal femur show evidence of ossifications in Aitken type A or B cases. At the present time there is no universally accepted surgical treatment for the unstable hip of types C and D PFFD. Attempts at surgical treatment by fusing the distal portion of the femur to the pelvis using the patients knee joint as a hip joint have been reported in the literature.[35] However, the procedure has never gained

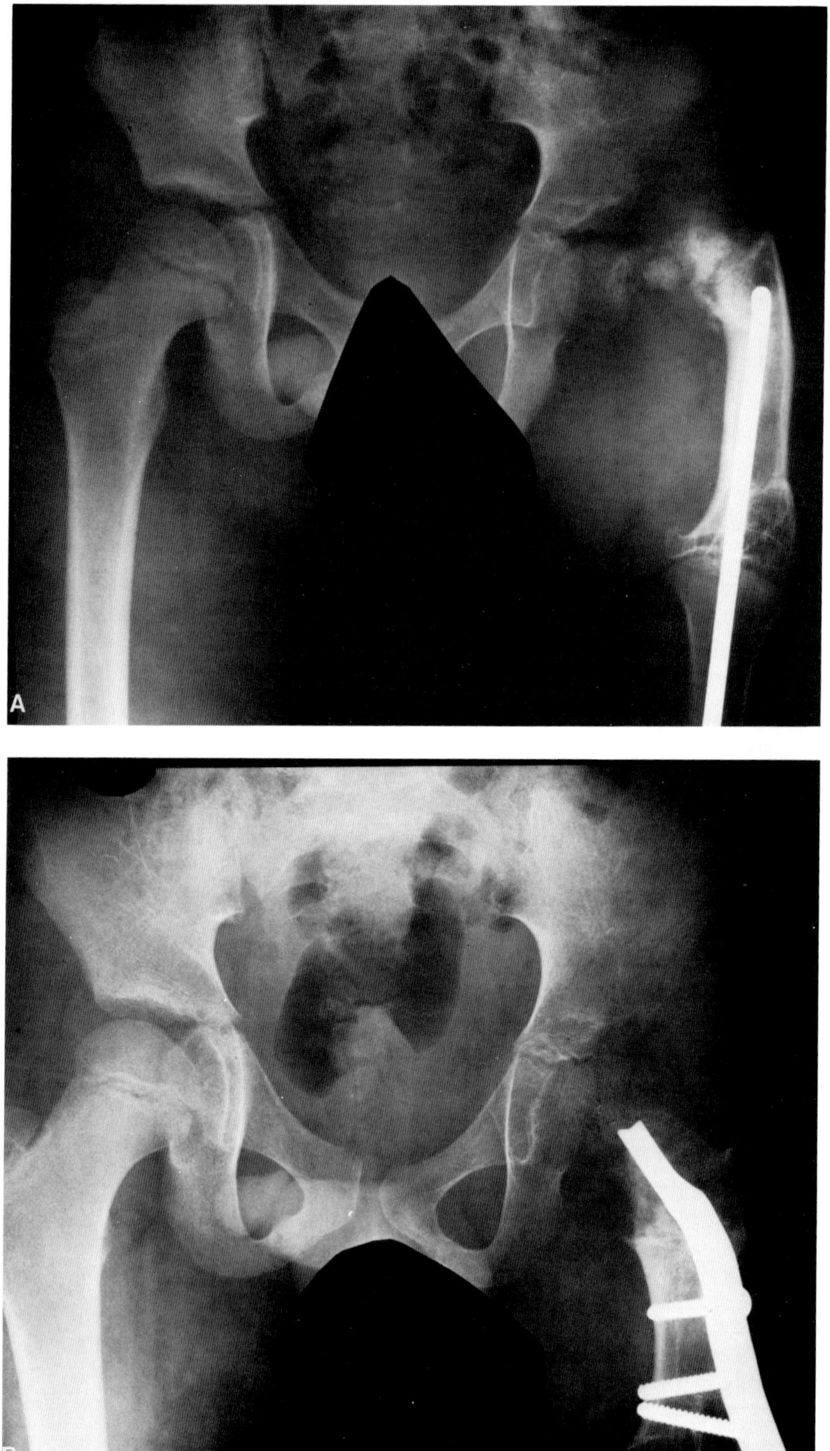
A
B

wide popularity, as it rarely results in functional improvement. It is not routinely practiced by us.

The importance of stabilizing the hip in lower grade PFFD may be further emphasized with the advent of dynamic methods of leg lengthening. With newer methods it may be possible that in the future some of these patients may benefit from leg-length equaling procedures. At this stage, however, it would be very much an experimental undertaking.

At the present time all unilateral PFFD patients ultimately need prosthetic fitting for bipedal locomotion. Appropriate prosthetic fitting is then of paramount importance. It is here that the patient with this complicated and serious deformity is in need of expert management by an experienced prosthetic team—be it patients treated by knee fusion and Syme's amputation; by knee fusion in Van Nes rotation-plasty; or even patients who had no surgery and the prosthetic fitting is accomplished around the untreated limb. It is progress in the field of prosthetics, with modern sockets and new foot designs, that allow these patients to enjoy the active life of children and teenagers together with their peers.

References

1. Aitken GT: Amputation as a treatment for certain lower-extremity congenital abnormalities. J Bone Joint Surg Am 41-A: 1267–1285, 1959.
2. Aitken GT: Proximal femoral deficiency, in: *Limb Development and Deformity: Problems of Evaluation and Rehabilitation,* Springfield Il, Charles C Thomas Publisher, 1969.
3. Aitken GT: Proximal femoral deficiency. Definition, classification and management, in: *A Symposium on Proximal Femoral Focal Deficiency—A Congenital Anomaly.* National Academy of Sciences, 1969.
4. Amstutz HC, Wilson PD Jr: Dysgenesis of the proximal femur (coxa vara) and its surgical management. J Bone Joint Surg Am 44-A: 1–24, 1962.
5. Amstutz HC: The morphology, natural history, and treatment of proximal femoral focal deficiency, in: *A Symposium on Proximal Femoral Focal Deficiency—A Congenital Anomaly.* National Academy of Sciences, 1969.
6. Badger VM, Lambert CN: Differential diagnosis of an apparent proximal femoral focal deficiency. InterClin Inform Bull 5(1): 3, 1965, New York: Committee on Prosthetic Research and Development.
7. Bevan-Thomas WH, Millar EA: A review of proximal focal femoral deficiencies. J Bone Joint Surg Am 49A: 1378, 1967.
8. Bochmann D. Prosthetic devices for the management of proximal femoral focal deficiency. Ortho-Pros 1980:4.
9. Borggreve J: Kniegelenksersatz durch das in der Beinlangachse um 180 degree gedrehte Fussgelenk. Arch Orthop Chir 28: 175–178, 1930.
10. Burgess E: The surgical means of obtaining hip stability with motion in

FIGURE 6.9. **A:** Aitken Class A PFFD with adequate femoral head and acetabulum. Note previous knee arthrodesis and van Nes rotation-plasty. **B:** Same patient 6 months following valgus osteotomy. Child is a hockey goalie on his school team.

congenital proximal femoral focal deficiency. InterClin Inform Bull 1(3):1, 1961, New York: Committee on Prosthetic Research and Development.
11. Epps CH Jr: Proximal femoral focal deficiency J Bone Joint Surg Am 65A: 867–870, July 1983.
12. Fixsen JA, Lloyd-Roberts GC: The natural history and early treatment of proximal femoral dysplasia. J Bone Joint Surg Am: 56-B: 86–95, 1974.
13. Gillespie R, Torode IP: Classification and management of congenital abnormalities of the femur, J Bone Joint Surg Am 65-B, No 5, 557–568, 1983.
14. Hall JE: Rotation of congenitally hypoplastic lower limbs to use the ankle joint as a knee. InterClin Inform Bull 6(2): 3, 1966, New York: Committee on Prosthetic Research and Development.
15. Hall JE, Bochmann D: The surgical and prosthetic management of proximal femoral focal deficiency, in: *A Symposium: Proximal Femoral Focal Deficiency—A Congenital Anomaly*. National Academy of Sciences, 1969.
16. Hamanishi C: Congenital short femur: clinical, genetic and epidemiological comparison of the naturally occuring condition with that caused by Thalidomide. J Bone Joint Surg Am 62-B 307–320, 1980.
17. Hussain T, Emmerson A: Conservative management of bilateral proximal femoral focal deficiency. InterClin Inform Bull 13(9): 9, 1974, New York: Committee on Prosthetic Research and Development.
18. Kalamchi A, Cowell HR, Kim KI: Congenital deficiency of the femur. J Pediatr Orthop 5:129–134, 1985.
19. King RE: Concepts of proximal femoral focal deficiencies. InterClin Inform Bull 1(2):1, 1961, New York: Committee on Prosthetic Research and Development.
20. King RE: Surgical correction of proximal femoral focal deficiency. InterClin Inform Bull 4(11):1, 1965, New York: Committee on Prosthetic Research and Development.
21. King RE: Providing a single skeletal lever in proximal femoral focal deficiency. InterClin Inform Bull 6(2):23, 1966, New York: Committee on Prosthetic Research and Development.
22. King RE: Some concepts of proximal femoral focal deficiency, in: *A Symposium: Proximal Femoral Focal Deficiency—A Congenital Anomaly*. National Academy of Sciences, 1969.
23. King RE, McCraney T: Proximal femoral focal deficiency—Quo vadis? InterClin Inform Bull 12(8):1, 1973, New York: Committee on Prosthetic Research and Development.
24. King RE, Marks TW: Follow-up findings on the skeletal lever in the surgical management of proximal femoral focal deficiency. InterClin Inform Bull 11(3):1, 1971, New York: Committee on Prosthetic Research and Development.
25. Korman LA, Meyer LC, Warren FH: Proximal femoral focal deficiency: A 50-year experience. Dev Med Child Neurol 24:344, 1982.
26. Kostuik JP, Gillespie R, Hall JE, et al: Van Nes rotational osteotomy for treatment of proximal femoral focal deficiency and congenital short femur. J Bone Joint Surg 57A:1039, 1975.
27. A. Kritter AE: Tibial rotation-plasty for proximal femoral focal deficiency. J Bone Joint Surg 59A:927, 1977.
28. Kritter AE, Gillespie T: Bilateral proximal femoral focal deficiency and

bilateral paraxial fibular hemimelia. InterClin Inform Bull 11(12):1, 1972, New York: Committee on Prosthetic Research and Development.
29. Lloyd-Roberts GC, Stone KH: Congenital hypoplasia of the upper femur. J Bone Joint Surg 45B:557, 1963.
30. Marotz RJ: Pregnancy and maternal proximal focal femoral deficiency. A case report. J Reprod Med 28(11): 798–800, 1983.
31. Meyer LC, Friddle D, Pratt RW: Problems of treating and fitting the patient with proximal femoral focal deficiency. InterClin Inform Bull 10(12):1, 1971, New York: Committee on Prosthetic Research and Development.
32. Morgan JD, Somerville EW: Normal and abnormal growth at the upper end of the femur. J Bone Joint Surg 42B:264, 1960.
33. O'Rahilly R: Normal development of the human embryo, in: *Normal and Abnormal Embryologic Development*. National Research Council. 1967.
34. Panting AL, Williams PF: Proximal femoral focal deficiency. J Bone Joint Surg 60B:46, 1978.
35. Steel Howard H, Lin Paul S, Betz Randal R, et al: Iliofemoral fusion for proximal femoral focal deficiency. J Bone Joint Surg 69-A, 6 (July), 1987.
36. Van Nes CP: Rotation-plasty for congenital defects of the femur. Making use of the ankle of the shortened limb to control the knee joint of a prosthesis. J Bone Joint Surg 32B:12, 1950.
37. Wagner H: Operative Beinverlangerung. Chirurg 42:260, 1971.
38. Wenzlaff EF: Surgical ablation of the remaining femoral segment in proximal femoral focal deficiency. InterClin Inform Bull 9(1):1, 1969, New York: Committee on Prosthetic Research and Development.
39. Westin GW, Gunderson GO: Proximal femoral focal deficiency—A review of treatment experiences. In deficiency—A review of treatment experiences, in: *A Symposium on Proximal Femoral Focal Deficiency—A Congenital Anomaly*. National Academy of Sciences, 1969.

7
Congenital Deficiency of the Fibula

ALI KALAMCHI

Introduction

Congenital deficiency of the fibula and associate anomalies of the lower limb represent a well-recognized clinical entity. The orthopedic literature has numerous reports describing mostly the severe forms, as fibula hemimelia.[4–6,9,13] Classification and treatment in the past were largely confined to the severe forms of the fibular deficiency.[4,10,16] Recent reports have outlined a clinical spectrum ranging from partial deficiency to complete absence.[1,3,8,12]

Fibular deficiency is not an isolated entity. In addition, there is shortening of the affected limb, involvement of both tibial and femoral segments, bowing of the tibia, and deformity of the foot.[1,2] In this chapter, the features of both complete and incomplete fibular congenital deformities are discussed.

Fibular hypoplasia is classified into Types I and II. Type I includes limbs in which at least part of the fibula is present. This group is also noted to have two subgroups. In Type IA (Fig. 7.1) the entire fibula is present with the proximal fibular epiphysis hypoplastic. The fibula is short, with the proximal growth plate distal to the level of the tibial growth plate. Conversely, the distal fibula growth plate is proximal to the dome of the talus. In Type IB (Fig. 7.2) there is partial absence of the proximal fibula (usually one half to one third). Routinely, the distal fibula is short and does not support the ankle joint.

In Type II (Fig. 7.3) there is complete absence of the fibula or, at times, a nonfunctional distal, vestigial fragment.

Clinical Features

The fibular hypoplasia reported by Achterman and Kalamchi,[1] Type I, is essentially as common as Type II. They had three patients with bilateral involvement where on one side there was complete absence and on the

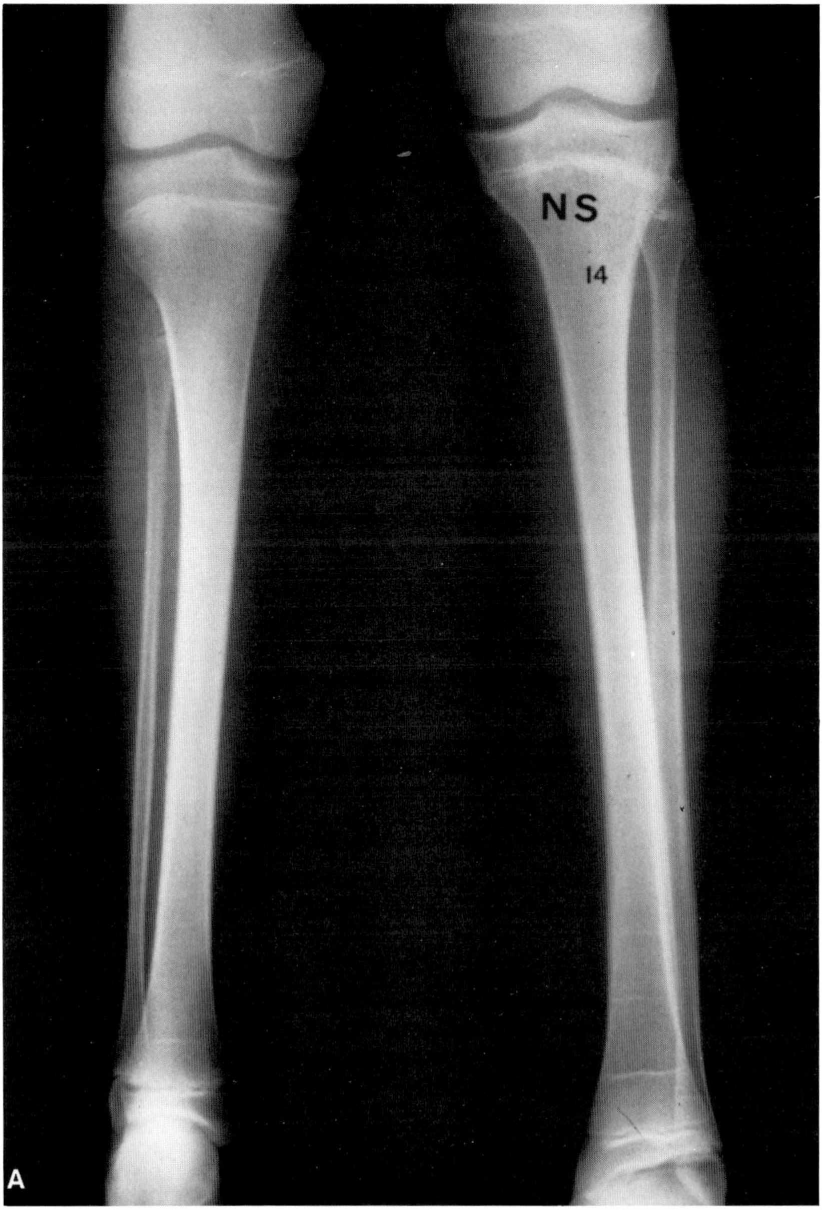

FIGURE 7.1. Type 1A fibular hypoplasia. Note the proximal shortening and the presence of the fibular epiphysis.

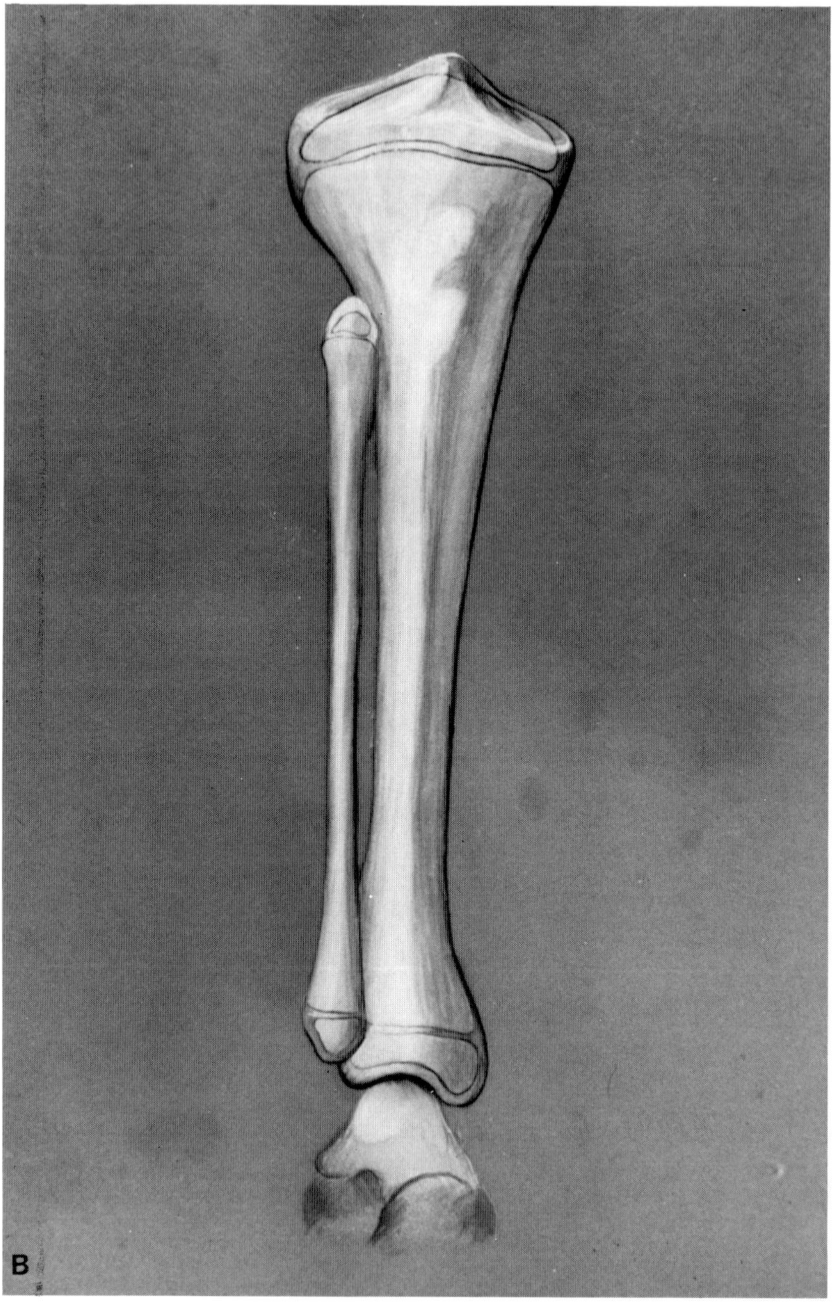

FIGURE 7.1. *Continued*

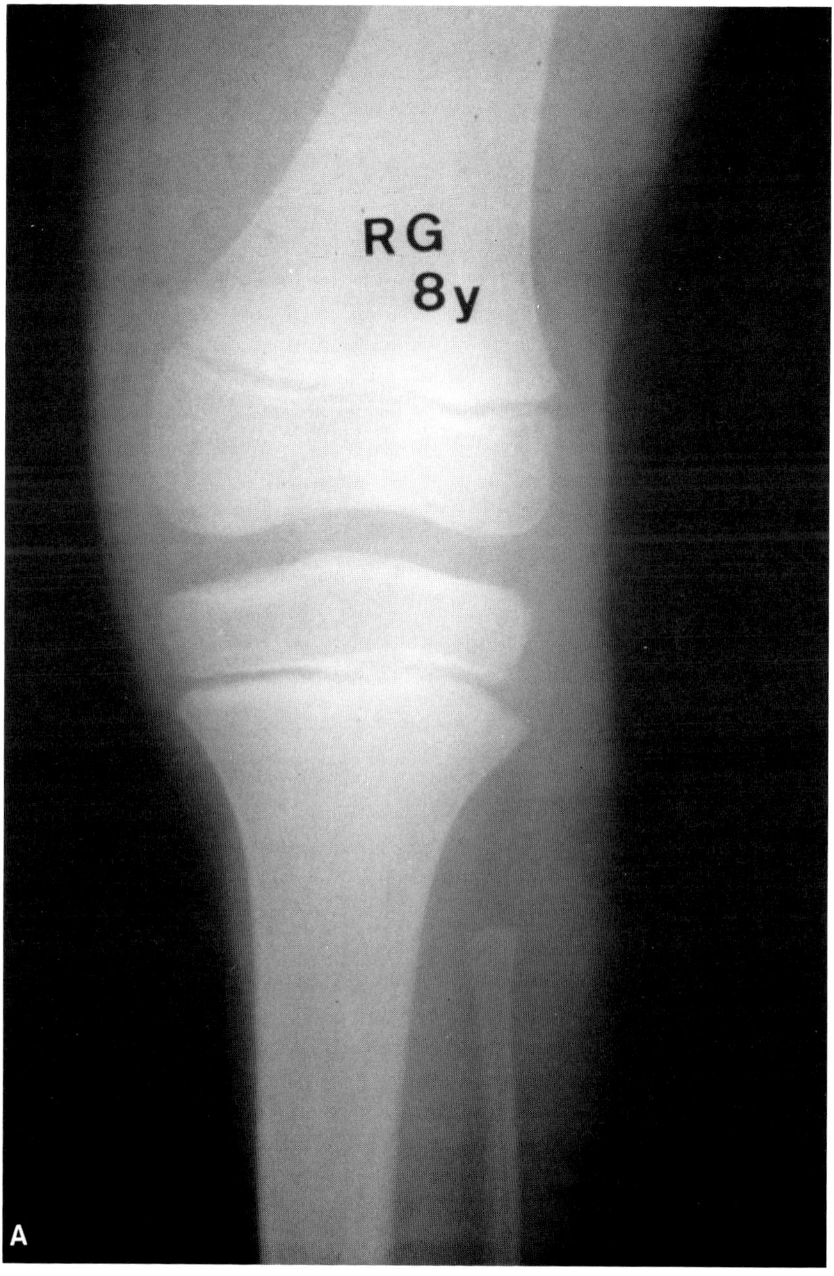

FIGURE 7.2. Type 1B fibular hypoplasia with the absent upper fibula and the valgus inclination of the distal tibia.

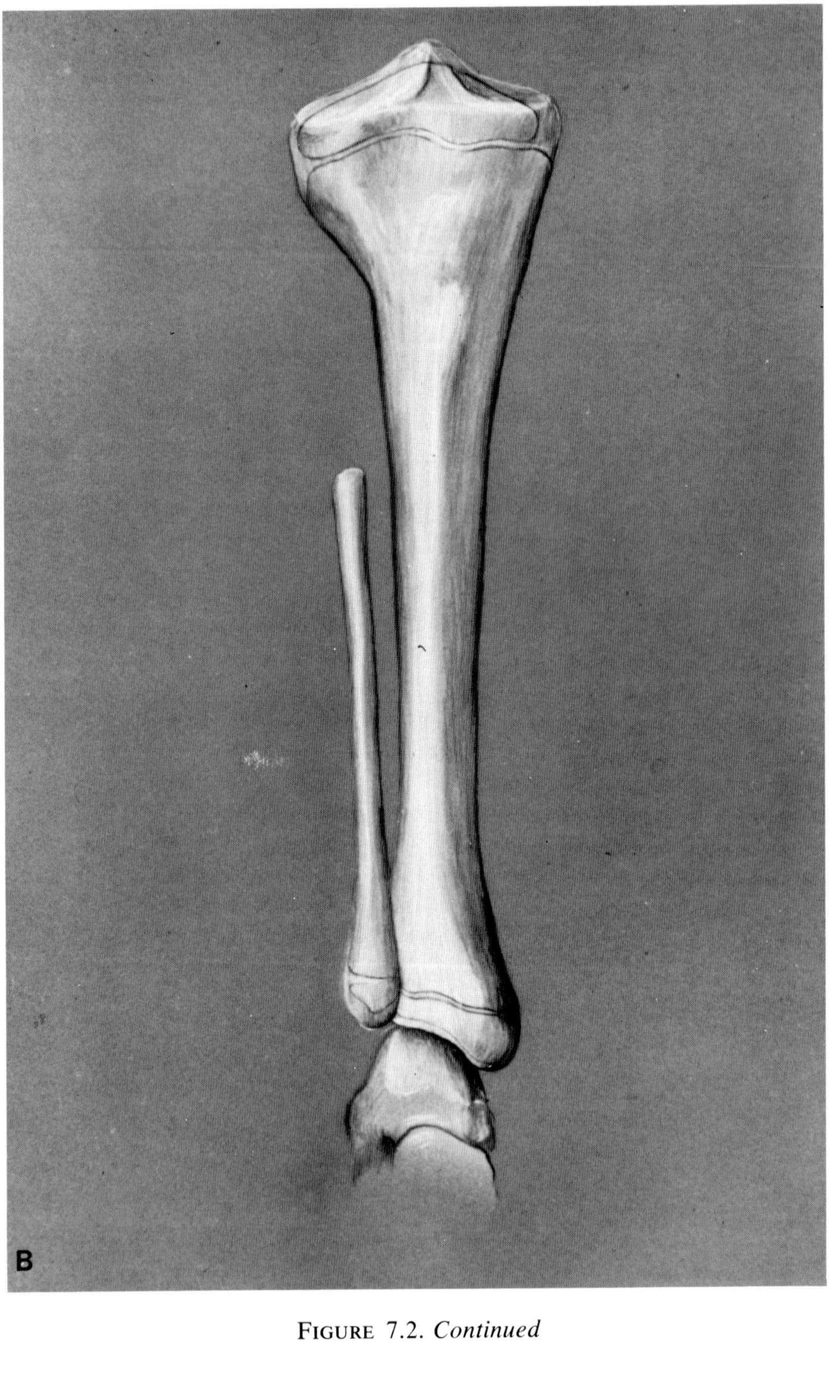

FIGURE 7.2. *Continued*

other side, fibular hypoplasia. This pattern of involvement had been reported previously by Bohne and Root.[3]

The incidence of Type I fibular hypoplasia in males and females is equal, and femoral abnormalities are common. In the Bohne and Root study, femoral anomalies were present in 66 of the 97 limbs and ranged from congenital shortening to classic proximal focal femoral deficiency. In congenital fibula deficiency Type I, there is increased valgus at the knee, and in most cases the patella is small and high riding. There is a high incidence of symptomatic patellar subluxation in this group. The combination of hypoplasia of the lateral femoral condyle and valgus deformity of the knee contribute to the subluxation. In both Type I and II, there is a high incidence of anterior instability of the knee, as noted by a positive drawer test, owing to anterior cruciate deficiency. Anteromedial bowing of the tibia is classically described in Type II deficiency.[1,2] In Type I it is usually present to some degree, with a classic dimple at the site of the maximum bowing of the tibia.

At the ankle, two general patterns of deformity have been noted. Ball-and-socket ankle is present in more than two thirds of the patients (Fig. 7.4). The ankle joint is usually in moderate valgus owing to the lack of fibula support due to shortening. In rare cases the tibiotalar joint is stable with an apparently normal distal tibia, despite fibular absence. Tarsal coalitions and associated anomalies of the hindfoot are extremely common in these patients. Achterman and Kalamchi noted that 50% of the patients with Type I deficiency had talocalcaneal coalition (Fig. 7.5). Absence of the lateral ray had been regarded as the hallmark of this group.[9]

Leg-length discrepancy is the key issue in the management of these patients, along with the degree of foot deformity. It is advisable that the discrepancy for the long bones be converted to percentages for easier future comparison. In my experience, the percentage of shortening is constant over the child's growth years, and the degree of shortening noted earlier is usually the expected percentage of shortening at skeletal maturity. In these patients, the added femoral shortening, varus of the femoral neck, and other hip deformities need to be considered when evaluating the overall leg-length discrepancy.

Other associated anomalies such as defects of the hand, absent ulnar rays, and syndactyly of the remaining digits have been reported. Cardiac and renal anomalies have also been described in these patients.

Discussion

Extensive studies of complete fibular absence and associated anomalies have been reported in the past.[4,6,9,14] It has always been apparent that a related condition of fibular hypoplasia existed.[1,3,7] Coventry and Johnson

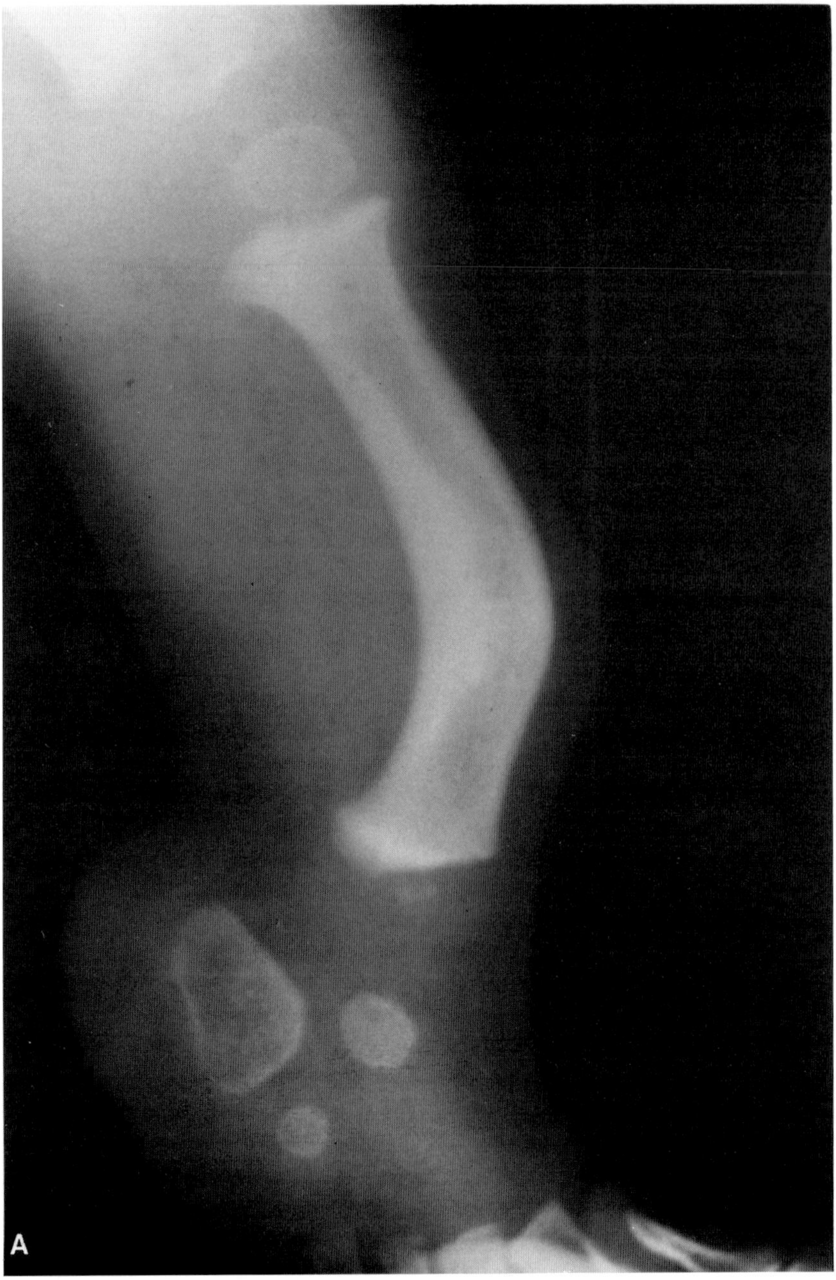

FIGURE 7.3. Type 2 fibular deficiency with complete absence of the fibula. Note the marked anterior bowing of the tibia and the deformity of the ankle joint.

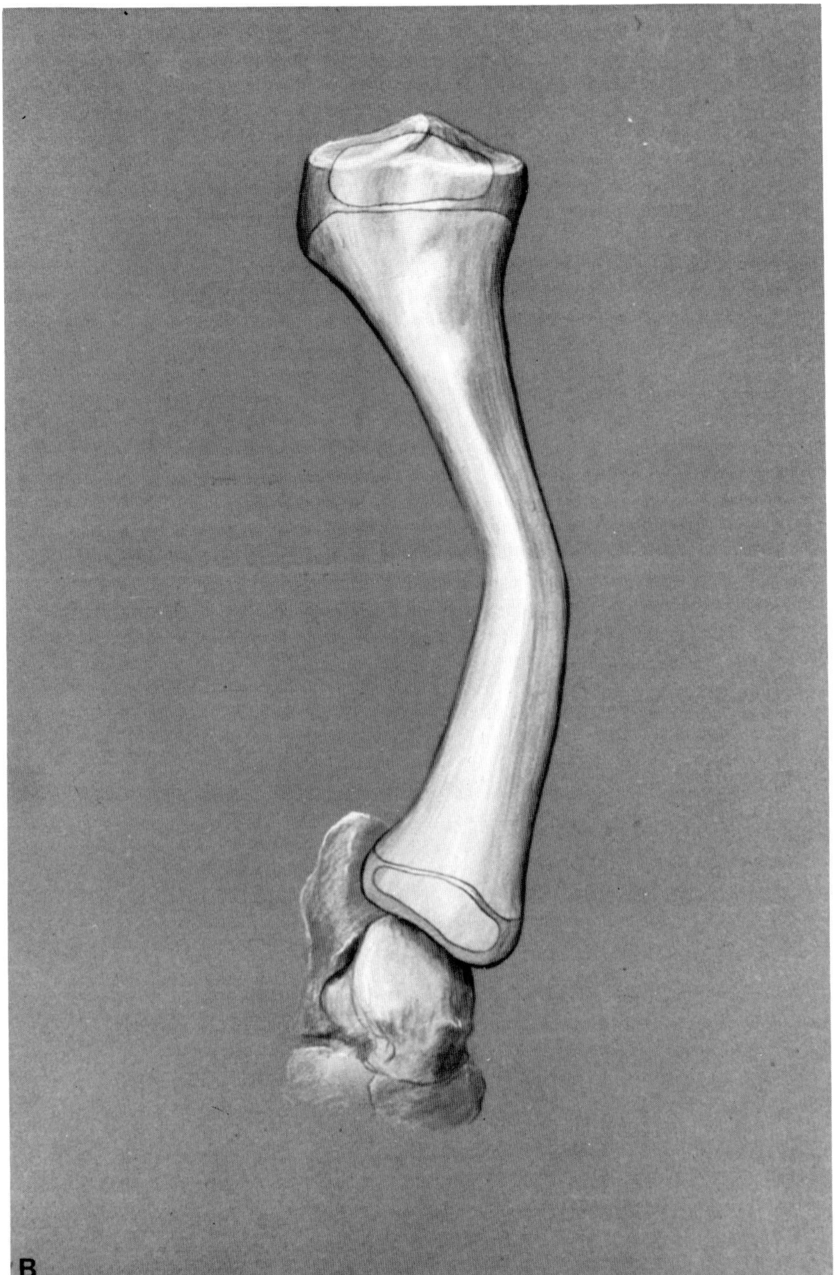

FIGURE 7.3. *Continued*

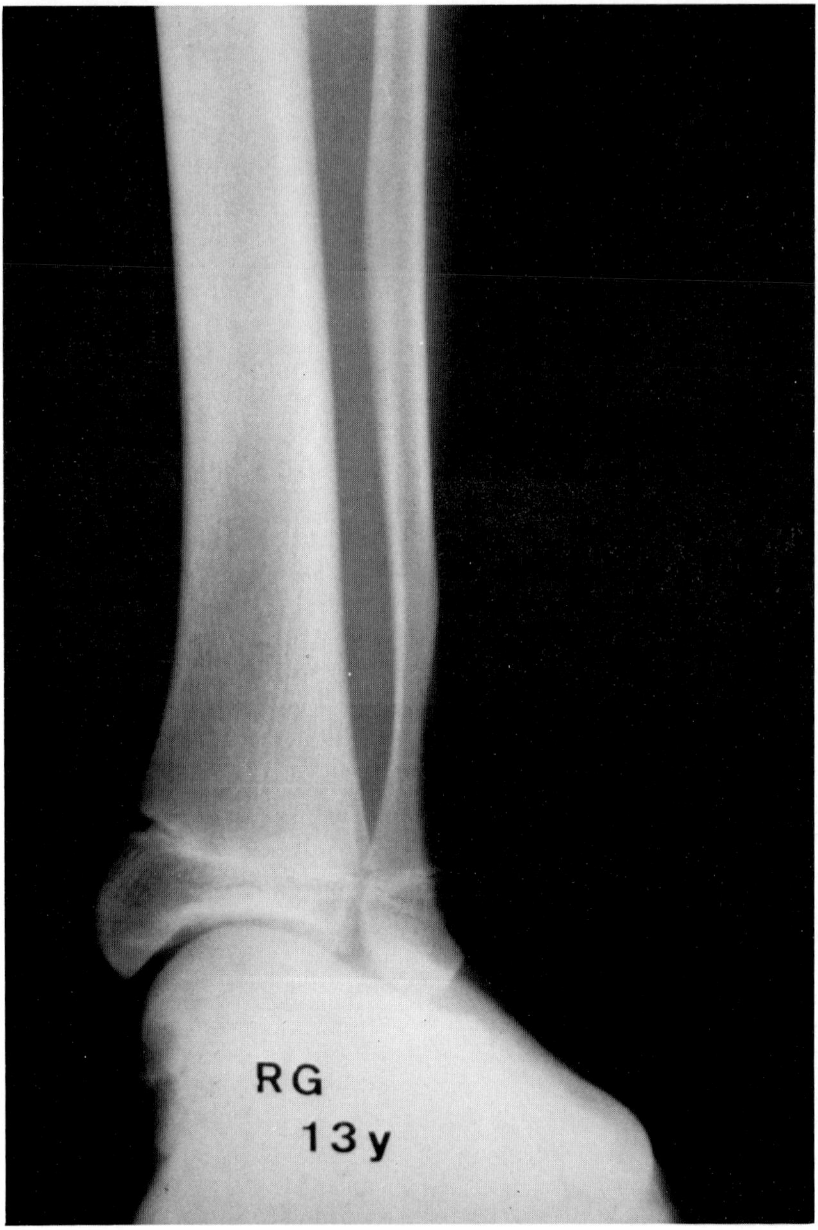

FIGURE 7.4. Ball-and-socket ankle in a patient with fibular hypoplasia.

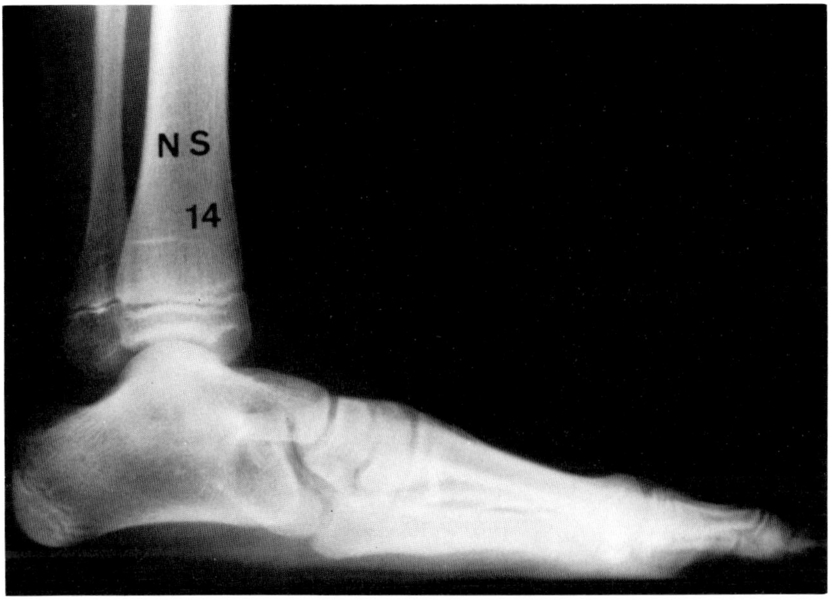

FIGURE 7.5. Talocalcaneal coalition as part of the complex abnormality in a patient with fibular hypoplasia.

reported three such cases and classified them as Type I. Other authors have reported similar cases.[2,6,7,10,14,16] Bohne and Root presented a series of 14 cases isolated from a larger study. By carefully examining their series of patients with congenital inequality of leg length, it became apparent that this deformity was perhaps more common than complete absence of the fibula.

The spectrum of abnormalities involving the lower limb is usually present whether the deficiency was complete or incomplete. The features of the two groups were similar; in most cases differences were a matter of degrees. In our series there were four common features. First, associated shortening or deformity of the femur was present in 70% of Type I limbs and in 50% of Type II. Second, increased valgus at the knee was present in approximately 30% of both Type I and Type II patients. Third, absence of the lateral rays of the foot and the presence of tarsal coalition were features of both groups, although both changes were more common in patients with complete fibular absence. Associated anomalies of the upper limb were seen in 15% of Type I and in 26% of Type II. Fourth, leg-length discrepancy was a constant feature, shortening averaged 13% for Type I and 19% for Type II.

The two types of fibular abnormalities were differentiated by three factors: Type I deficiency showed a low incidence of tibial bowing, a stable configuration of the ankle, and a plantigrade foot. Tibial bowing was seen in only 9% of Type I cases, compared with 96% of Type II cases. Three configurations of the ankle joint occurred in Type I deficiency: (1) In some limbs the ankle appeared normal, but 75% had a ball-and-socket ankle, classically seen in the Type IA groups. (2) In 14% there was a tibiotalar articulation in which the fibula was present but did not reach the joint, a characteristic finding in Type IB group. (3) When the fibula was completely absent, there was always a tibiotalar articulation with variable degrees of stability. The position of the foot distinguished the two types of fibular deformity. In the Type I group the foot was plantigrade in 66% of the cases, equinovalgus in 25%, and equinovarus in 8%. In the Type II group all feet were in varying degrees of equinovalgus.

Summary

The manifestations of fibular hypoplasia have been noted in the literature. In his original article describing the congenital ball-and-socket ankle, Lamb[11] noted that in two of five cases the lateral malleolus was poorly developed, and the involved limb was congenitally short; in two other cases tarsal coalitions were present. Thus, in two, and possibly four, of these five cases, hypoplasia of the fibula and the associated anomalies were present. In a radiographic review of cases, Schreiber[13] found a congenital ball-and-socket ankle in 4 of 18 cases with fibular hypoplasia and in 10 of 26 cases with congenital inequality of limb length. Both the Lamb and Schreiber reports emphasized that the tarsal coalition explained the existence of the ball-and-socket ankle. In our series, a tarsal coalition was seen in 18 of the 38 ball-and-socket ankles.

Examination of the treatment used in our series demonstrates further the similarities and differences between the patients with fibular hypoplasia and those with complete absence of the fibula. In Type IA the lesser degree of shortening and the relatively stable foot and ankle have led to the successful use of epiphysiodesis to balance leg lengths in 50% of the cases, while another 25% were followed without treatment. In the Type IB group, six of seven feet were in the severe equinovalgus position, and epiphysiodesis alone was not enough: Two patients walked with custom-made prostheses without limitation, and another two patients underwent leg-lengthening procedures. Treatment of patients with complete absence of the fibula has been discussed extensively by others.[1,5,10,15,16] Amputation of the foot with preservation of the heel pad for weight-bearing is the currently favored treatment.

References

1. Achterman CA, Kalamchi A: Congenital deficiency of the fibula. J Bone Joint Surg 61-B:133–137, 1979.

2. Amstutz HC: Natural history and treatment of congenital absence of the fibula. J Bone Joint Surg 54-A:1349, 1972.
3. Bohne WHO, Root L: Hypoplasia of the fibula. Clin Orthop 125:107–112, 1977.
4. Coventry MD, Johnson EW: Congenital absence of the fibula. J Bone Joint Surg 34-A:941–955, 1952.
5. Eilert RE, Jayakumar SS: Boyd and Syme ankle amputations in children. J Bone Joint Surg 58-A:1138–1141, 1976.
6. Farmer AW, Laurin CA: Congenital absence of the fibula. J Bone Joint Surg 42-A:1–12, 1960.
7. Frantz CH, O'Rahilly R: Congenital absence of the fibula. J Bone Joint Surg 42-A:1202–1224, 1961.
8. Hootnick D, Boyd NA, Fixsen JA, et al: The natural history and management of congenital short tibia with dysplasia or absence of the fibula: A preliminary report. J Bone Joint Surg 59-B:267–271, 1977.
9. Jansen K, Anderson KS: Congenital absence of the fibula. Acta Orthop Scand 45:446–453, 1974.
10. Kruger LM, Talbott RD: Amputation and prosthesis as definitive treatment in congenital absence of the fibula. J Bone Joint Surg 43-A:625–641, 1961.
11. Lamb D: The ball and socket ankle joint—A congenital abnormality. J Bone Joint Surg 40-B:240–243, 1958.
12. Pappas AM, Ranawalt BJ, Anderson M: Congenital defects of the fibula. Orthop Clin North Am 3:187–198, 1972.
13. Schreiber RR: Congenital and acquired ball and socket ankle joint. Radiology 84:940–944, 1965.
14. Thompson JC, Straub LE, Arnold WD: Congenital absence of the figula. J Bone Joint Surg 39-A:1229–1236, 1957.
15. Westin GW, Sakai DN, Wood WL: Congenital longitudinal deficiency of the fibula: Follow-up of treatment by Syme amputation. J Bone Joint Surg 58-A:492–496, 1976.
16. Wood WL, Zlotsky N, Westin GW: Congenital absence of the fibula: Treatment by Syme amputation—indications and technique. J Bone Joint Surg, 47-A:1159–1169, 1965.

8
Congenital Deficiency of the Tibia

ALI KALAMCHI

Introduction

Congenital deficiency of the tibia (tibial hemimelia, tibial aplasia, and dysplasia) is a rare longitudinal deficiency of the lower limb. In this type of congenital deformity, the fibula is usually intact and the deformity is confined to the tibia. There is usually total aplasia or marked dysplasia of the tibia. The limb involved is short and usually bowed. There is marked foreshortening of the whole lower limb.[2,9] The foot is rigid and in marked supination. There is also marked foreshortening of the first metatarsal with associated medial ray defects (Fig. 8.1). There is accompanying traits such as flexion contractures of the knee and a skin dimple overlying the proximal tibial region.

The incidence of congenital tibial deficiency in the United States is approximately 1 in 1 million live births.[4] Familial incidence of this condition has been reported. It was Otto[12] who first reported the condition in 1841. In 1877 Albert[3] described transfer of the fibula underneath the femur to serve as a weight-bearing strut. This concept was brought to North America by Myers,[11] who created a functional fibulofemoral arthroplasty, and was reintroduced and popularized by Brown[4] in the mid-1960s. In 1961 Frantz and O'Rahilly[7] were the first to classify lower-limb deficiency. In 1978 Jones et al[9] devised a means of classification specifically for congenital deficiency of the tibia with an intact fibula based on initial x-ray findings. Kalamchi and Dawe[10] introduced their anatomic classification in 1985 based on the deficiency present on initial examination. This latter classification was also used in predicting the natural history of the deformity and helped in planning of the treatment program early on.

Classification

In this chapter I will be using the classification that we devised and used at our clinic at the Alfred I. duPont Institute in Wilmington, Delaware. The classification is simple and of clinical help in delineating the extent of the deformity and in assisting the planning for future management.

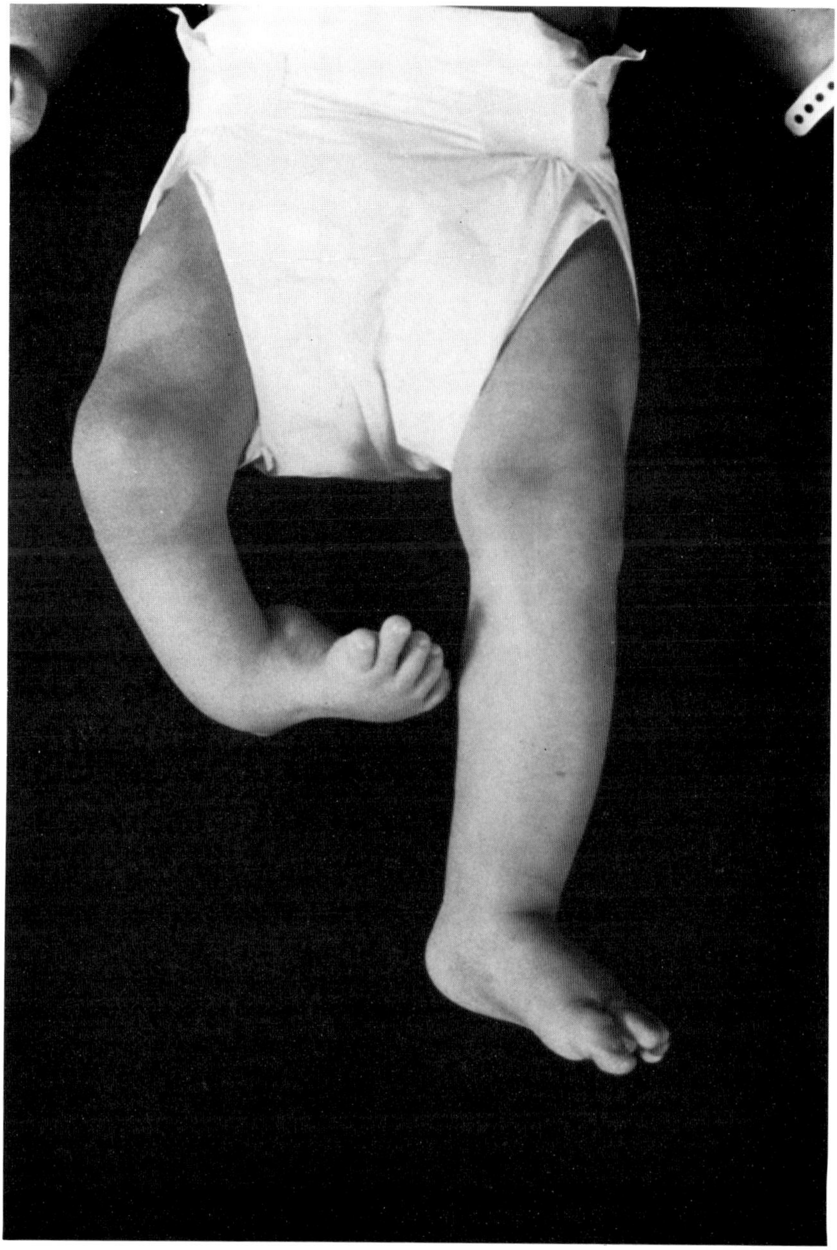

FIGURE 8.1. Child with classic congenital tibial deficiency demonstrating knee contracture and varus deformity of the foot with a markedly prominent distal fibula.

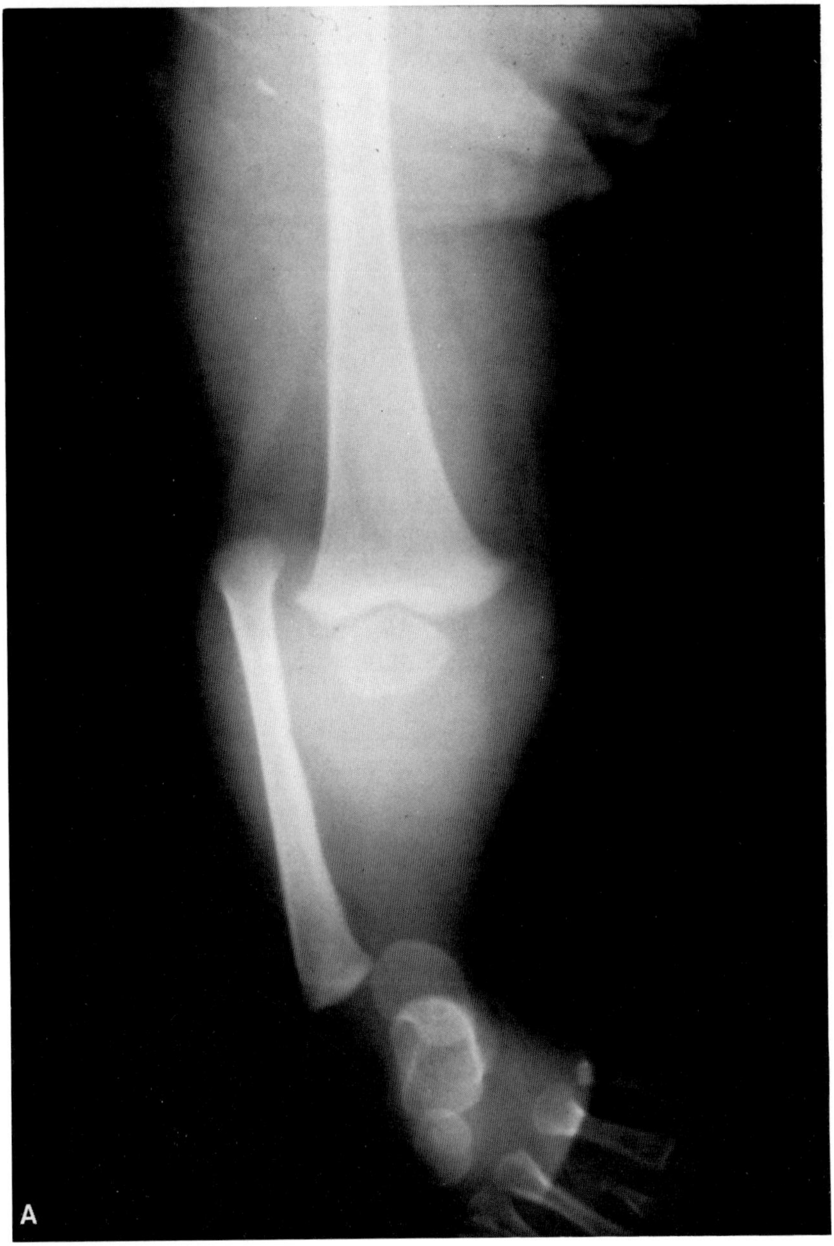

FIGURE 8.2. (**A** and **B**) Demonstration of the classic findings of a patient with total absence of the tibia.

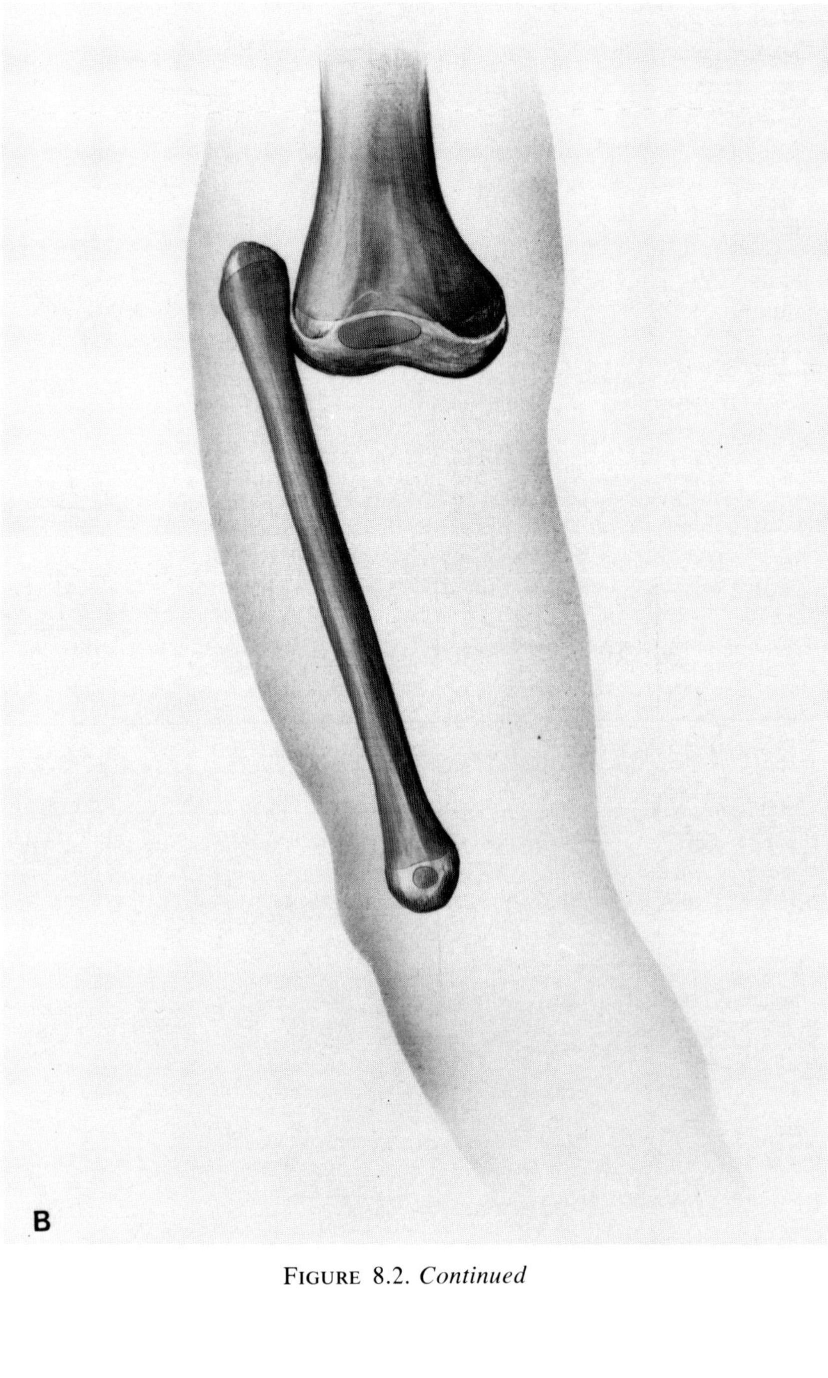

FIGURE 8.2. *Continued*

Type I: Total Absence of the Tibia

The children in this group are born with marked knee flexion contractures, variable rotation of the leg, and marked inversion and adduction of the foot, with occasional deficiency of the medial rays (Fig. 8.1). Clinically, there is a knee flexion contracture of more than 45 degrees with no active quadriceps mechanism. The radiographs show total absence of the tibia (Fig. 8.2A,B). Other features commonly seen are proximal migration (dislocation) of the fibular head and marked hypoplasia of the distal femur. The hypoplasia of the distal femoral condyle include definite reduction in the width of the distal metaphysis and marked retardation of the ossification of the femoral epiphysis. This was noted initially by Jones et al[9] in their comprehensive review in 1977, and we found it to be an excellent guide to the degree of involvement of the tibia and the quadriceps deficiency.

Type II: Distal Tibial Aplasia

The proximal tibia is usually present at birth and with further growth will develop and lead to a fairly normal articulating tibial plateau. Active quadriceps function can be detected early in life. The average knee contractures are between 25 and 45 degrees and correlate well with the degree of the proximal tibial development. Initial radiographic evaluation reveals the proximal tibia with its normal relationship to the distal femur. When the proximal tibial segment is underdeveloped and mostly cartilaginous, it can not be visualized on regular x-rays. In the early stages, if there is concern, a knee arthrogram will outline the cartilaginous plateau clearly. (Recently M.R.I. has been used to visualize the cartilagenous proximal tibia.) The clue for the presence of the proximal tibial anlage is the presence of an active quadriceps and the normal development of the distal femur as seen on plain radiograph. This usually includes a normal width of the distal femoral metaphysis and a normal ossification of the distal epiphysis at birth (Fig. 8.3A,B). The proximal fibular migration is usually not as severe as in Type I.

Type III (Dysplasia of the Distal Tibia with Diastasis of the Tibiofibular Syndesmosis)

This was the rarest form in our initial series. There is a normally formed knee joint and a well-developed quadriceps mechanism. The deformity is usually limited to the distal third of the tibia, with hypoplasia and shortening being the rule. Usually the talus is subluxed proximally with varying degrees of diastasis. The distal fibula is usually prominent on the lateral side of the ankle and the foot is tilted in varying degrees of varus (Fig. 8.4).

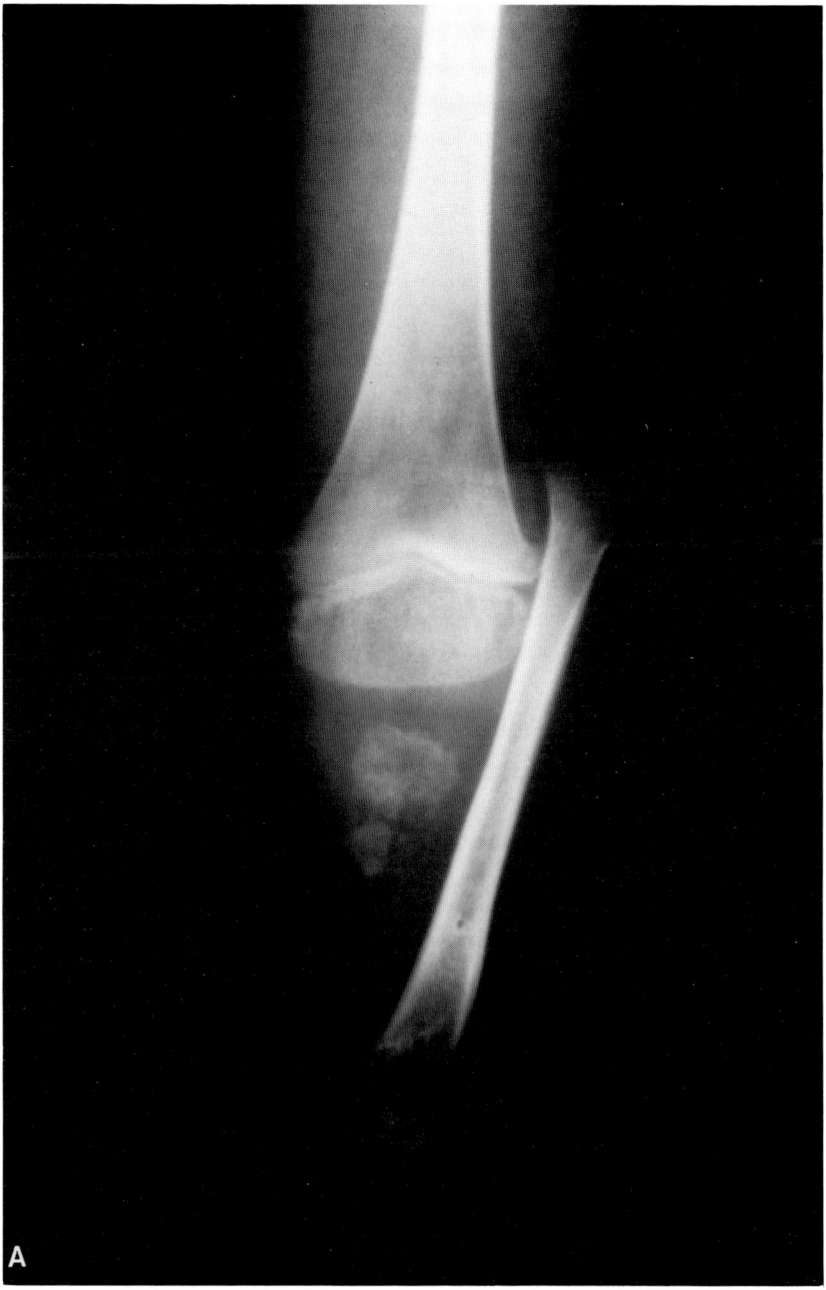

FIGURE 8.3. **A:** Illustration of the findings of a patient with type II deficiency. Note the proximal tibia articulating with the distal femur, forming a stable knee joint. **B:** Radiograph of same type II deficiency where the proximal tibia is present. The knee is well preserved. Also note the minimal proximal migration of the fibula.

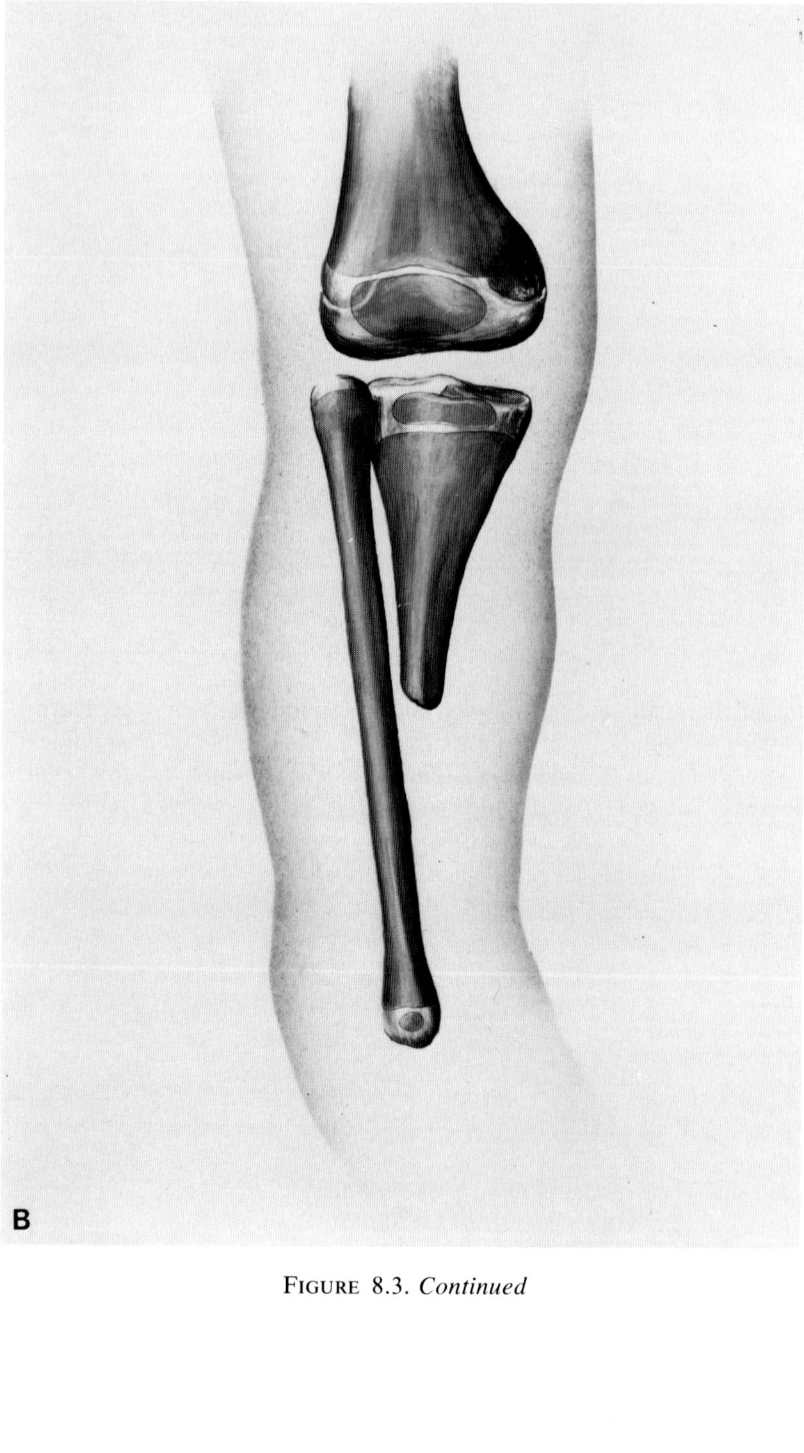

Figure 8.3. *Continued*

There is another form of tibial deficiency that was noted by Jones et al[9] in 1978. They described two cases of a deficient proximal tibia with variable dysplasia of the remaining tibia. This entity must be extremely rare for it has not been reported in the recent North American literature.

Associated Anomalies

Children with tibial deficiencies were noted to have a high incidence of associated congenital anomalies.[2,6,9,13] In Kalamchi and Dawe's series, two thirds of their patients had evidence of additional anomalies.[10] The most frequent ones were anomalies of the hand (43%), male gonadal anomalies (43%), anomalies of the other foot (39%), and ipsilateral femur anomalies (29%). Of the hand anomalies, the most frequently seen were "lobster claw" hand and anomalies of the thumb. The foot anomalies included four cases of severe equinovarus deformities.

Management Recommendations

The initial radiographs of children with congenital tibial deficiency can be used to delineate the presence or absence of a tibial anlage, as well as the status of the distal femoral metaphysis and epiphysis. The clues learned from careful evaluation of the initial radiographs can be the best guide to the knowledge of the functional integrity of the intra-articular knee structures. The presence of the proximal tibia and a structural knee joint correlates with a functional quadriceps mechanism.

I feel that the clinician can make, with some accuracy, a distinction between the various degrees of tibial deficiency on the initial visit. It is critical to these children and their parents that plans for treatment are made early. Our classification of three types of deficiency is simple and functional and can aid the clinician in accurately selecting the appropriate surgical procedure.

In Type I patients we recommend early knee disarticulation, which enables the patient to begin early ambulation with a pylon type of prosthesis. Reconstructive surgical procedures to salvage the knee in this group of patients did not yield good results. The lack of proximal tibia and active quadriceps function lead to persistence of marked knee contractures and the inability to gain functional range of motion. In rare cases a femoral fibular fusion can be considered if the ipsilateral femur is markedly hypoplastic. This procedure adds length to the existing stump, giving a better lever arm, and allows proper prosthetic fitting. In Type I patients, above-knee amputation is contraindicated primarily because of bony overgrowth in children.

In Type II patients the ideal procedure is tibiofibular fusion to obtain

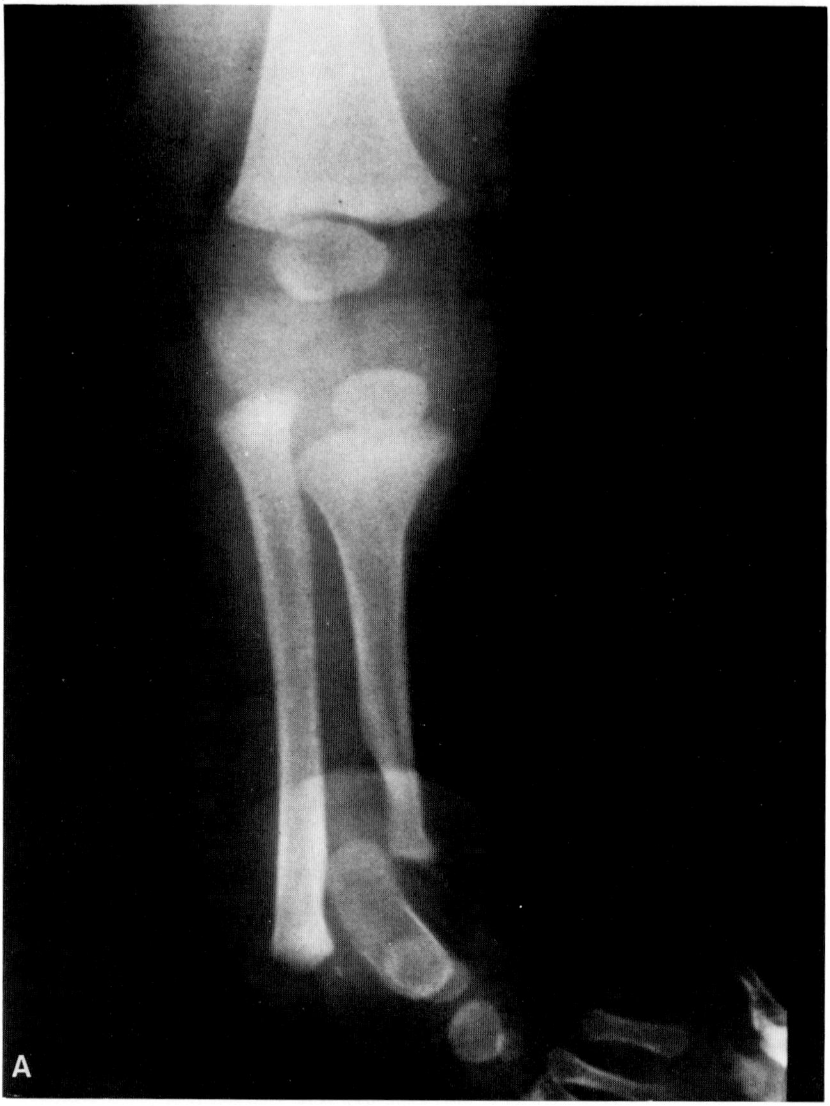

FIGURE 8.4. Illustration **(A)** and radiograph **(B)** of hypoplasia of the distal tibia with diastesis of the distal tibiofibular syndesmosis.

stability. This procedure can be done in two fashions. When it is performed early, the proximal fibula can be embedded in the tibial cartilaginous anlage (modified Brown[5] procedure). If the patient is seen at later stages, a classic side-by-side tibiofibular synostosis can be accomplished to obtain stability. These children will usually have excellent function of the knee. Therefore, it is of the utmost importance to

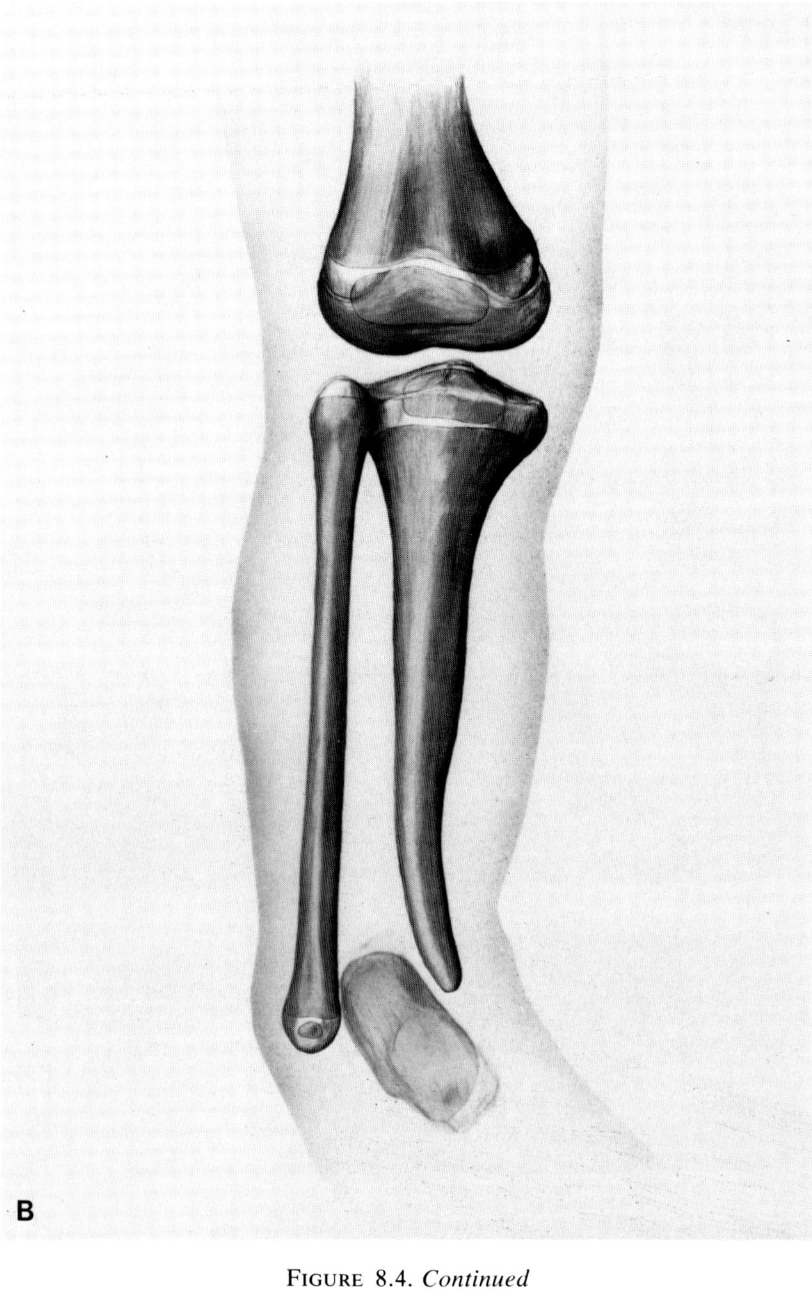

FIGURE 8.4. *Continued*

recognize this group early, and the goal is to preserve their knee joint. Because of the pronounced leg-length discrepancy and/or abnormality of the foot, these children benefit from foot-ablation procedures.[1,8,14] We prefer to carry out a modified Boyd amputation by implanting the distal fibula within the os calcis body. The arthrodesis helps to maintain stability of the stump and longitudinal growth is preserved by salvaging the distal fibular growth plate. This procedure results in an excellent end-bearing stump. I strongly believe that below-knee amputation should be avoided in this group of patients because of the overwhelming difficulties with bony overgrowth, as well as the constant skin breakage of the stump.

In Type III patients the ideal procedure is a talofibular fusion to stabilize the hindfoot and to improve the function of the foot. If this is not possible, talectomy and modified Boyd procedures should be performed. If there is marked instability between the distal tibia and figula, synostosis should be achieved.

References

1. Achterman CA, Kalamchi A: Congenital deficiency of the fibula. J Bone Joint Surg Br 61133–137, 1979.
2. Aitken GW: Tibial hemimelia, in: Aitken GT (ed): Selected Lower Limb Anomalies. National Academy of Sciences, 1971, pp. 1–19.
3. Albert E: Wein Med Presse 1877, p 111.
4. Brown FW: The Brown operation for total hemimelia tibia, in Aitken GT (ed): Selected Lower Limb Anomalies. National Academy of Sciences, 1971, pp 21–28.
5. Brown FW: Construction of a knee joint in congenital total absence of the tibia (paraxial hemimelia tibia). A preliminary report. J Bone Joint Surg 47-A:695–704, 1965.
6. Clark MW: Autosomal dominant inheritance of tibial meromelia. Report of a kindred. J Bone Joint Surg 57-A:262–264, 1975.
7. Frantz CH, O'Rahilly R: Congenital skeletal limb deficiencies. J Bone Joint Surg 43-A:1201–1224, 1961.
8. Hootnick D, Boyd NA, Fixen JA, et al: The natural hisotry and management of congenital short tibia with dysplasia or absence of the fibula. J Bone Joint Surg Br 59-B:267–271, 1977.
9. Jones D, Barnes J, Lloyd-Roberts GC: Congenital aplasia and dysplasia of the tibia with intact fibula. Classification and management. J Bone Joint Surg Br 60-B:31–39, 1978.
10. Kalamchi A, Dawe RV: Congenital deficiency of the tibia. J Bone Joint Surg 67-B:581–584, 1985.
11. Myers TH: Further report on a case of congenital absence of the tibia. Am J Orthop Surg 8:398–400, 1910.
12. Otto AW: Monstorum sexcentorum descripto anatomica, in: *Sumptibus Ferdinandi Hirt*. Breslau, 1841.

13. Pashayan H, Fraser FC, McIntyre JM, et al: Bilateral aplasia of the tibia, polydactyly, and absent thumb in father and daughter. J Bone Joint Surg Br 53-B:495–499, 1971.
14. Wehbe MA, Weinstein SL, Ponseti IV: Tibial agenesis. J Pediatr Orthop 1:395–399, 1981.

Section III—Treatment Modalities

9
Tibial Rotation-Plasty for Proximal Femoral Focal Deficiency

Alfred E. Kritter

Introduction

Management of patients with proximal femoral focal deficiency (PFFD) presents a unique challenge to orthopedic surgeons. In general, children with lower extremity skeletal deficiencies suffer four major biomechanical losses: limb-length inequality, malrotation, inadequacy of proximal musculature, and instability of proximal joints.[1] In PFFD patients these losses are particularly well exemplified; therefore, efforts to correct, or compensate for, these biomechanical losses should constitute the basis of a treatment program.

When patients present themselves to an orthopedist or an amputee clinic team, they are typically classified into one of two groups: class 1, which includes patients with congenital short femurs with coxa vara, and class 2, which includes PFFD patients. For patients in class 1, treatment primarily involves equalizing leg lengths; however, various treatment alternatives, such as amputation, knee fusion, or tibial rotation-plasty,[3,8,10] should be considered for class 2 patients.

As Koman et al[10] pointed out, many factors must be considered when grouping these patients. For example, class 1 patients with greater than 60% of predicted femoral length, evidence of pelvic-femoral stability, less than 17 cm of projected extremity shortness, and a good, stable plantar-grade foot should be considered for equalization procedures. Class 2 patients with less than 60% of predicted femoral length or greater than 17 cm of predicted extremity shortness are candidates for the various reconstructive procedures.

All the variable factors of the hip, knee, and foot must be considered when designing a treatment program for unilateral PFFD patients. Aitken's classification of PFFD hips into four groups[1] is a helpful guide for determining a treatment program. Amstutz[2] found that proportional shortening of the femur remains the same except for the proximal migration of the femur with time. And, as Panting and Williams[16] point out from Drachman and Sokoloff's 1966 study,[7] if an acetabulum is present in infancy, a femoral head and neck will be evident on x-ray studies taken later in the patient's life.

Tibial rotation-plasty, the "van Nes procedure," is one alternative in the treatment of PFFD patients; however, it is not appropriate treatment for all PFFD patients. This procedure offers a more reasonable probability of obtaining a functional end motor unit in an abnormally shortened and externally rotated lower limb with reconstructive surgery, than does amputation. The concept of rotating the foot to produce a functioning end motor unit was first reported in 1930 by Borggreve.[5] Since then, it has gained in popularity for the treatment of congenital PFFD patients and even more frequently used for enbloc resection of osteosarcoma of the distal femur.*

A successful rotation-plasty provides a better end result than an above-knee amputation.[15] Furthermore, it can functionally approach the results obtained with a below-knee amputation. In addition, retention of the foot at the end of the extremity gives patients a sense of position, which is lacking with more proximal amputations.

Tibial rotation-plasty has been rejected by some orthopedists because of complications, such as ischemia, postoperative derotation, prolonged hospital stays, and difficult prosthetic fitting.[2,4,14,20] However, an 8-year study[13] of seven patients from the Milwaukee Children's Hospital Juvenile Amputee and Congenital Limb Deficiency Center has shown that this technique is both safe and satisfactory. Furthermore, the procedure has been performed on many other patients without reports of ischemia, prolonged hospitalization, or derotation.

Patients aged 1 or 2 years old are usually treated with an extension-aid-type prosthesis. This provides adequate length, controls rotation, and prevents progression of the flexion deformity of the anatomic knee and hip (Fig. 9.1). It is often preferable to perform the tibial rotation-plasty before a child enters nursery school, since the extension aid is not cosmetically acceptable because of the presence of the highly visible foot at the contralateral knee-joint level.

One technique[13] will be presented, recognizing there are other techniques for tibial rotation-plasty available.[11,17]

Indications for Use of Tibial Rotation-Plasty

A patient with a unilateral PFFD, a predicted deficiency of the involved femur of 60% or more and a normal foot and ankle is an ideal candidate for tibial rotation-plasty. Patients with the most stable hip, such as Aitken's

* References 4–6, 9, 11, 12, 14, 18, 19.

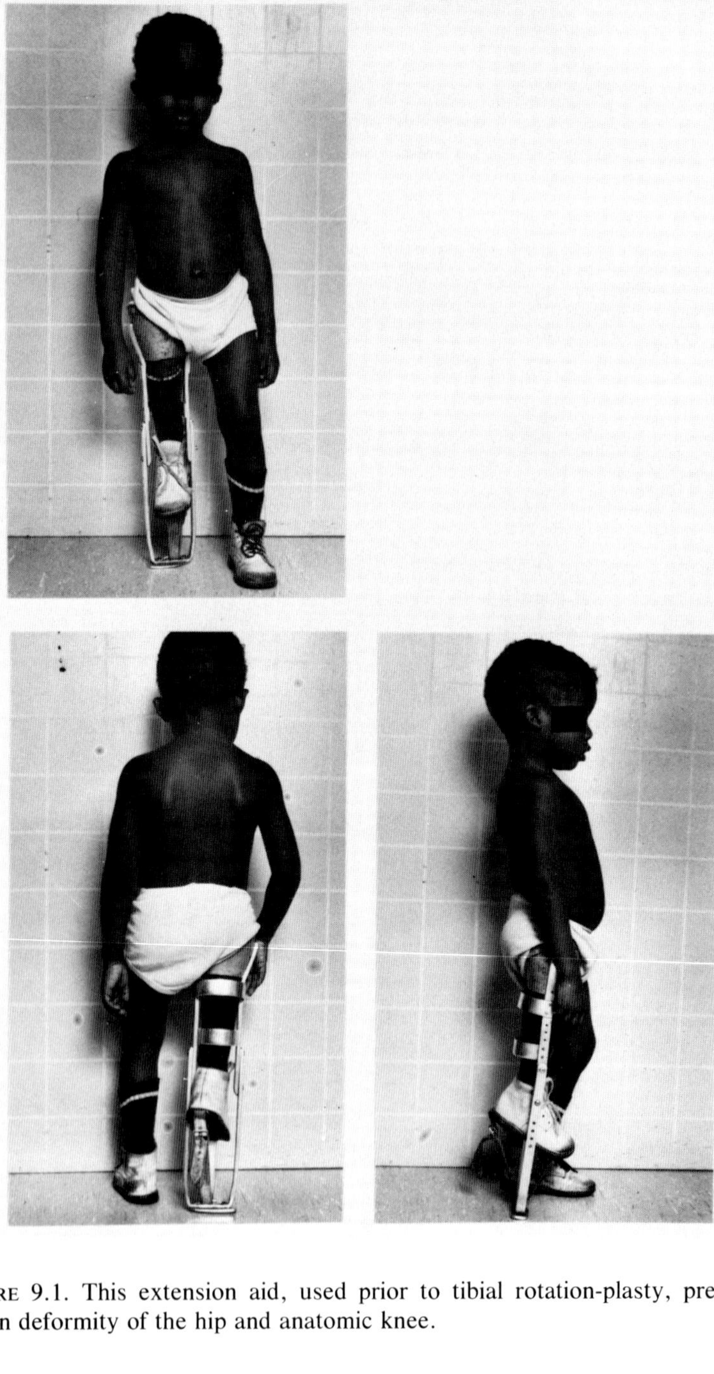

FIGURE 9.1. This extension aid, used prior to tibial rotation-plasty, prevents flexion deformity of the hip and anatomic knee.

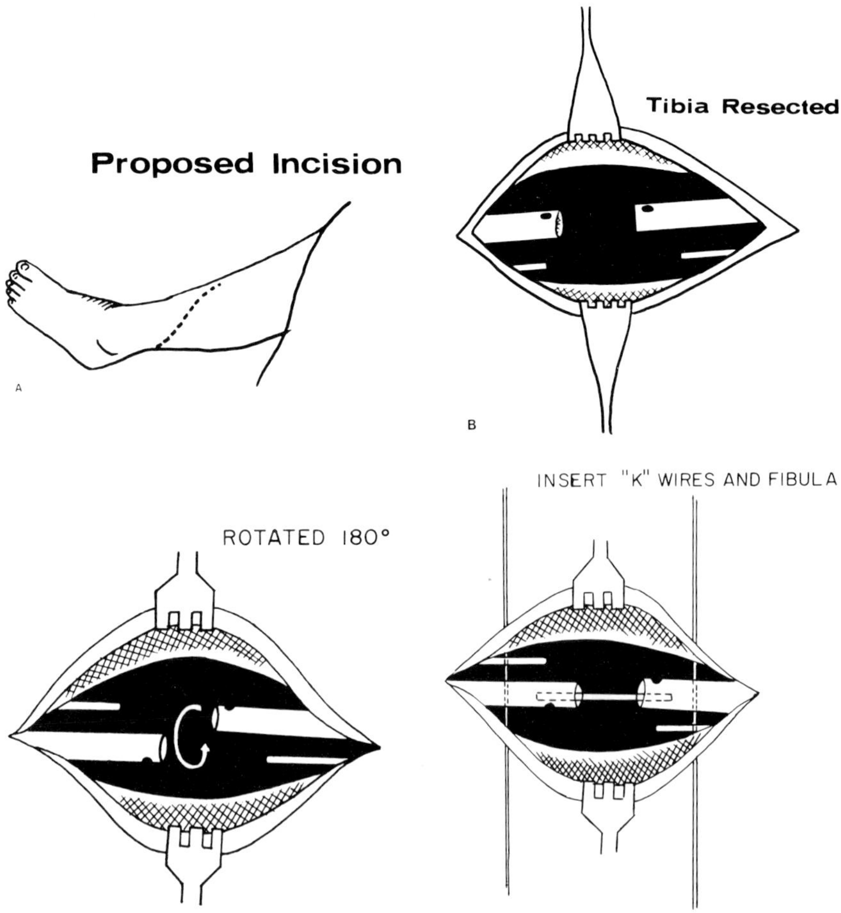

FIGURE 9.2. **A:** The oblique incision. **B:** The tibia is marked proximally and distally as a landmark so that the surgeon will know how much rotation has been obtained. **C:** A generous resection of tibia and fibula allows 180-degree rotation, as determined by the marks on the tibia. **D:** Rotation is complete. A strut graft is in place and two Kirschner wires are drilled.

Class A, will have the best gait,[1] whereas those with Class B, C, or D hips will have proportionally poorer gaits owing to hip instability.

Candidates for this procedure should have a femoral segment of such length that after tibial rotation-plasty and subsequent knee fusion, the center axis of the ankle will be at the same level as the center axis of the contralateral knee. When the femoral segment is too long, the rotated ankle cannot be placed at the same level as the contralateral knee; therefore, tibial rotation-plasty would be contraindicated.

Tibial rotation-plasty is also contraindicated if the foot is severely

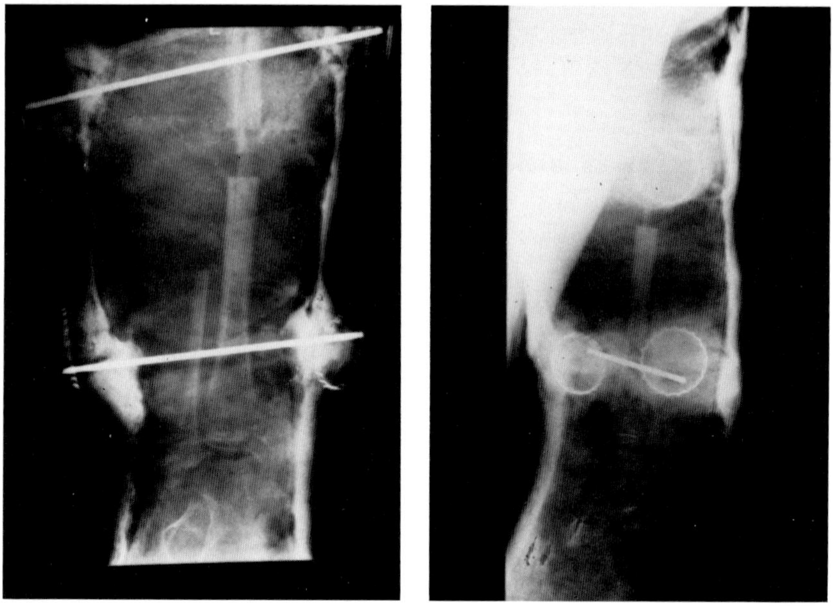

AP LAT

FIGURE 9.3. Anteroposterior **(A)** and lateral **(B)** roentgenograms, taken at the completion of surgery, show satisfactory alignment and continuity of the tibial rotation-plasty maintained in plaster with Kirschner wire fixation.

deformed and the ankle lacks the active range of movements necessary to function as a knee joint. It can be used with a mildly abnormal foot, such as one with a partial absence of the fibula and a diminished fifth ray, if the foot is in a reasonable anatomic position and not in a severe valgus deformity.[1] If the tibial rotation-plasty fails, it can be converted easily by a Syme's amputation and fusion of the anatomic knee.

A Tibial Rotation-Plasty Technique

Under general anesthesia, with the patient supine and without the use of a tourniquet, an oblique incision is made from the proximal anteromedial aspect of the leg distal to the anterolateral aspect of the leg (Fig. 9.2A). The tibia is then marked proximally and distally with an osteotome so that the surgeon has a good reference point for determining the amount of rotation achieved. The marking of the tibia is essential because the unstable knee and hip joints, with surgical drapes over them, do not provide stable anatomic landmarks for determining exactly when 180 degrees of rotation have been obtained. The diaphysis of the tibia and fibula is generously exposed subperiosteally. Approximately 10 cm of

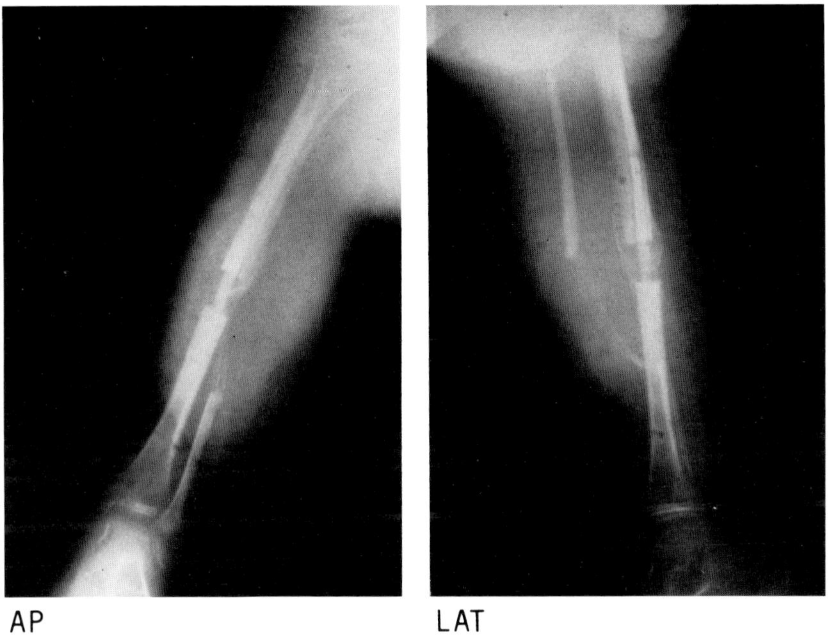

FIGURE 9.4. Anteroposterior **(A)** and lateral **(B)** roentgenograms show good callus formation 6 weeks after surgery.

fibula is removed and saved. Depending on the femoral length, approximately 8 cm of tibia is removed (Fig. 9.2B). The distal segment can then be rotated externally a full 180 degrees, as determined by the mark previously placed on the tibia (Fig. 9.2C).

Generous resection of fibula and tibia is the most important aspect of the operation because it prevents ischemia, which is caused by undue soft-tissue tension resulting from the 180-degree rotation. The resected fibula should be placed intramedullarly in the proximal and distal segments of the tibia[9] for use as a strut graft to maintain the alignment and stability of the tibia. This strut graft, which has a much smaller circumference than the original tibia, reduces the tension on the soft tissues by reducing the linear distance that the soft tissues must stretch as they turn during the rotation-plasty. Surgical absence of the fibula also reduces the soft-tissue tension. If ischemia occurs after the rotation, soft-tissue tension can be reduced by telescoping the tibial fragments on the fibular graft.

After the rotation has been completed, Kirschner wires (K wires) are inserted in the same coronal plane, through the proximal and distal segments of the tibia (Fig. 9.2D). It is important to insert these K wires after the full rotation to avoid soft-tissue distortion on the wires. The stab wounds for the K wires should be generous enough to provide adequate

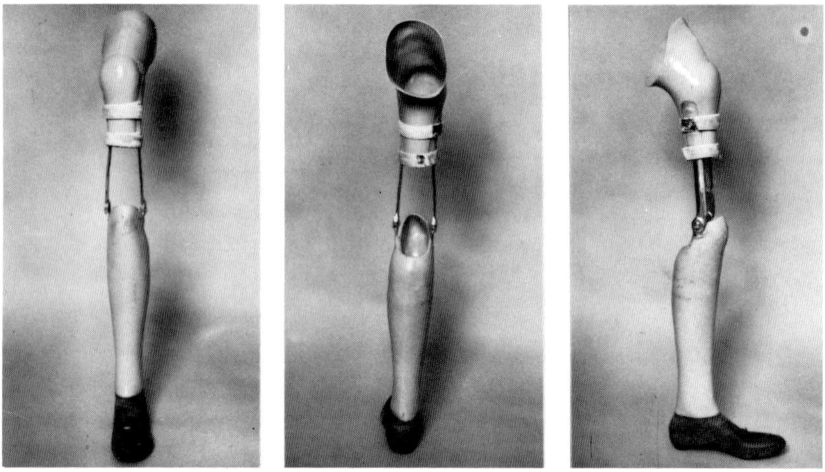

FIGURE 9.5. This tibial rotation-plasty prosthesis has a quadrilateral plastic socket, optional pelvic band, outside-knee hinges, and a socket for the foot that has a high trim line over the heel of the rotated foot.

drainage without tension on the adjacent soft tissues. These wires, placed parallel after the full 180-degree rotation, give the surgeon a landmark for maintaining the complete rotation during closure of the wound and application of a plaster case, which incorporates the wires.

If necessary, the overall length of the tibia can be adjusted by telescoping the tibial segments on the fibular graft. This makes it easy to adjust the level of the ankle joint to match the contralateral knee level. The fibular graft provides excellent alignment and continuity, minimizing the chance of position loss either intra- or postoperatively.

After the procedure, only the skin layers are closed. Attempting to close the periosteum or fascia can cause ischemia of the leg and foot. Adequate hemostasis is easily obtained and tube drainage of the wound is appropriate. A cast is then applied from just proximal to the knee joint down to the toes. The cast should be open over the plantar surface of the foot, which is now facing anteriorly. This permits easy inspection of the foot to determine its viability and readiness for an early exercise program. Postoperative roentgenograms are then made to confirm the proper alignment of the rotation-plasty (Fig. 9.3).

If physically capable, the patient is allowed to walk with crutches a few days after surgery and is then discharged. The K wires and cast are removed after 6 weeks (Fig. 9.4), and a model limb is made for prosthetic fitting. A second cast is then applied to maintain the position of the foot until the prosthesis is fitted 8 to 10 weeks after surgery.

The prosthesis consists of a quadrilateral plastic socket with an optional

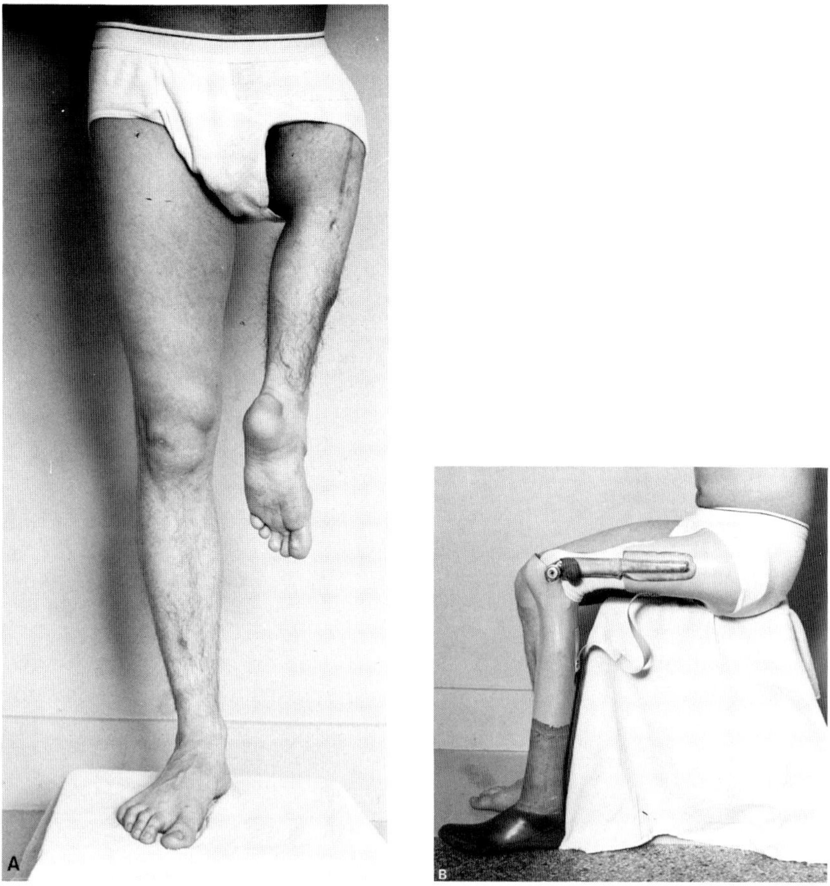

FIGURE 9.6. **A:** Patient with rotation-plasty shows the ideal positioning of the foot and ankle, which is at the level of the contralateral knee. **B:** Side view of a patient sitting shows the excellent functional range of the rotated foot at the level of the contralateral knee.

pelvic band, outside knee hinges, and a socket for the foot that has a high trim line over the heel of the rotated foot (Fig. 9.5). This design provides stability for the hip and anatomic knee, enables rotary control of the leg, an permits active use of the turnaround foot as a knee joint.

In addition to the tibial rotation-plasty, an integral part of the overall treatment of these patients is the fusion of the anatomic knee. When anatomic knee fusion is performed at the time of skeletal maturity, the orthopedist can "fine tune" the rotation-plasty surgery by placing the ankle exactly at the level of the contralateral knee (Figs. 9.6A,B). The residual knee-flexion deformity of the anatomic knee is corrected at the

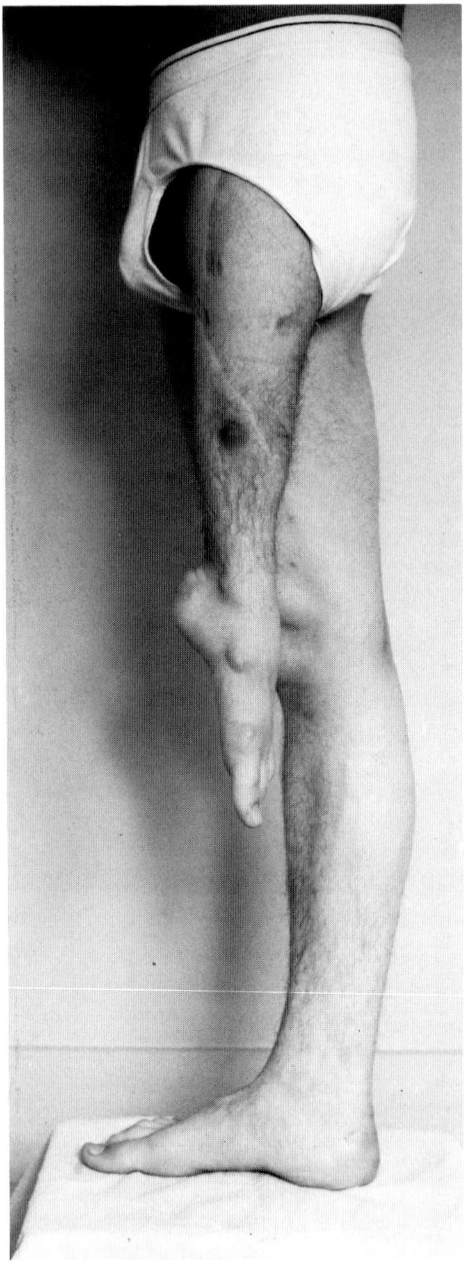

FIGURE 9.7. Side view of rotated foot and fused anatomic knee with hip flexion contracture completely stretched out.

time of fusion. Following the fusion, the hip flexion contracture stretches out well (Fig. 9.7).

Summary

A recent study of functional performance in children after tibial rotation-plasty in resections of malignant tumors was conducted by Murray et al.[15] Despite some gait abnormalities, the rotation-plasty subjects walked at speeds comparable to those of normal children. Improved function after rotation-plasty has been noticed by many PFFD patients, particularly in activities such as stair climbing and bicycle riding. In addition, training these patients to use the ankle dorsiflexors as knee flexors and the ankle and foot plantar flexors as knee extensors has been very successful. When properly executed, rotation-plasty can provide many PFFD patients with superior functionality compared with through-knee amputations.

References

1. Aitken GT: Proximal femoral focal deficiency—definition, classification, and management, in: Aitken GT (ed): *Proximal Femoral Focal Deficiency. A Congenital Anomaly*. National Academy of Sciences, 1969, pp. 1–22.
2. Amstutz HC: Prognosis for growth and development of congenital anomalies of the lower extremities. J Bone Joint Surg Am 49:1011, 1967.
3. Amstutz HC, Wilson PD Jr: Dysgenesis of the proximal femur (coxa vara) and its surgical management.J Bone Joint Surg Am 44:1–24, 1962.
4. Bevan-Thomas WH, Millar EA: A review of proximal focal femoral deficiencies. J Bone Joint Surg Am 49:1376–1388, 1967.
5. Borggreve J: Kniegelenksersatz durch das in der beinlangasachse um 180° gedrehte fussgelenk. Arch Orthop Unfallchir 28:175–178, 1930.
6. Chapchal G, Van de Kerkhove W: Die umdrehplastik des sprunggelenkes bei der behandlung des kongenitalen femurdefektes. Arch Orthop Unfallchir 41:109–115, 1941.
7. Drachman DB, Sokoloff L: The role of movement in embryonic joint development. Dev Biol 14:401–420, 1966.
8. Gillespie R, Torode IP: Classification and management of congenital abnormalities of the femur. J Bone Joint Surg Br 65:557–568, 1983.
9. Hall JE: Rotation of congenitally hypoplastic lower limbs to use the ankle joint as a knee. Interclin Inf Bull 6:2, 1966.
10. Koman LA, Meyer LC, Warren FH: Proximal femoral focal deficiency: natural history and treatment. Clin Orthop 162:135–143, 1982.
11. Kostuik JP, Gillespie R, Hall JE, et al: Van Nes rotational osteotomy for treatment of proximal femoral focal deficiency and congenital short femur. J Bone Joint Surg Am 57:1039–1046, 1975.
12. Kotz R, Salzer M: Rotation-plasty for childhood osteosarcoma of the distal part of the femur. J Bone Joint Surg Am 64:959–969, 1982.

13. Kritter AE: Tibial rotation-plasty for proximal femoral focal deficiency. J Bone Joint Surg Am 59:927–934, 1977.
14. Murat JE, Guilleminet M, Descamps R: Long-term results of rotation-plasty in two patients with subtotal aplasia of the femur. Am J Surg 113:676–679, 1967.
15. Murray MP, Jacobs PA, Gore DR, et al: Functional performance after tibial rotation-plasty. J Bone Joint Surg Am 67:392–399, 1985.
16. Panting AL, Williams PF: Proximal femoral focal deficiency. J Bone Joint Surg Br 60:46–52, 1978.
17. Torode IP: Rotation-plasty of the lower limb for congenital defects of the femur. J Bone Joint Surg Br 65:569–573, 1983.
18. Van Nes CP: Rotation-plasty for congenital defects of the femur. Making use of the ankle of the shortened limb to control the knee joint of a prosthesis. J Bone Joint Surg Br 32:12–16, 1950.
19. Watts HG: Introduction to resection of musculoskeletal sarcomas. Clin Orthop 153:31–38, 1980.
20. Westin GW, Gunderson FO: Proximal femoral focal deficiency—a review of treatment experiences, in Aitken GT (ed): *Proximal Femoral Focal Deficiency. A Congenital Anomaly*. National Academy of Sciences, 1969, pp. 100–110.

10
Syme and Boyd Amputations in Children

S. JAY KUMAR

Introduction

Amputation through the ankle with or without retention of the os calcis is a useful procedure for children with severe congenital anomalies of the lower extremity where the foot is so deformed as to preclude weight-bearing and wearing of normal shoes, or where limb inequality is of such magnitude that standard equalizing procedures are of no avail and walking is possible only with the use of an unappealing prosthetic extension to the shortened extremity (Figs. 10.1 and 10.2).[1,2,7,11,17] Amputation through the ankle, as opposed to amputation through the distal tibia, has the distinct advantage of preserving growth in an already shortened extremity, since the distal tibial growth plate remains undisturbed (Fig. 10.3). It also avoids the problem of bony overgrowth, which is common when amputations are done through the diaphysis or metaphysis of growing bones (Fig. 10.4).

Two types of amputations performed on children through the ankle have now become synonymous with the names of the authors who first described them: James Syme, who reported his procedure in 1843, and Harold Buhaltz Boyd, whose work appeared in 1939. Neither of these procedures was initially intended for children, rather, they were done for adults with badly traumatized feet.[6,15] Syme's amputation was done before the advent of antisepsis, anesthesia, asepsis, or antibiotics, and the results, according to the report published in the London and Edinburgh Monthly Journal of Medical Sciences, were quite good. Burghard credits Gordon Watson with being the first to describe amputation of the foot with a calcaneotibial fusion.[6] Similar procedures were described by Ricard and Kofmann without calcaneotibial fusion, but ultimately these joints proved to be unstable on weight-bearing.[6] Harold Boyd, who first described amputation of the foot and concomitant calcaneotibial fusion, performed this technique on an adult whose foot had been crushed by a train.[6] After World War II, greater attention was paid to the treatment of limb deficiencies in children, and the Syme amputation became the preferred method when foot ablation was needed.

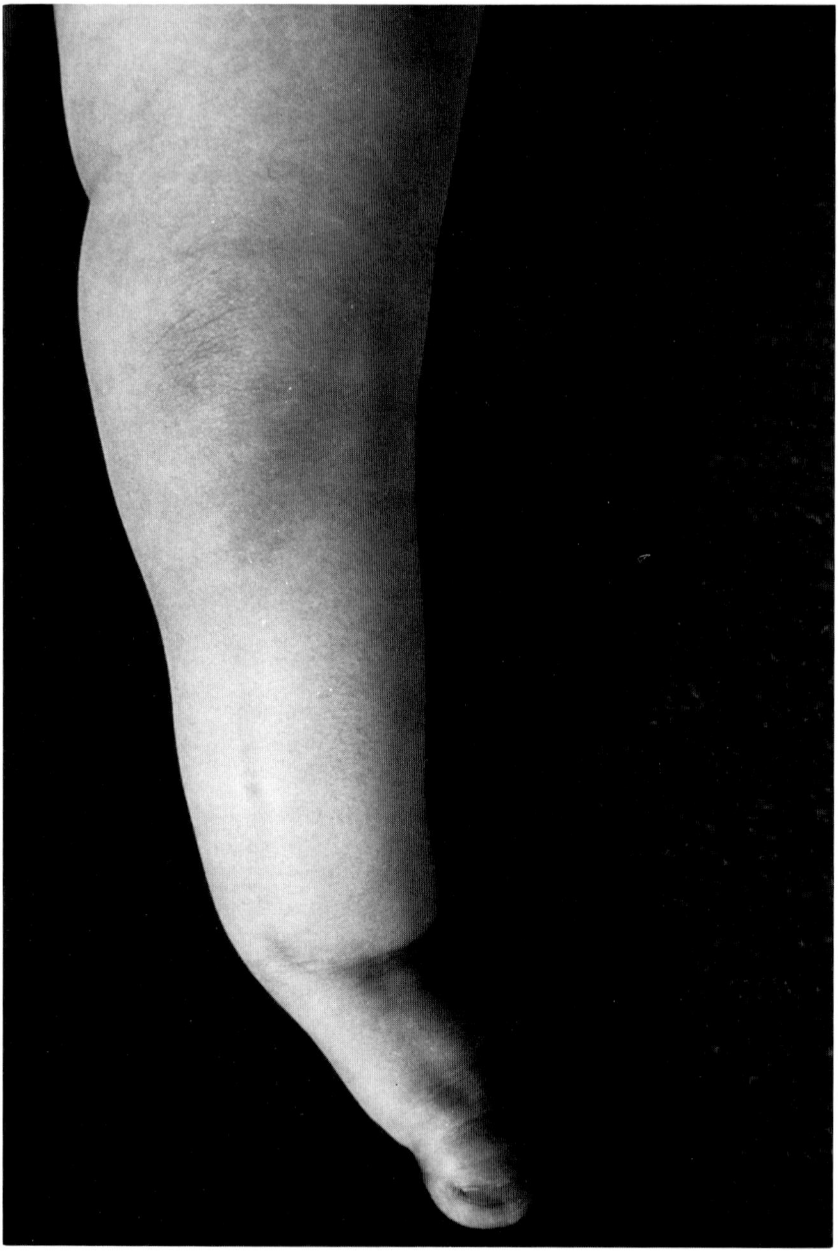

FIGURE 10.1. A single-digit foot in a markedly shortened lower extremity. Normal shoes could not be worn, and a Syme amputation was performed.

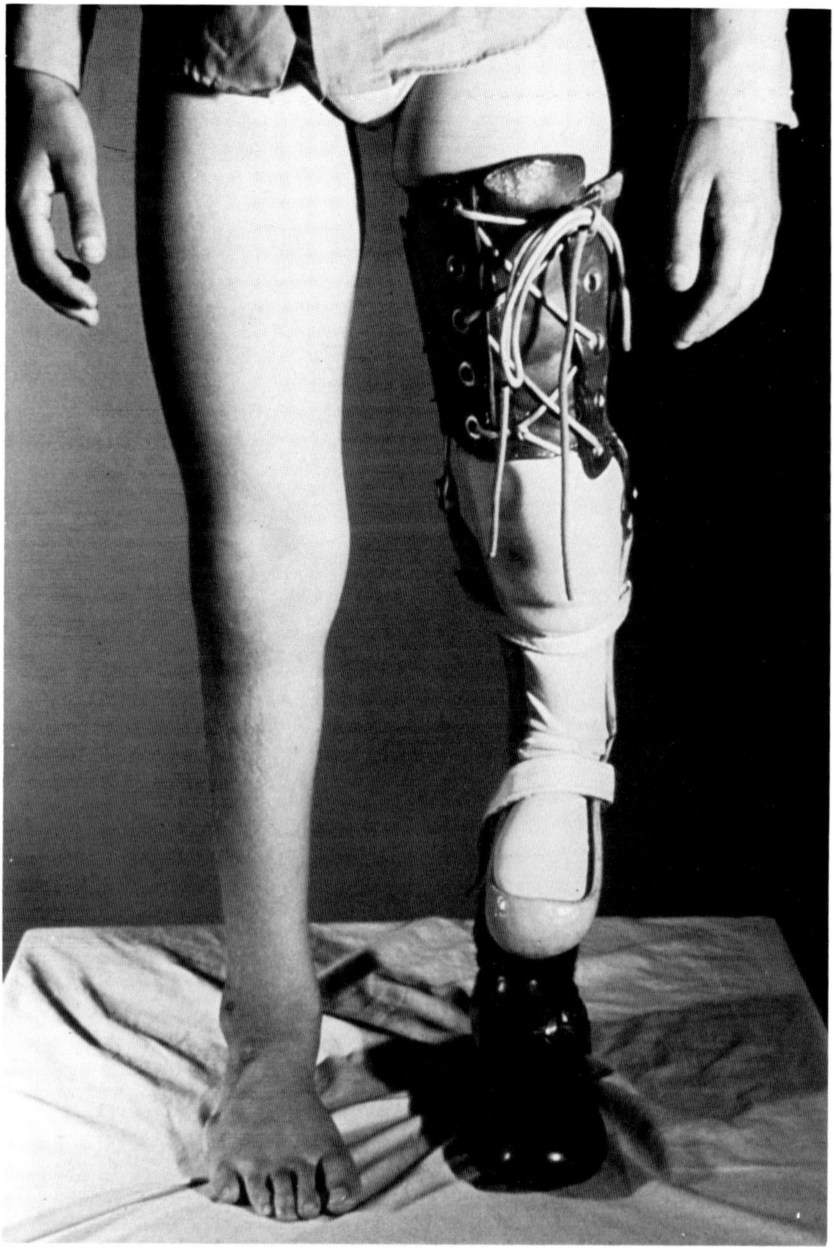

FIGURE 10.2. Patient with an absent fibula and a shortened lower extremity. Since the foot was left intact, an unappealing prosthetic extension had to be fitted to the lower extremity. The patient subsequently underwent Boyd-type amputation as a salvage procedure.

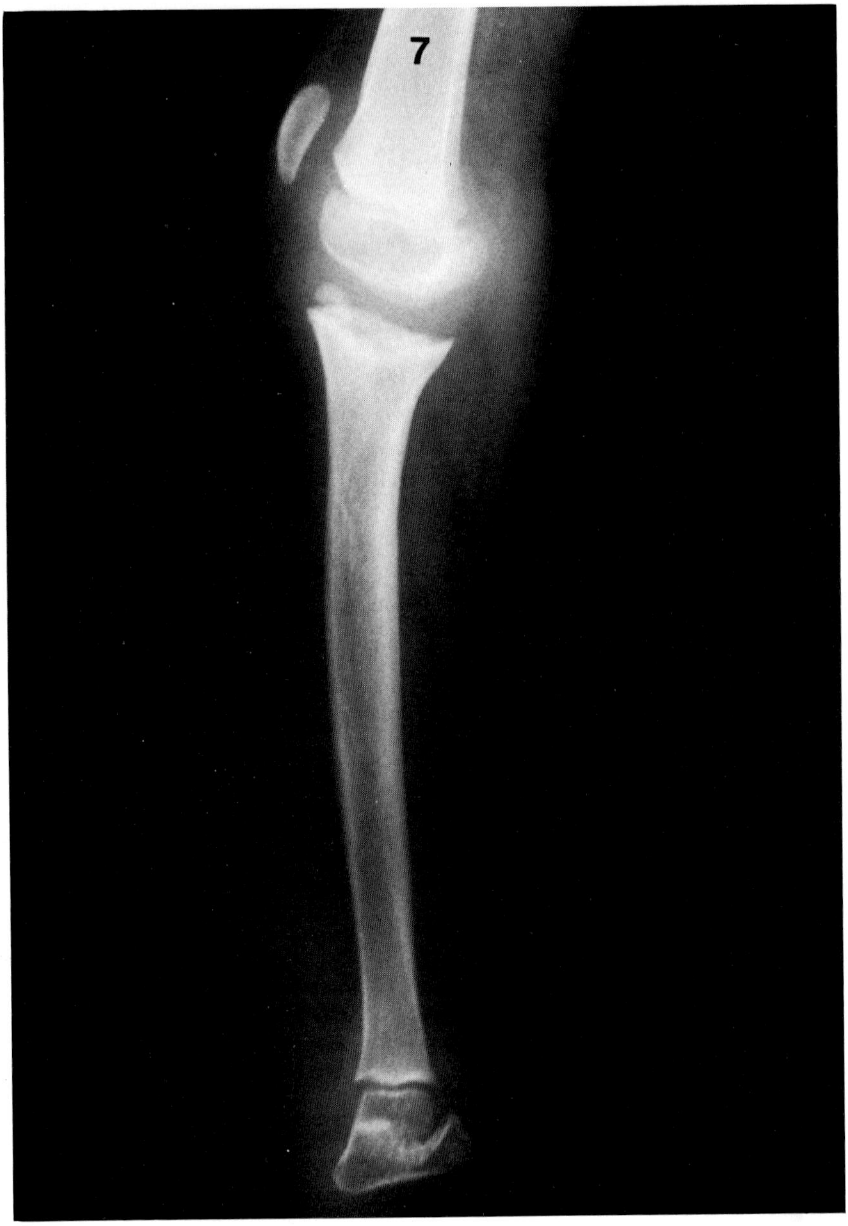

FIGURE 10.3. Radiograph of a 7-year-old child, demonstrating an open growth plate at the distal tibia 6 years following a Boyd amputation.

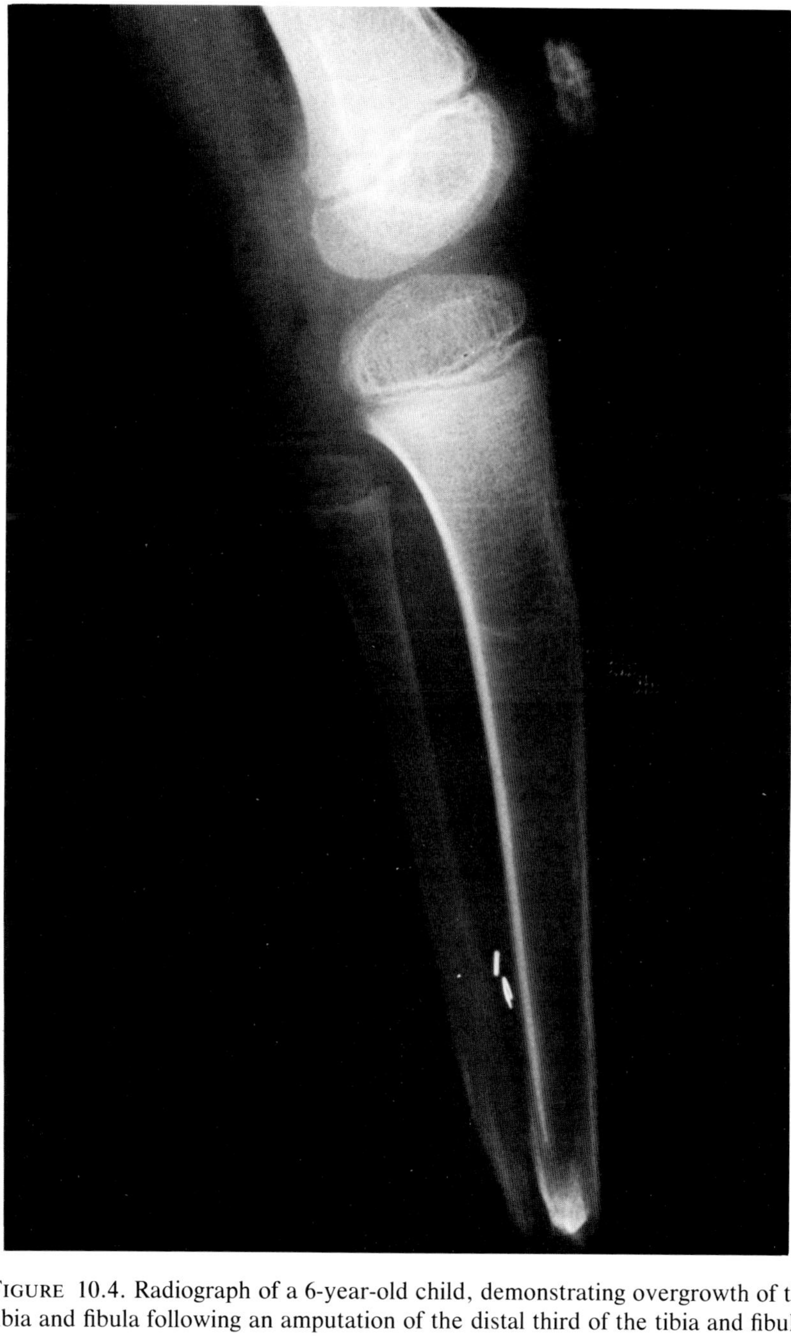

FIGURE 10.4. Radiograph of a 6-year-old child, demonstrating overgrowth of the tibia and fibula following an amputation of the distal third of the tibia and fibula.

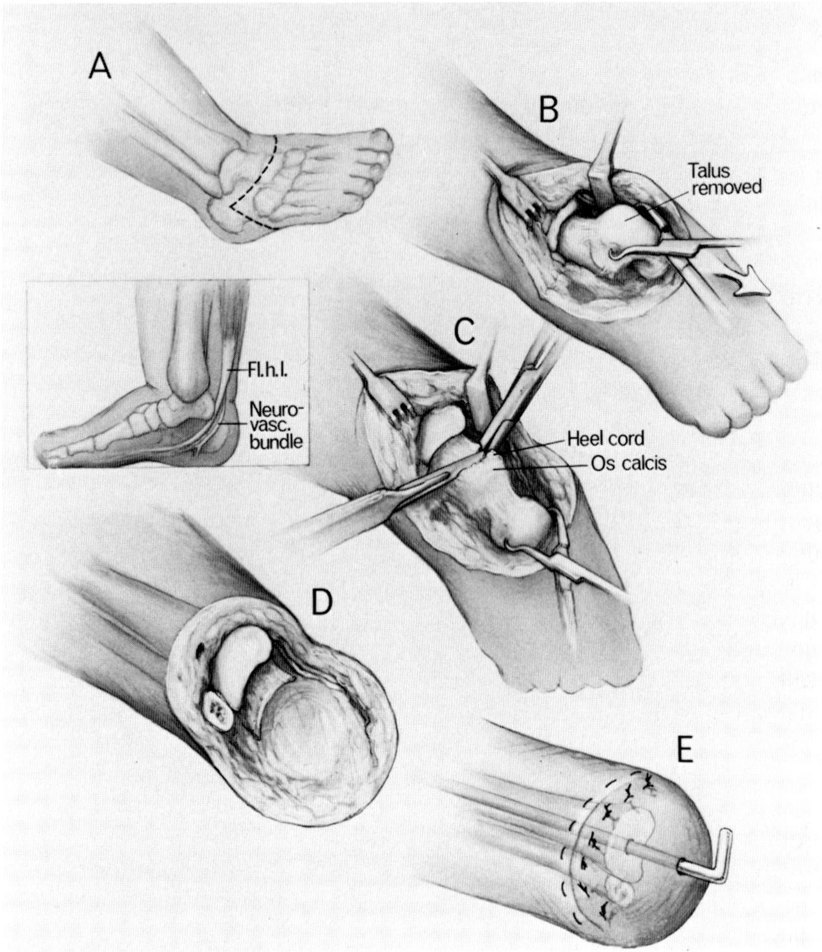

FIGURE 10.5. **A:** Technique of Syme amputation. This is performed through a fishmouth skin incision. **B:** The foot is plantar flexed and the talus is removed. **C:** With the foot plantar flexed, the heel cord is sectioned and the os calcis is dissected subperiosteally. Care should be taken not to violate the fat pad of the heel during this procedure. **D:** The plantar flap is shown with an intact fat pad. **E:** The skin is closed. If there is a problem maintaining the position of the skin, a Steinmann pin may be used to stabilize it. A Penrose drain (not shown) should be used to drain the wound. Inset shows the position of the flexor hallucis longus and the neurovascular bundle.

There are only a few reports about the Boyd amputation prior to 1964. Newton McCollough and his group reported favorable results from this procedure in three cases.[13] In 1976, Eilert and Jayakumar compared the results of the Boyd amputation with those of the Syme amputation in children at the Alfred I. duPont Institute and concluded that the Boyd amputation provided a surer method of obtaining an intact plantigrade heel pad.[8]

Indications for the Boyd and Syme Amputations

The indication for either amputation is severe shortening of the lower extremity not amenable to the standard equalizing procedures, or severe deformity of the foot. Since Heinz Wagner described a method of leg lengthening with fewer problems, and Colin Moseley devised a chart that could predict the discrepancy at maturity with a reasonable degree of accuracy, the indications for amputation on the basis of limb inequality alone have declined.[14,16]

Although both the Syme and Boyd amputations can be done at any age, the ideal time to do these in the limb-deficient child is between 12 and 18 months of age. This would enable the child to use the prosthesis to start walking and follow the normal milestones of development. At this age, adaptation to the prosthesis is very rapid and psychological acceptance is optimum.

Technique of Syme Amputation

The technique of Syme amputation is similar to that described by Alldredge and Harris, and later modified by Wood and coworkers (Fig. 10.5).[3,4,9,10,12,18] Under tourniquet control, a fishmouth incision is used with the apices at the level of the lateral malleolus and slightly distal to the medial malleolus. To avoid tension on the skin following the amputation, generous skin flaps should be created, especially on the plantar aspect. The dissection proceeds from the dorsal surface toward the plantar surface. Division of the deltoid and fibular collateral ligaments facilitates plantar flexion of the foot and isolation of the talus. While dissecting on the medial side, the flexor hallucis longus tendon is retracted along with the neurovascular bundle. This will prevent injury to the neurovascular bundle. The foot is plantar flexed and the talus is removed. The Achilles tendon is completely sectioned, and care should be taken not to injure the overlying skin. The os calcis is then removed by careful subperiosteal dissection to avoid rupturing the partitions of fat in the heel pad. This is the most critical part of the procedure, and, as Harris has emphasized, the hydraulic cushioning of the heel pad should be preserved (Fig. 10.6). The

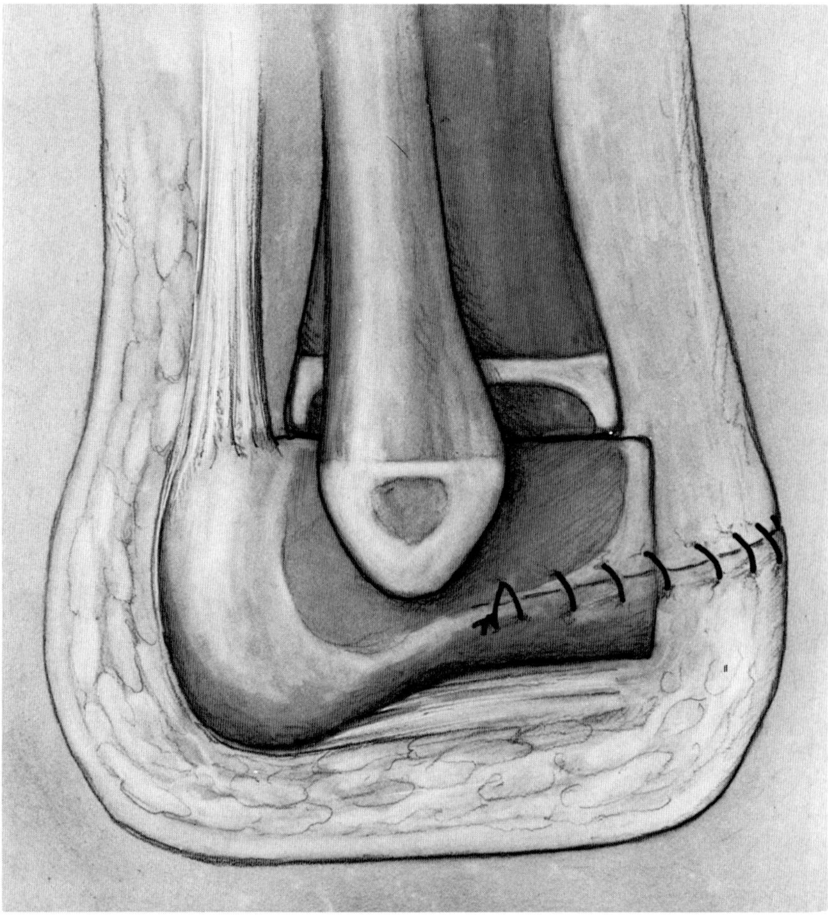

FIGURE 10.6. Lateral view of the Boyd stump, illustrating the fat pad under the heel, which should not be violated while performing either the Syme or Boyd amputation.

cartilaginous calcaneal apophysis is also left intact with the volar flap. If the malleoli are prominent, they are cut flush with the tibia. The heel pad is drawn squarely beneath the end of the tibia and held there with skin tapes or bandages. If there is difficulty in maintaining the heel pad in its proper position, a smooth Steinmann pin is used to fix the heel pad to the tibia. This pin passes from the plantar aspect into the medullary canal of the tibia. The wound is closed over a Penrose drain, which is removed after 48 hours. In young children, a hip spica cast is applied over the dressings. A long-leg cast will suffice in older patients. If a pin has been used to stabilize the flap, it is removed at the end of 6 weeks. A new cast is worn for an additional six weeks and ambulation is encouraged in this cast. At the end of this period, the stump will be ready for prosthetic fitting (Fig. 10.7).

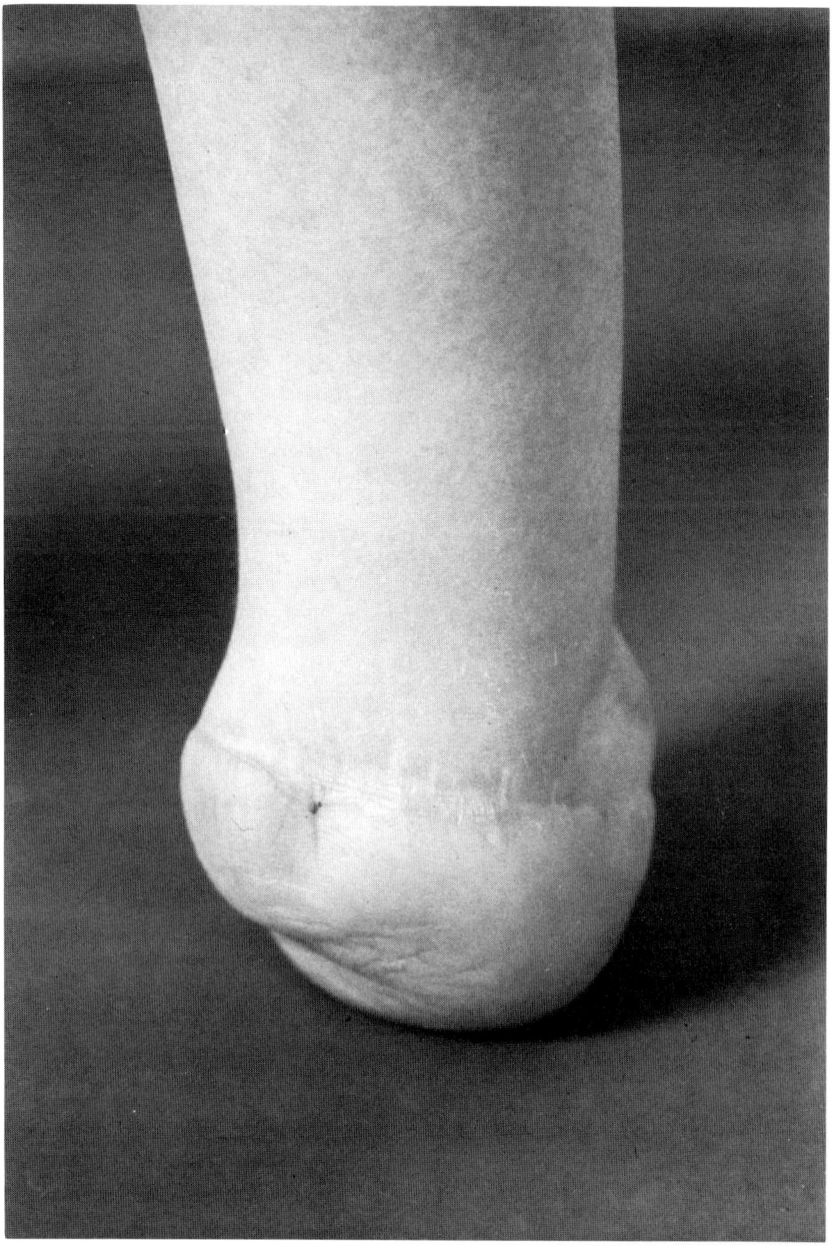

FIGURE 10.7. An end-bearing Syme stump.

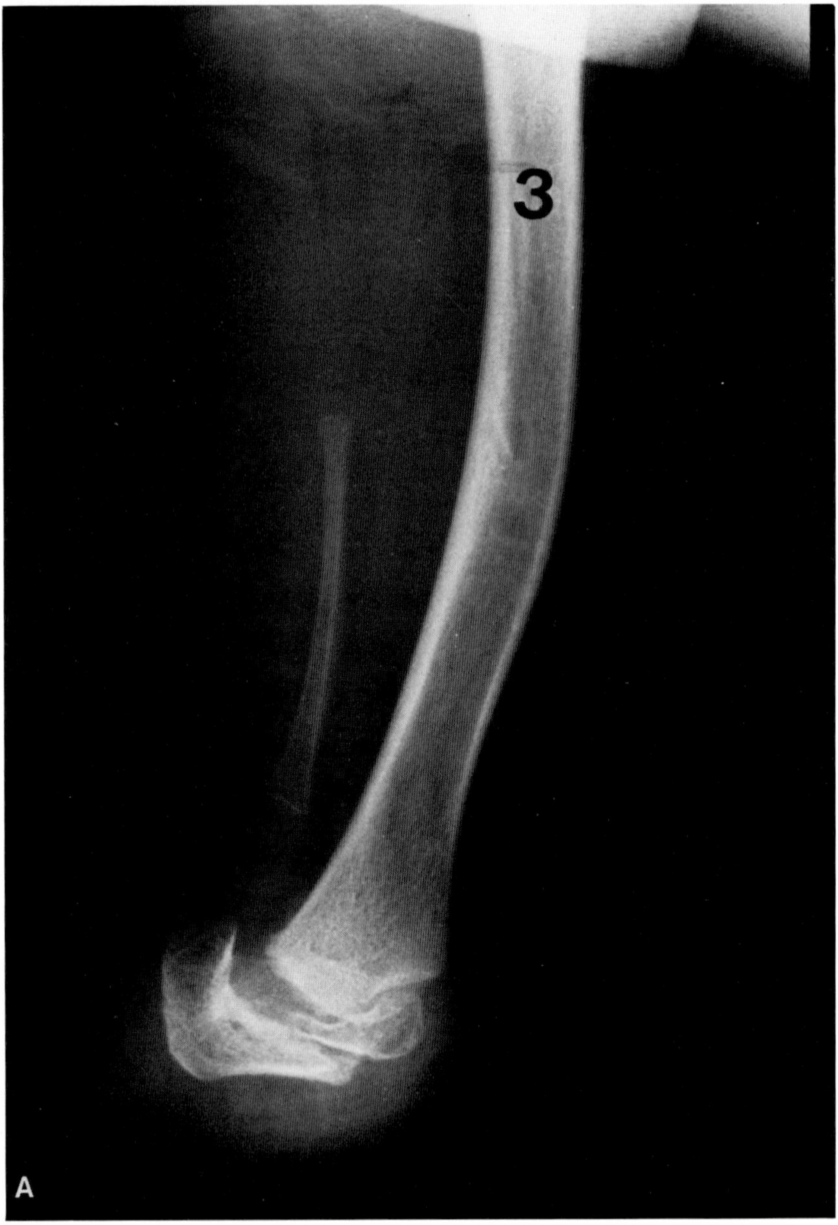

FIGURE 10.8. **A–B:** Radiographs of a patient who had a Syme amputation. A big sliver of the os calcis was left in place, along with the apophysis, and, in time, the os calcis regenerated to resemble a normal os calcis.

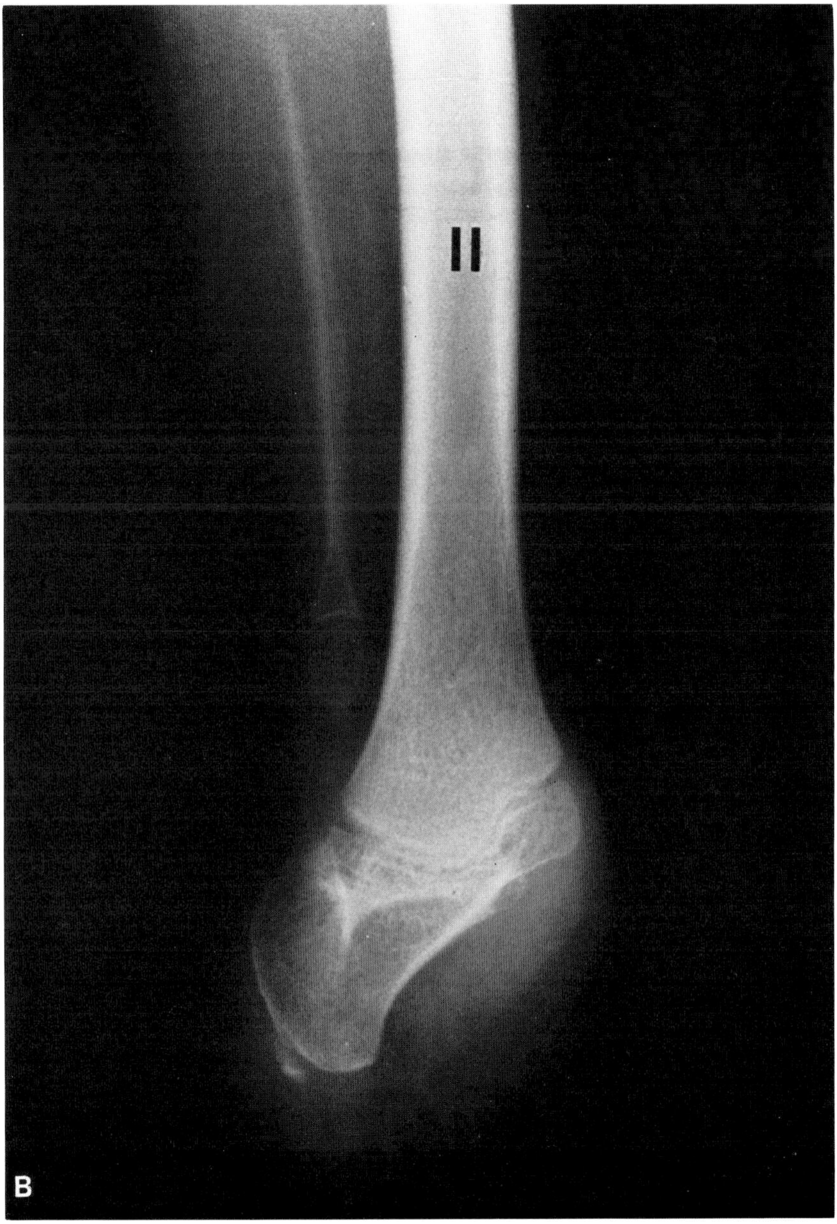

FIGURE 10.8. *Continued*

Retention of the calcaneal apophysis has not caused any problems in our series of patients. The os calcis regenerates with time, and in two of our patients it looked like a normal os calcis. Thus, a Syme stump eventually might be converted to a Boyd stump (Fig. 10.8).

Technique of Boyd Amputation

Refinements of the technique of the Boyd procedure were described by Blum and Kalamchi.[5] The technique is illustrated in Figure 10.9.

Under tourniquet control, a fishmouth incision is used, similar to the Syme procedure. The dissection should be carried directly to bone with no undermining. The dissection progresses from the dorsal surface toward the plantar surface. First, the talus is excised very carefully. Care should be taken not to injure the neurovascular bundle on the posteromedial aspect. The foot is then amputated. The articular cartilage lining the distal tibia is removed, so the underlying cancellous bone is visible. Care must be taken not to injure the growth plate during this procedure. The anterior portion of the os calcis is osteotomized just distal to the peroneal tubercle. The articular cartilage from the superior surface of the os calcis is resected so as to form a flat surface which fits congruously under the inferior surface of the tibia. If this fit is properly done, the os calcis will not be in calcaneus or equinus. The os calcis should also be shifted forward to sit squarely under the tibia. If the heel cord is tight, it is sectioned by reaching posteriorly through the space left by the enucleation of the talus. One of the critical parts of the procedure is preparing the distal tibia, especially in very young children. Sufficient cartilage should be removed to expose the cancellous nucleus. This is best achieved by serially slicing the cartilage with a sharp scalpel. When the fit of the os calcis on the distal tibia is satisfactory, a smooth Steinmann pin is inserted percutaneously into the os calcis across the fusion site and into the medullary canal of the tibia. Radiographs are taken in the anteroposterior and lateral projections to assess the alignment. The skin is closed loosely over a drain. The postoperative management is similar to that of the Syme amputation. Depending on the stability of the calcaneotibial fusion, the stump will usually be ready for prosthetic fitting 2 to 3 months following surgery (Fig. 10.10).

Once again, it is stressed that the os calcis should fit at right angles to the tibia, with no equinus. In patients where the os calcis is displaced posteriorly and is in marked equinus, proper alignment of the heel pad may not be possible and a Syme procedure may be preferred.

In both the Syme and Boyd amputations, the distal tibial growth plate is not violated; hence, the growth of the tibia is preserved. Unlike the adult patient with Syme amputations, the end of the stump is not bulbous, because in the limb-deficient child either the tibia or fibula is absent. However, even if both bones are present, the malleoli are usually

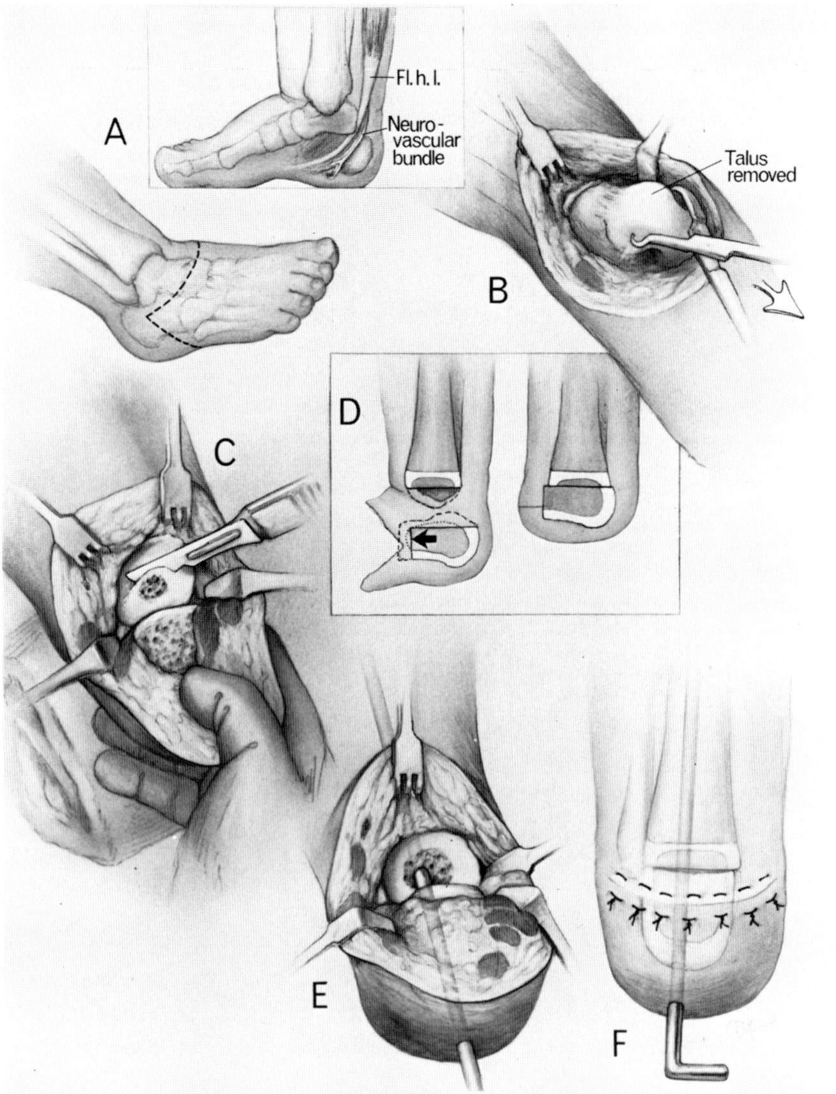

FIGURE 10.9. **A:** Technique of Boyd amputation. This is also performed through a fishmouth incision. **B:** The foot is plantar flexed and the talus is removed. **C:** Using a sharp knife, a thin sliver of cartilage is removed from the distal end of the tibia until the cancellous nucleus is visible. Care should be taken not to violate the growth plate. **D:** Bone is removed from the superior and anterior aspects of the os calcis to form a perfect fit. **E:** The os calcis is translated anteriorly and fitted under the inferior surface of the tibia and is stabilized with a smooth Steinmann pin. **F:** The wound is closed loosely, with a Penrose drain (not shown) in place.

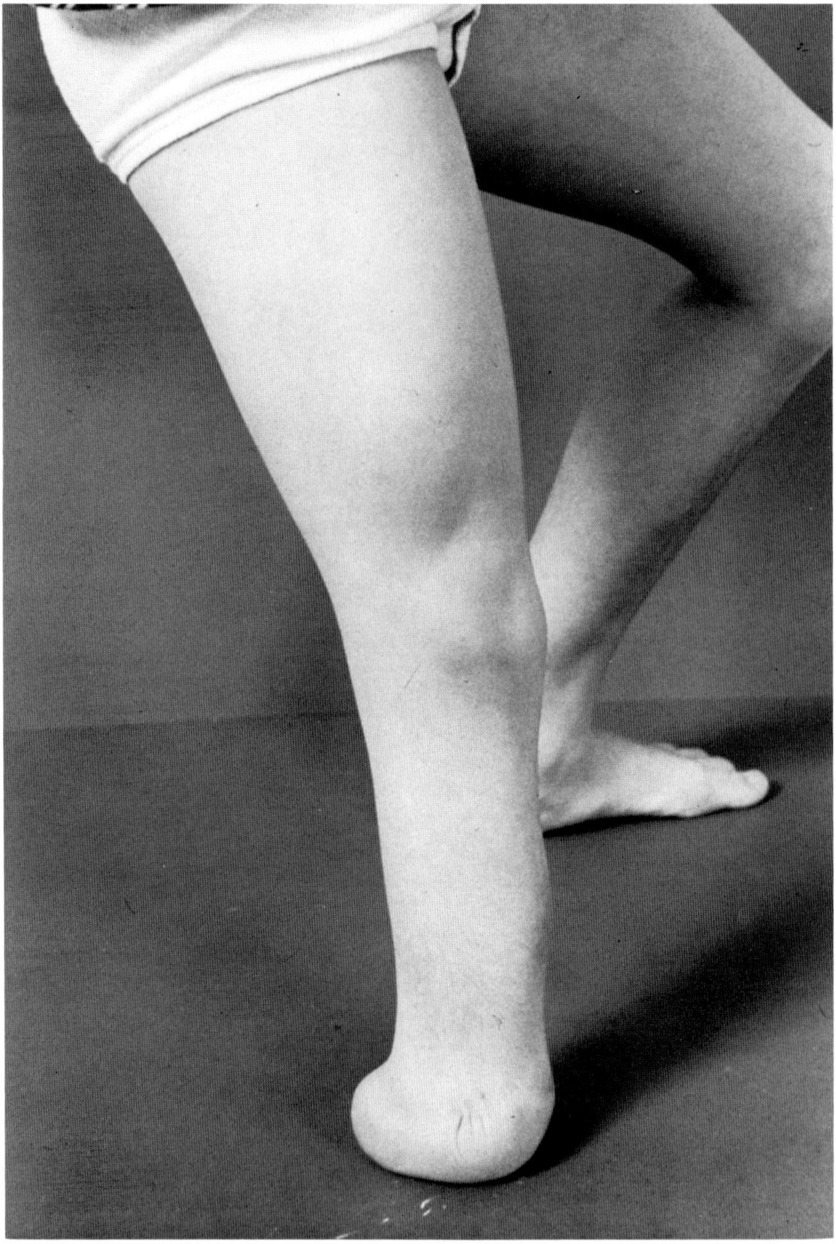

FIGURE 10.10. A functional weight-bearing Boyd stump is illustrated.

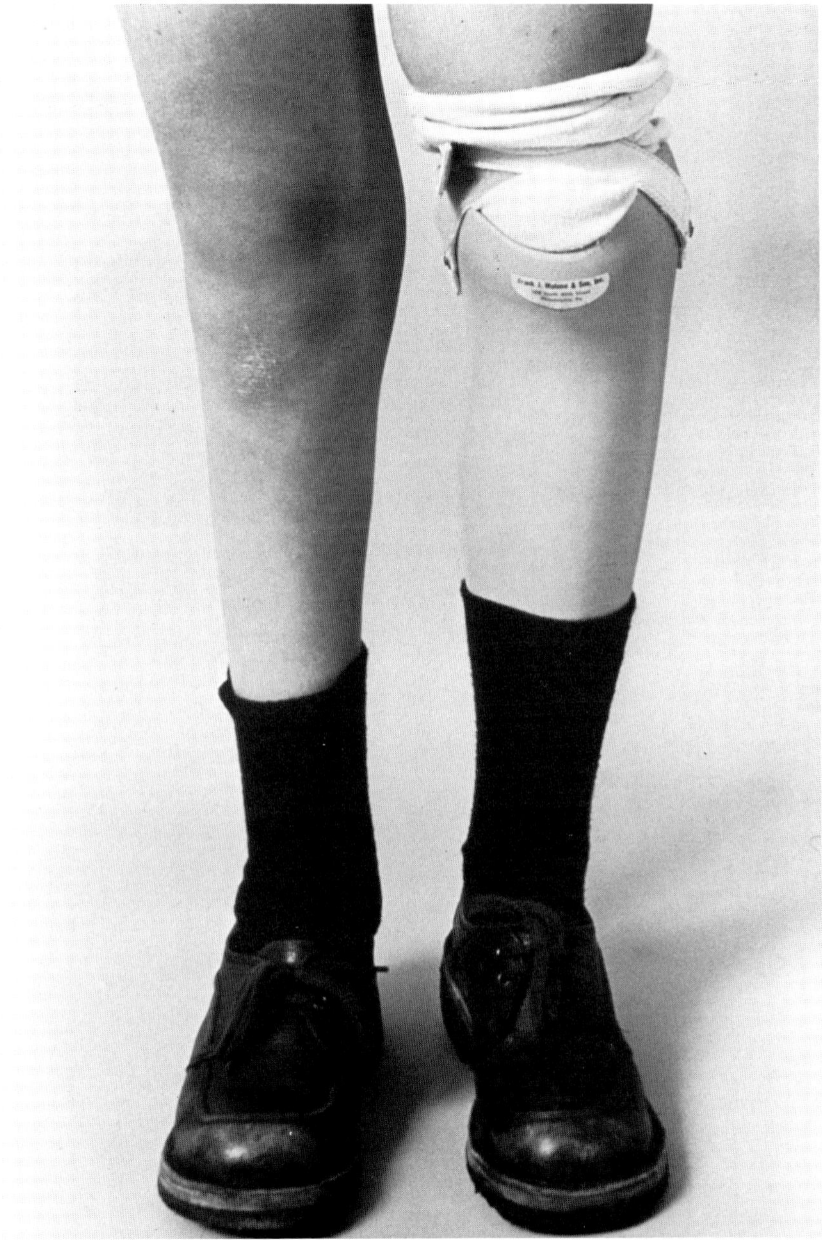

FIGURE 10.11. A 10-year-old boy with a Boyd amputation wearing a below-knee prosthesis with a supracondylar T-strap, showing an excellent cosmetic result.

hypoplastic and the stump is non-bulbous; hence, the prosthesis is cosmetically acceptable. Small children are initially fitted with a standard below-knee prosthesis with a thigh corset, which helps in suspension. At about 8 to 10 years of age, this is changed to a below-knee prosthesis with a sash foot and only a supracondylar "T" strap (Fig. 10.11).

At our institution, we prefer the Boyd procedure to that of Syme because of the ease of aligning the heel flap with the tibia and the extra length that it provides the stump. In the occasional case where the os calcis is in equinus, proper alignment of the heel flap may not be possible and the Syme amputation should be performed.

References

1. Achterman CA, Kalamchi A: Congenital deficiency of the fibula. J Bone Joint Surg 61-B:133–137, 1979.
2. Aitken GT: Amputation as a treatment for certain lower extremity congenital abnormalities. J Bone Joint Surg 41-A:1267–1285, 1959.
3. Alldredge RH, Thompson TC: The technique of Syme amputation. J Bone Joint Surg 28:415–426, 1946.
4. Anderson L, Westin GW, Oppenheim WL: Syme amputations in children: Indications, results and long-term follow-up. J Pediatr Orthop 4:550–554, 1984.
5. Blum CE, Kalamchi A: Boyd amputations in children. Clin Orthop 165:138–143, 1982.
6. Boyd HB: Amputation of the foot with calcaneotibial arthrodesis. J Bone Joint Surg 21:997–1000, 1939.
7. Davidson WH, Bohne WD: The Syme amputation in children. J Bone Joint Surg 57-A:905–909, 1975.
8. Eilert RE, Jayakumar SS: Boyd and Syme amputations in children. J Bone Joint Surg 58-A:1138–1141, 1976.
9. Harris RI: Syme amputation: the technical details essential for success. J Bone Joint Surg 38-B:614–634, 1956.
10. Harris RI: The history and development of Syme amputation. Artif Limbs 6:4–43, 1961.
11. Kruger LM, Talbot RD: Amputation and prosthesis as definitive treatment in congenital absence of the fibula. J Bone Joint Surg, 43-A:625–642, 1961.
12. Mazet R, Jr.: Syme's amputation: A follow-up study of fifty-one adults and thirty-two children. J Bone Joint Surg 50-A:1549–1563, 1968.
13. McCollough NC, Matthews JG, Traut A, Caldwell CP: Early opinions concerning the importance of bony fixation of the heel pad to the tibia in the juvenile amputee. NYU Interclin Inf Bull, 3:1–16, 1964.
14. Moseley CF: A straight-line graph for leg-length discrepancies. J Bone Joint Surg 59-A:174–179, 1977.
15. Syme J: Amputation at the ankle joint. London and Edinburgh, J Med Sci, 3:93–96, 1843.
16. Wagner H: Surgical lengthening or shortening of femur and tibia. Technique and indications. Prog Orthop Surg, Springer-Verlag, 1:71–96, 1977.

17. Westin GW, Sakai DN, and Wood WL: Congenital longitudinal deficiency of the fibula: Follow-up of treatment by Syme amputation. J Bone Joint Surg 58-A:492–496, 1976.
18. Wood WL, Zlotsky N, Westin GW: Congenital absence of the fibula. Treatment of Syme amputation—Indications and technique. J Bone Joint Surg 47-A:1159–1169, 1965.

11
Lower Limb Lengthening

J. RICHARD BOWEN AND IN HO CHOI

Introduction

Treatment of congenital lower-limb length discrepanices by lengthening procedures is complex, time-consuming, and has a high incidence of complications. To achieve satisfactory results in surgery, the surgeon must have a comprehensive understanding of the complexity of the deformity and the limitations of treatment modalities.

Most congenital lower-limb length discrepancies are obvious at birth, and parents are often extremely anxious to understand the eventual outcome of the disability. The idea of lengthening a congenitally short and deformed extremity may create feelings of enthusiasm in patients or their families that may lead to unrealistic expectations and anticipation of correction of the deformities. The extent of the deformity needs to be clearly defined very early in the treatment process so that realistic expectations can be developed.

A reasonable prognosis of the natural history of most congenital deformities can be made during infancy, and families need to be given information about the anticipated deformity, its cosmetic implications, and a general timetable for scheduled treatment modalities. If the family has adequate expectations and understands the nature of each treatment modality, the severe anxieties and frustrations that force many parents to seek numerous medical opinions and choose unorthodox treatment methods can be prevented. Many frustrated parents will desire several medical opinions, and when consultations are appropriately chosen, patient care generally can be enhanced. However, if treatment is fragmented among many physicians with different timetables and goals, results are likely to be unsatisfactory.

To be successful in lengthening a congenitally shortened extremity, it is essential to understand the principles of leg lengthening. Once these principles are understood, the various techniques of lengthening can be altered to meet the patient's specific needs. There appears to be no single technique that is best suited for each patient, and multiple techniques may be necessary to achieve satisfactory results.

The basic principles of mechanical lengthening of an extremity were first outlined by Codivilla in 1905.[14] These include osteotomizing the bone to be lengthened, distraction of the osteotomy site, and healing or osteosynthesis of the lengthened segment. The object of the lengthening is to achieve this phenomenon without inflicting permanent injury to the extremity or substantial risk to the patient. The biological capacity of the tissue to undergo such a process is paramount in selecting a patient to undergo a leg-lengthening procedure. These biological capacities include stability of the adjacent joints, adequate vascular supply to the extremity, pliable soft tissue that is capable of undergoing lengthening, and an extremity that would be acceptable both cosmetically and functionally once the lengthening has been achieved. Joint stability is an extremely important factor in lengthening procedures. When the femur is lengthened, considerable forces are applied to both the hip and the knee joint, whereas when the tibia is lengthened, the forces generally are applied to the knee and ankle joints. Most patients with congenital shortening of the extremities will have some joint deformity. If instability is present, subluxation or dislocation of a joint can result in a severe discrepancy. Specific areas of concern are dysplasia of the hip associated with coxa vara, anteroposterior instability of the knee, valgus deformity of the knee with lateral displacement of the patella, knee flexion contractures, and ankle instability or contractures. If the joint instability is associated with an angular deformity, a preoperative osteotomy may be necessary in order to align the joint better, resulting in a reduced chance of complications.

Adequate and pliable soft tissue about the lengthened area is exceedingly important because the nerves, vessels, tendons, and other soft tissue must obviously be stretched during the lengthening process. If these tissues are nonpliable, adequate lengthening cannot be achieved. Forced distraction of nonpliable tissue may result in exceedingly high transarticular forces that result in joint contractures or subluxation and dislocation of the articular surfaces. Although many patients may have adequate biological tissue for lengthening purposes, the overall cosmetic and functional aspects of the extremity may be inappropriate for lengthening. For example, if a patient has an adequate femur for lengthening but a deformed foot that will not be an acceptable weight-bearing structure, lengthening would achieve the desired equalization of the leg-length discrepancy, but would not result in an improved function. Therefore, in this instance, leg lengthening would be contraindicated.

Prediction of Limb-Length Discrepancy

Adequate prediction of the anticipated limb-length discrepancy at maturity is essential to formulate treatment plans and time schedules. In general, congenital deformities result in a relatively proportional discrepancy with growth.* The percentage of inhibition can be determined shortly after birth, and at maturity most congenital deformities will have a relatively similar percentage of deformity; however, the absolute leg-length discrepancy increases as the patient grows. Methods to predict relative adult leg-length discrepancy may be derived by extrapolating the percent inhibition from the anticipated adult leg length. Shortly after birth, the physician can inform the parents of the anticipated deformity by comparing the shortened extremity with the more normal extremity. For example, if the foot of the shorter extremity is at the midtibial area of the longer extremity, the foot will maintain a similar relationship to the more normal extremity and be at the midtibial area at maturity. This fact is extremely important when initially counseling the parents.

Documentation of growth of the patient, the extremity, and bone age is essential when developing precise predictive data. At the time of initial evaluation, shortly after birth, the physician needs to determine if the patient will be a suitable candidate for limb lengthening. This involves a thorough history, physical, and social evaluation with specific attention to deformities in the involved extremity; stability of the joints of the involved extremity; soft-tissue abnormalities such as contractures, paralysis, or weakness; and specific data related to leg lengths. These specific leg-length data include the overall length of both extremities, the length of the femurs and tibiae, the bone age, and the patient's height. It is useful to consider the average height of the family, although in specific terms, this is only informational in predicting the overall height of the patient. In the authors' experience, many patients with congenital shortening of an extremity tend to be relatively shorter than other normal family members.

Measurement of the patient's height generally has been determined by utilizing the longer extremity. At birth the patient is placed supine and the length is determined as the distance between the point of the tip of the crown of the head to the sole of the heel of the longer extremity. In ambulatory patients the height is measured with the patient standing on the longer leg.

Clinical Measurement

The length of the leg is measured clinically and radiographically. There are many clinical methods to measure limb length; however, there is considerable confusion regarding the significance of the measurements. Currently, there is no generally acceptable standard clinical method of measuring limb length, although the authors prefer measuring the distance between the points of the anterosuperior iliac spine and the distal aspect

---

* References 2, 5, 19, 32, 40, 50, 51, 56.

of the medial malleolus with a tape measure. There are obvious inaccuracies in this method, such as genu varus, genu valgus, and contractures of the hip and knee. The most important clinical measurement is the difference between the two extremities, and the authors prefer the wooden block method. The patient is asked to stand on wooden blocks of premeasured heights until the pelvis is level. The discrepancy between the extremities is the height of the wooden blocks. The functional and cosmetic appearance can be evaluated more thoroughly when the patient is examined by this method.

Radiographic Measurement

Radiographic determination of leg-length discrepancies is exceedingly important. In the past, multiple papers have been written demonstrating errors in radiographic measurements that involve magnification factors, false positioning of the patient, inadequate target-film distances, and difficult patient positioning specifically related to joint contractures. All these factors must be considered when evaluating the radiographic measurements of a patient's extremities. Currently, orthopedic radiographs utilizing a 6-ft target-to-film distance is becoming the accepted standard.[26] In this technique, a radiopaque calibrated ruler is placed beside the extremity to be measured, and exposures are made at the hip, knee, and ankle areas. It is important that the patient does not move between each of the exposures for considerable error can occur. Other methods used to accurately measure bone length are slit scanography,[23] computed tomography (CT) scanning,[30] and low-dose digital scanograms.[4]

There is confusion about which bony landmarks to select when determining the length of the extremity. The superior aspect of the femoral head, the distal aspect of the medial femoral condyle, and the midpoint of the distal tibia at the ankle commonly are selected. In certain congenital anomalies, these radiographic points cannot be determined or utilized adequately for they may give inappropriate information. For example, in proximal femoral focal deficiency, the femoral head may be entirely absent and the hip may be dislocated, resulting in a significant elevation of the femoral head; frequently, a substantial limb-length discrepancy exists in the foot that may be hypoplastic and not accounted for by these methods. When anatomical deformities occur that compromise orthoroentgenographic measurements, clinical correlation of the deformity is exceedingly significant.

Determination of the patient's skeletal maturity is important in predicting femoral and tibial length and subsequent extremity length. Classically, an anteroposterior (AP) radiograph of the left hand has been used to determine skeletal age by utilizing the Greulich and Pyle[27] or Tanner[52] systems. In patients with congenital anomalies, there may be marked skeletal maturation differences between the right and left extremities and between the upper and lower extremities. This may result in extreme difficulty in determining the individual's true skeletal maturation. Generally, hypoplastic extremities show a delay in skeletal maturation. The authors are unaware of any exact standard used to determine true skeletal maturation when marked anomalies of the upper extremity exist. Clinical correlation of maturity is often necessary, such as evaluation of secondary sexual characteristics and chronological age. However, all of these conditions may result in a degree of error when making predictions. In all of the standard techniques used in determining bone age, there is a relatively wide standard deviation that also increases the potential for error. The Gruelich and Pyle[27] atlas has been the most accepted documentation of skeletal age; however, more recently the Tanner[52] scale has been introduced.

Height and extremity length data should be obtained at intervals so that adequate information is available to determine growth patterns and to predict adult height. A radiograph of the entire involved extremity is useful at the time of the initial evaluation in determining associated anomalies such as progressive coxa vara or angulatory deformities. In older patients, orthoroentgenograms are useful in prediction of leg-length discrepancies. Orthoroentgenograms are advised at approximately 2-year intervals until the prepubertal period in which yearly radiographs may be helpful. In the authors' experience, large numbers of orthoroentgenograms taken in young patients generally have not been helpful in decision making. In general, orthoroentgenograms should be taken at decisive times in order to allow adequate predictive data, and yet not exposure the patient to excessive radiation or the expense of unnecessary radiography.

The most common methods used for predicting leg-length discrepancies are those of Green and Anderson[6,25] and Moseley.[47] The Green-Anderson remaining growth method allows the physician to predict the expected normal growth of the distal femoral or proximal tibial physis at various skeletal ages, sexes, and relative heights. To use this method, the percent of growth inhibition of the shorter extremity is determined by subtracting the amount of growth of the normal extremity, divided by the growth of the normal extremity and then multiplying by 100.

$$\frac{\text{Normal growth} - \text{involved growth}}{\text{Normal growth}} \times 100 = \text{percent of growth inhibition}$$

From a standardized chart developed by Green and Anderson,[6] the remaining growth of the normal leg can be determined. The future increase in discrepancy is derived by multiplying the percent inhibition by the anticipated remaining growth of the normal leg. Therefore, the predicted discrepancy at maturity can be calculated by adding the present discrepancy to the future increase in discrepancy.

A more recent method of predicting leg-length discrepancy has been developed by Moseley.[47] Using this method, the growth is expressed graphically and limb length at maturity is expressed by linear extrapolation of straight lines. The advantages of using this straight-line method are that there are no mathematical calculations and the growth patterns are expressed visually, thus making the measurements more easily appreciable.

Biological Considerations of Lengthening

The principles of leg lengthening were first described by Codivilla[14] in 1905 and are divided into three parts: (1) osteotomy of the bone to be lengthened; (2) distraction (traction and countertraction); and (3) osteosynthesis (bone healing). Since then, many modifications of leg-lengthening techniques have been developed that use various apparatuses and techniques to achieve these principles. Osteotomies have been described in the diaphysis, metaphysis, and physis. Many distraction apparatuses are available that allow adequate gauging of the speed of distraction, provide control of the extremity, and encourage activities to preserve the function of joints, muscles, and nerves. Osteosynthesis has been enhanced by various forms of internal fixation, bone-grafting techniques, and callus distraction. Codivilla[14] first described a leg-lengthening technique consisting of an osteotomy of the shortened bone and traction applied to the extremity by a nail through the os calcis. The patient was placed in a cast from the umbilical area to the ankle, and the cast was cut circumferentially around the bone to be lengthened. The distraction pin was incorporated into the distal aspect of the cast and traction was applied through the pin to the os calcis by a windlass. Alignment of the extremity was maintained by the cast, and the windlass was turned on a regular basis to offer distraction. After adequate lengthening had been obtained, the patient was kept in a cast until healing occurred.

In 1921, Putti[49] enhanced the technique of lengthening by placing pins proximally and distally to the osteotomy, allowing traction and countertraction directly on the bone, and further emphasized the fundamental fact that gradual and continuous traction must be applied to overcome the elastic resistance of soft tissues. This apparatus was called an osteoton; it consisted of two large metal pins that were applied to the proximal and distal fragments of the osteotomized bone and a telescoping tube containing a strong, spring-loaded screw that controlled the degree of distraction.

Abbott[1] developed a distraction apparatus in 1927 in which pins were placed proximally and distally to the osteotomized bone, and continuous distraction was achieved by spring-loaded telescoping tubes connected between the pins. The patient's extremity was maintained in a properly aligned position by incorporating the spring-loaded expandable tubes to a Thomas splint by a stabilizing frame. Barr and Ober[9] used four transfixing pins in the bone to be lengthened (two above and two below the osteotomy) and developed a distraction apparatus using springs similar to those used in the Abbott device. In 1952 Anderson[7] developed a more versatile lengthening apparatus by using the Abbott frame, double-fixation pins above and below the osteotomy, transfixing the bone being incorporated, and a screw distraction that had a controlled rate of $\frac{1}{8}$ in./d. This results in lengthening controlled by a rate of distraction rather than a rate of force as previously applied by the spring-loaded apparatuses. In 1951 Ilizarov[33] developed an external fixation device that uses multiple transfixation wires above and below the osteotomy site that attach externally to a ring frame that, in turn, allows controlled distraction in multiple planes and axial movement to enhance bone healing. In 1971 Wagner[53] described a lengthening apparatus with the double pins above and below the osteotomy that exit on one side of the extremity (cantilever effect) and connect to a square telescoping apparatus (monolateral).

The biological demands of lengthening have led to a plethora of distractors, techniques of distraction, and methods to stimulate healings; however, there is little scientific information available about the biological consequences of lengthening.

During lengthening, the soft tissues gradually are distracted. This involves stretching of all tissue planes with specific reference to muscle, nerve, vascular supply, and periosteum. Changes in various tissues have been outlined by Kawamura and associates,[41] who demonstrated minimal damage to soft tissues when no greater than 3% of the bone length is reached initially, when the lengthening of the extremity is limited to approximately 10% of the initial length of the bone, and when lengthening is carried out gradually in short increments. However, rapid distraction or excessive lengthening results in severe tissue disruption.

The biological response still needs significant research to determine the effects of changes in the rate of distraction (mm/day), the rhythm of distraction (the number of increments of distraction per day), and bone healing (months/cm).

The exact method in which the muscle-tendon unit is lengthened is unclear, but the vascular clips above the muscle-tendon unit show that the muscle and not the tendon elongates (personal work). Experimental work at the Alfred I. duPont Institute in rats suggests that slow distraction stimulates the muscle polar cells to divide and become incorporated into the myocyte. Radioactive uptake of the dividing cells during lengthening is seen throughout the length of the muscle but appears to be more abundant at the muscle-tendon position.[42] Muscle biopsies in patients undergoing lengthening show a perivascular infiltration of lymphocytes and plasma cells. Biopsies taken years after lengthening typically show a mild increase in perifascicular fibrosis.

Adenosine triphosphatase (ATPase) enzyme staining typically demonstrates a normal pattern; however, occasional areas of grouped fiber typing is observed. The grouped fiber types probably indicate neurological changes with denervation followed by regeneration. Clinically, the muscles of patients with congenital abnormalities are harder to lengthen.

During lengthening procedures, there is an increased force transmitted across adjacent joints. During femoral lengthening, the predominant deformity at the hip is a flexion contracture and adduction contracture. Generally, these are mild and can be treated simply by physical therapy. The most pronounced contractures during femoral lengthening are at the knee. Most frequently, flexion contractures of the knee occur secondary to tightness of the hamstring muscles and the iliotibial band. The flexion contractures must be treated by intensive physical therapy to maintain an acceptable range of motion, and use of a splint between therapy sessions has been helpful. Occasionally, a patient will develop an extension contracture of the knee during the lengthening process secondary to tightness of the quadriceps muscle. Generally, there is tightness of both the hamstring muscle group and the quadriceps muscle group, resulting in limitation of full flexion and extension of the knee. During the lengthening procedure, physical therapy should be used to maintain near-full extension and at least 70° to 90° of flexion. If this degree of motion cannot be maintained, then lengthening should be temporarily delayed until adequate motion has been obtained. Frequently, many patients with a congenitally short leg tend to have anteroposterior ligamentous instability of the knee and a mild genu valgum with hypoplasia of the lateral femoral condyle. Frequently, the intercondylar area appears flattened on radiographs, and the patella may be smaller and laterally displaced (Fig. 11.1). Specific attention should be directed toward prevention of posterior subluxation of the tibia on the femur (Fig. 11.2) and lateral dislocation of the patella (Fig. 11.3) during lengthening.

Lengthening of the tibia has a greater tendency for a deformity to occur at the ankle than at the knee joint. With lengthening, tightness of the Achilles tendon may occur, resulting in an equinus deformity of the foot (Fig. 11.4). This should be treated aggressively by physical therapy, encouraging dorsiflexion and posterior splinting to maintain posture of the foot between therapy sessions. In many patients with congenital shortening of the tibia and fibula, ankle and foot deformities are frequent. Ball-and-socket ankle deformities and tarsal coalitions are also prevalent.

The exact mechanism by which nerves elongate has not been clearly demonstrated. Clinical experience has shown that gradual distraction at a rate of approximately 1 to 1.5 mm/d is clinically well tolerated until approximately 10% to 15% of the length of the original bone undergoing

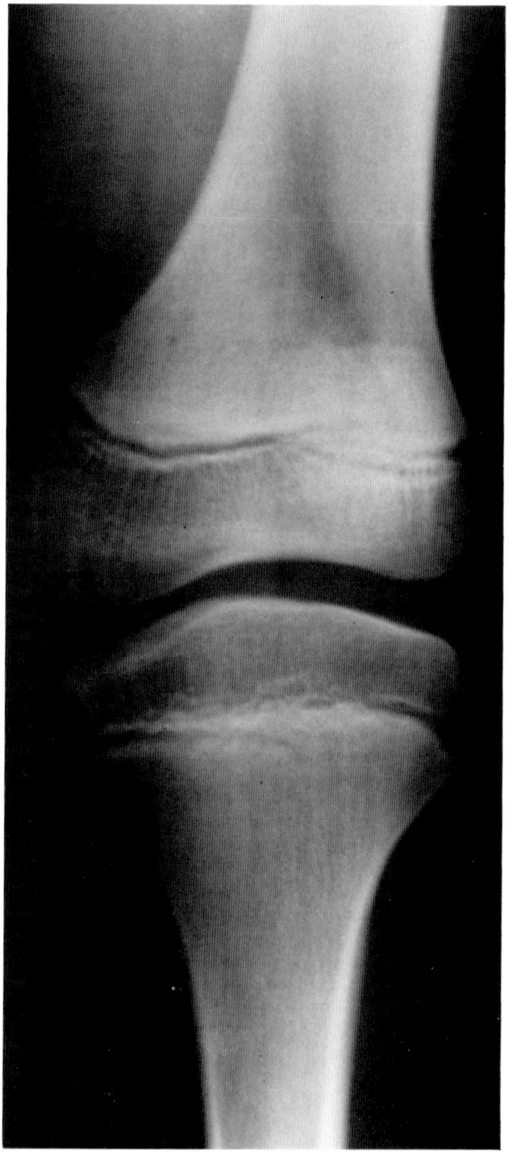

FIGURE 11.1. Hypoplastic lateral femoral condyle in a patient with congenital fibular hemimelia. Note the flattened intercondylar notch.

lengthening is reached.[41] The symptoms most reported during lengthening have been hyperesthesia or pain over a peripheral nerve distribution, most commonly the peroneal nerve. In a series of patients treated at the Alfred I. duPont Institute, these early sensory changes resolved when further distraction was delayed or tension relieved by a few millimeters. Clinically, the sensory changes precede any significant motor loss; however, an occasional muscle biopsy following lengthening has shown

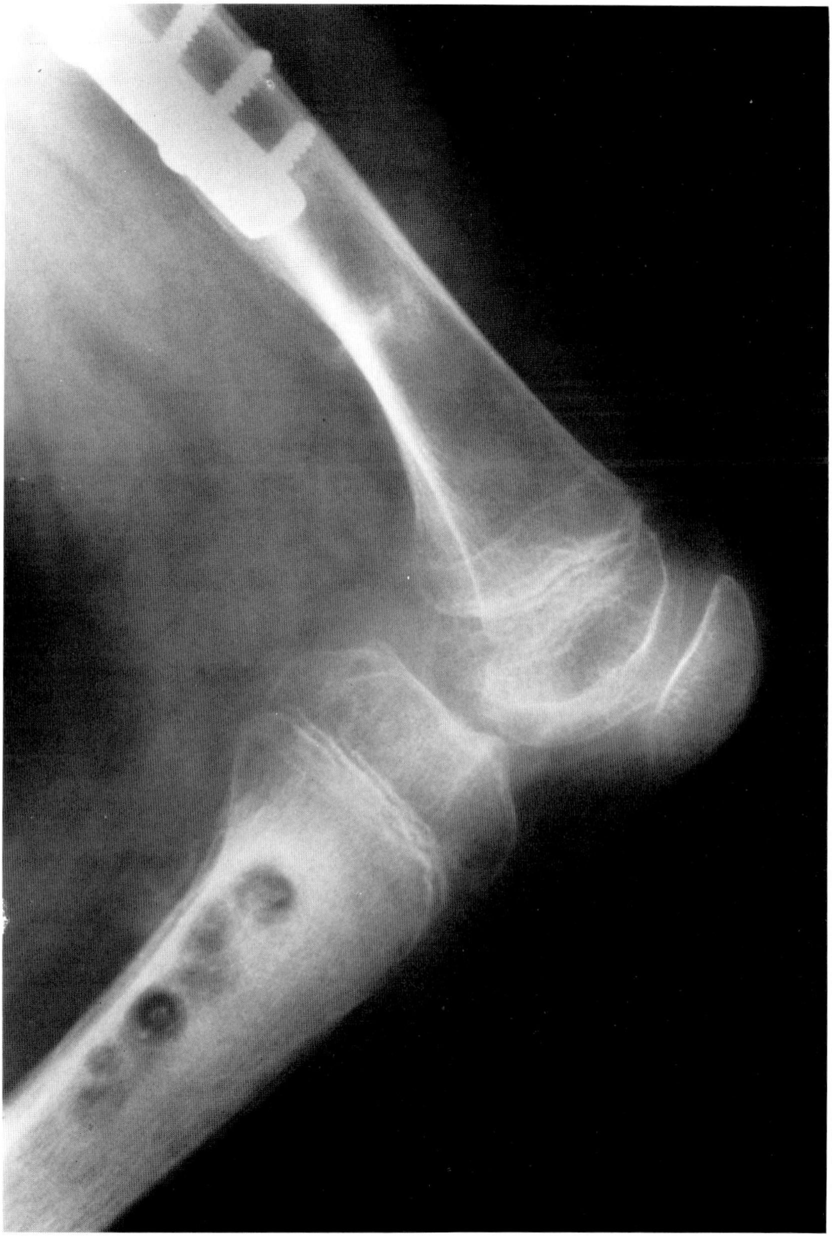

FIGURE 11.2. Posterior subluxation of the tibia on the femur occurred during Wagner lengthening of both femur and tibia.

fiber-type grouping changes characteristic of peripheral denervation and regeneration. Hypertension has occurred during the acute phase of lengthening, but the mechanism of the hypertension is unclear.[58,61] Hypertension appears to be more prevalent in femoral lengthenings than in tibial lengthenings. If hypertension occurs, a delay in distraction until the blood pressure returns to more normal values or a decrease in the tension of the distraction has resulted in a resolution of the problem. In the authors' experience, no patient has remained hypertensive after completion of the leg-lengthening procedure.

If contractures of specific muscle groups occur during lengthening, the lengthening of tendons frequently can facilitate reduction of contractures, although an intensive physical therapy program is necessary to maintain function. If at any time adequate joint motion is not achieved, the lengthening should be halted temporarily until adequate motion is regained by therapeutic means. When adequate motion is not maintained, severe contractures, stiffness, and joint subluxations may occur and are exceedingly difficult to treat. Once the lengthened bone has reached the desired lengthened distraction, osteosynthesis is necessary. Bony healing varies with the area and type of osteotomy and with the age of the patient. Typically, younger patients heal faster than older patients. By 6 to 8 years of age, patients are mature enough to tolerate the stress of lengthening. After 20 to 25 years of age, healing may be slow; however, this is only hypothetical.

Osteotomies may be performed in the diaphyseal area, the metaphyseal area, or by epiphyseal distraction. Diaphyseal osteotomies tend to heal at a slower rate than metaphyseal osteotomies or physeal distraction. After a diaphyseal transverse osteotomy and a distraction rate of 1.0 to 1.5 mm/d, a fibrous tube forms between the disrupted bone ends. This fibrous tube resembles periosteum, and with time, periosteal new bone and cartilage undergoing endochondral ossification are seen. The center

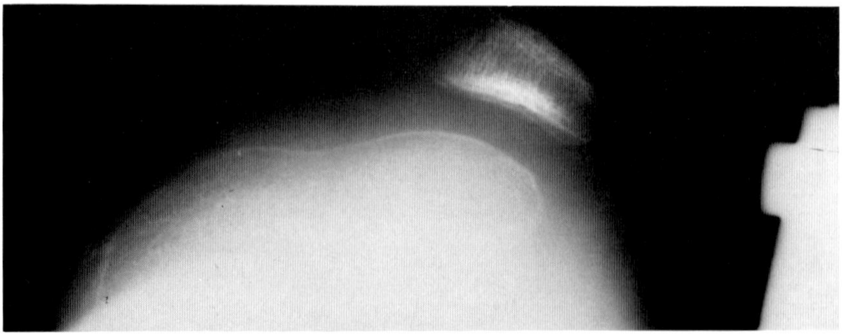

FIGURE 11.3. Lateral dislocation of the patella during femoral lengthening in a congenital short femur.

of the fibrous tube is filled with straw-colored serous fluid. The serous-filled cavity is gradually filled by fibrous tissue resembling periosteum, and eventually the new bone and cartilage undergo endochondral ossification. Subsequently, the bone remodels by almost 18 months, forming strong cortical bone with a medullary canal. Occasionally, this healing sequence is interrupted, and within the distraction area a nonunion may form or the bone in the distraction area may be insufficient to withstand the normal stresses of weight-bearing.

Many techniques have been described in performing the diaphyseal osteotomy to enhance healing, such as a long oblique osteotomy,[29] step-cut osteotomy,[3] transverse osteotomy with periosteal sleeve,[12,57] and osteotomy without incision of periosteum.[7] Because diaphyseal osteotomies with lengthening tend to heal slowly, internal fixation and grafting is frequently used to facilitate the speed of healing. If bone grafting and internal fixation are anticipated (as with the Wagner technique), the transverse osteotomy is advantageous, but if osteosynthesis is anticipated without grafting or internal fixation, then oblique osteotomy offers greater surface area and bony contact for union to occur. When performing diaphyseal osteotomies, the blood supply to the bone and periosteum should be preserved as much as possible. The periosteum should be incised minimally, and the authors prefer to drill the bone percutaneously through a single periosteal hole and use an osteotome to induce the osteotomy. A step-cut osteotomy is not preferred by the

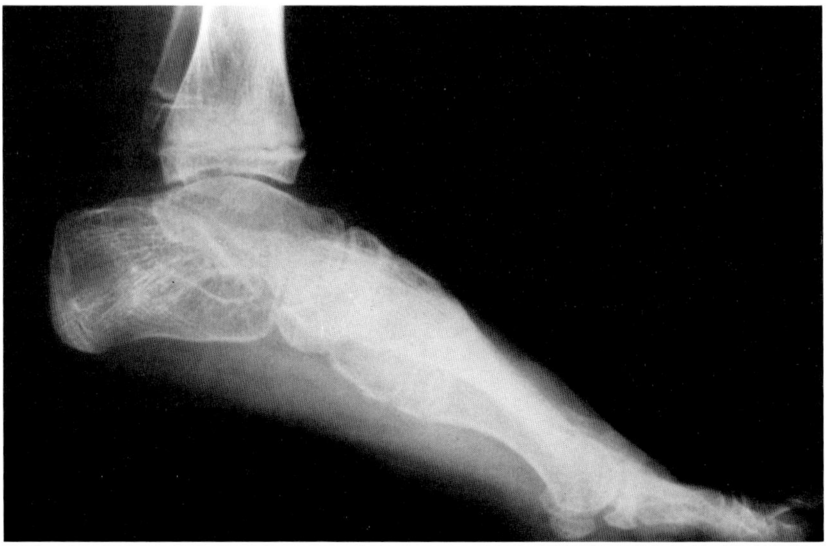

FIGURE 11.4. Severe equinus deformity can develop as a complication of tibial lengthening.

authors because a long periosteal incision is necessary, and bone necrosis in the step-cut segments may severely delay union. In patients with congenital shortened extremities, bone union is occasionally significantly delayed, and bone grafting as well as internal fixation is often necessary.

If the osteotomy is performed in the metaphyseal area, the distraction gap reossifies more rapidly than in the diaphyseal area. The metaphyseal osteotomies heal primarily by formation of cancellous bone if the rate of distraction is low (0.5 to 1.0 mm/d) and the rhythm is multiple times per day (2 to 4 times/d).

Preservation of the blood supply at the osteotomy site appears to be a major biological factor. In 1927 Abbott[1] suggested waiting 10 days after the osteotomy until revascularization and callus formation have begun before distraction. Ilizarov[33] developed a concept of a "corticotomy" in which the periosteum is preserved: the cortex is cut gently, and the medullary bone's vascularity is preserved. By lengthening at a slow rate (0.5 to 1.0 mm/d) in multiple, small increments per day, the blood supply of the medullary area is preserved. De Bastiani et al[21] combined the corticotomy and delayed callus formation before lengthening to further enhance healing and referred to this technique as "callus distraction or callotasis." Currently, the authors prefer (1) oblique subperiosteal osteotomy in the metaphysis performed by multiple drill holes and osteoclasis; (2) a delay in initial distraction of 10 days to 2 weeks to allow for callus formation; and (3) slow distraction to allow the callus formation to nearly match the distraction rate, such as 0.25 mm every 6 hours.

Physeal distraction was reported in patients by Monticelli and Spinelli[46] as "distraction epiphysiolysis." The growth plate is distracted gradually until the sudden rupture occurs, and distraction is continued until the desired length is achieved. The acute epiphysiolysis frequently results in a premature physeal arrest. De Pablos[22] demonstrated in sheep that the rate of distraction is an important factor in premature growth plate closure and that a 0.5 mm/d-distraction rate results in a healthy physis. Although technically possible, physeal distraction is currently limited in clinical use and should possibly be limited to patients who are near skeletal maturity. Physeal lengthening may be most appropriate in patients with asymmetric physeal growth disturbances near skeletal maturity. The bony bridge across the growth plate is osteotomized and the angulation is corrected during lengthening.

Fixators

Many distraction devices are available for achieving leg lengthening. Currently, internal devices—expanding plates or intramedullary rods—are not developed satisfactorily.[10,11,24,50,59,60] External distractors use two methods of bone fixation, either the cantilever-type fixator or the thin pin transfixator. In the cantilever types, large pins nearly 5 mm in diameter are placed into the bone and typically are secured to a monoaxial (monolateral) expandable fixator (e.g., Wagner and Orthofix techniques). In the transfixation types, a pin or wire is placed through the bone and extremity (e.g., Ilizarov and Anderson techniques) and connected to a multiaxial (multilateral, multilinear) distractor.

In the cantilever system, the stiffness of the pins serve as a cantilever and as a means to transmit distraction from a monolateral fixator to the bone; the threads in the screws allow for bone fixation. These monoaxial fixators are less bulky and adapt more easily to the anatomy of the femur, but have the disadvantage of concentrated stress at the base of the junction, which may cause osteolysis (Fig. 11.5) or subsequent infection. This is probably caused by a big difference of elasticity between bone tissue and pins. The monolateral fixators are strong in the plane of the pins but less stable in bending and torsion.[47] Generally, ambulation is poorly tolerated with monolateral fixators until callus fills the distraction area.

In contrast to this, the distractors that use transfixation rely on pins or wires that traverse the extremity. Tension on and the criss-cross positioning of the wires in the bone offer stability. The small wires have little skin

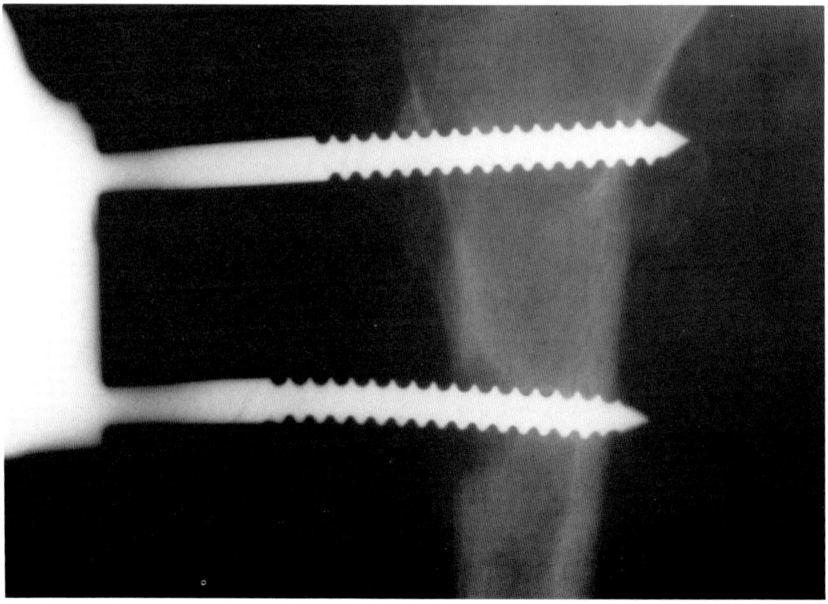

FIGURE 11.5. Osteolysis at the junction between the lateral femoral cortex and Shanz screw in a femoral lengthening using the Wagner device. This seems to be the result of the stress concentration at the base of the junction when a monolateral cantilever-type fixator is used.

or bone reaction. Ambulation is possible several days after osteotomy, resulting in cyclic axial compression of callus in the distraction area. This stimulates bone remodeling because the transfixation system permits axial microelastic movement, eliminating sliding or torsional movement. But these distractors are often bulky and circumferential around the extremity, and transfixator pins are poorly tolerated in the femur by the patient. The authors have used the Wagner method since 1977 and the Ilizarov technique in recent years for leg lengthening of congenital short limbs.

Technique of Diaphyseal Lengthening (Wagner Method)

One of the most common techniques of diaphyseal lengthening is that developed by Wagner.[16,17,31,53–55] This methods involves a transverse osteotomy of the diaphysis of the bone to be lengthened, subsequent distraction using paired Shanz pins above and below the osteotomy, and the Wagner external fixator for leg lengthening. Once the acquired distraction is achieved, a second operation is performed in which the lengthened bone is secured by a neutralization plate, the distraction gap is filled with bone graft, and the Wagner external fixator and the Shanz screws are removed. Some years later, after adequate bone healing has occurred, the neutralization plate is removed (Figs. 11.6).

The leg to be lengthened is prepared and draped, creating a sterile field from the iliac crest superiorly distal to the foot and medially to the peroneal area. An image intensifier is used to document adequately the bony landmarks. For femoral lengthening, paired Shanz pins are applied proximally and distally in the femur. Generally, the first pin is placed distally approximately 1 to 2 cm cephalad to the physeal growth plate. The area for the placement of this first pin is identified under the image intensifier, and 1 ml of 1% lidocaine with 1 : 100,000 epinephrine is injected subperiosteally using a 21-gauge spinal needle. This injection reduces postoperative periosteal pain and hematoma formation. A 3-mm skin incision is made laterally along the anterior aspect to the iliotibial band. A 3-mm periosteal elevator is inserted through the subcutaneous fat and vastus lateralis to the periosteum. The periosteum is elevated percutaneously anteriorly and posteriorly to allow adequate identification of the width of the femoral shaft. A 4.5mm drill hole is placed parallel to the articular surfaces of the femoral condyles 1 to 2 cm cephalad to the physeal growth plate. In order to aid in positioning of this drill hole, the drill bit is placed against the lateral margin of the femur and the contour of the bone is felt by raising and lowering the bit to the midaspect of the bone. Specific attention should be directed toward not placing the drill hole more posteriorly, and toward the fact that the distal femur is oval and the neurovascular structures must be protected. After the drill hole has been made, the bit is removed and a 5-mm Shanz screw is inserted. This screw should be inserted so that the tip penetrates the far cortex by approximately two or three threads.

The next Shanz pin is placed approximately at the level of the lesser trochanter. A 3-mm skin incision is made laterally over the leg at the level of the lesser trochanter. The periosteum is injected with 1 ml of 1% lidocaine with epinephrine 1 : 100,000 to minimize postoperative pain and hematoma formation. A 3-mm-wide periosteal elevator is inserted through the skin incision along the subcutaneous fat and vastus lateralis to the periosteum. The periosteum is elevated superiorly and inferiorly, and a 4.5-mm drill hole is placed laterally to medially at the midlateral line of the femur to the lesser trochanter.

Using an appropriate drill guide, the third and fourth pins are placed in the same fashion, thus resulting in paired pins proximally and distally. The distraction apparatus (Wagner apparatus, etc.) is secured to the Shanz pins. In the femur, the distraction apparatus is applied superiorly to the Shanz screws to allow better access to the posterolateral aspect of the leg, which will be necessary for subsequent application of the neutralization plate at the next stage of the operative procedure.

The diaphyseal osteotomy is performed midway between the paired Shanz pins. The osteotomy may be performed percutaneously when the anticipated lengthening will be less than 6 to 7 cm. In the case of more extensive lengthening procedures, open transection of the iliotibial tract and lateral intermuscular septum may be necessary. For the percutaneous osteotomy, a 3-mm incision is placed posterolaterally at the level of the lateral intramuscular septum. Using a 21-gauge spinal needle, 2 ml of lidocaine is injected subperiosteally. A 3-mm-wide periosteal elevator is inserted through the subcutaneous fat, vastus lateralis, and the periosteum is elevated anteriorly and posteriorly. A 4.5-mm drill bit is directed through a drill sleeve to the femoral shaft. The femoral shaft is multiply drilled percutaneously under the guidance of image intensification. The external fixator is then distracted approximately 0.5 cm, which places tension across the Shanz pins. A 3-mm osteotome is introduced through the 3-mm incision to the area of the drilled diaphysis. The osteotomy is then completed by using image intensification verification. The previously applied tension through the distraction device will cause separation of the osteotomy.

Next, a percutaneous iliotibial band lengthening is performed. A #15 scalpel is inserted through the distal pin incision, and the anterior half of the iliotibial tract is incised percutaneously. A scalpel of the same size is then inserted into the incision where the femur was osteotomized and the middle of the iliotibial tract transversed. The scalpel is inserted into the incision of the proximal Shanz pin, and the remainder of the iliotibial tract

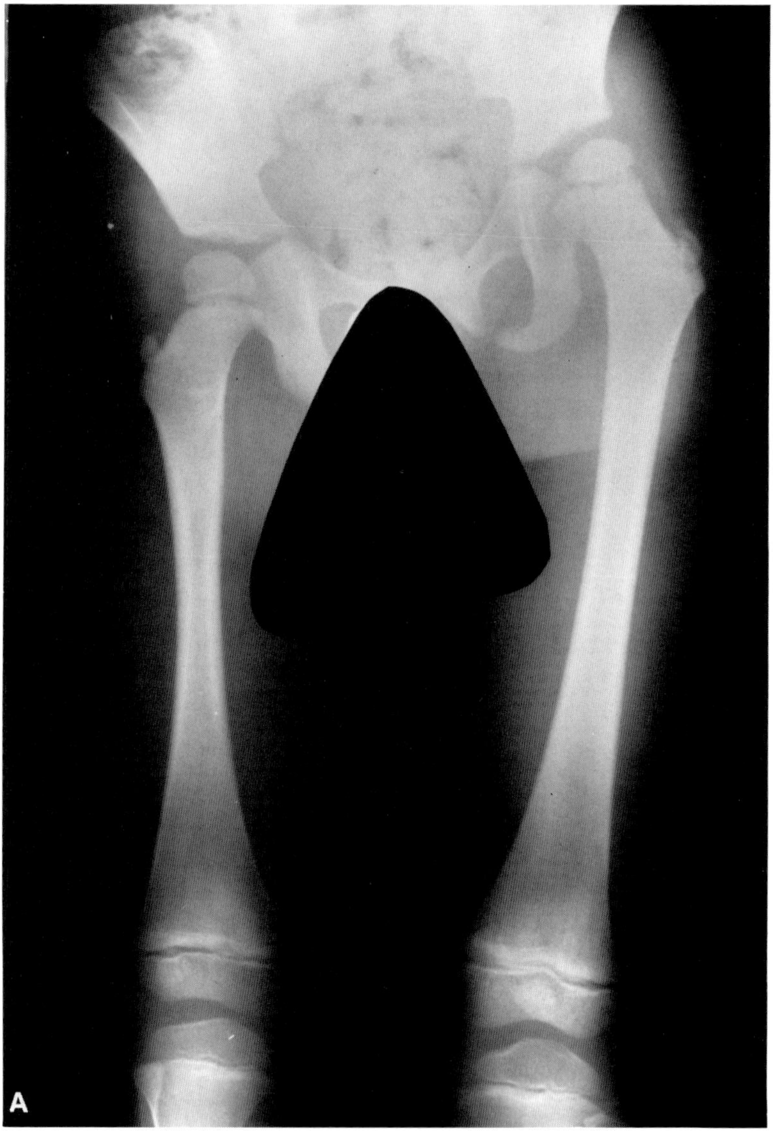

FIGURE 11.6. **A:** A 4-year-old boy with a congenital short femur on the right side. **B:** Sixty-nine days after diaphyseal osteotomy (Wagner stage I) of the femur, 8 cm of lengthening was obtained. An indistinct ossification shadow is seen in the distraction gap. Osteolysis at the bases of junction of lateral cortex and screws was noted. **C:** Bone remodeling is complete at 2.5 years after Wagner stage I. At this point, plate and screws were removed.

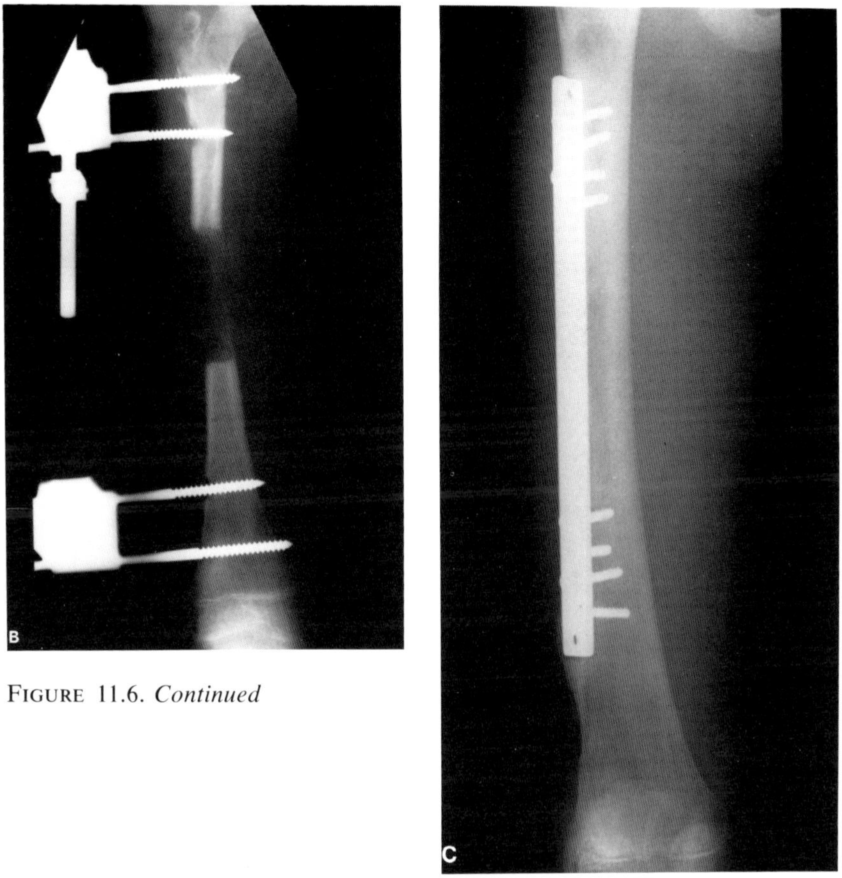

FIGURE 11.6. *Continued*

is incised percutaneously. During the percutaneous incision of the iliotibial tract, specific care should be taken to ensure that no neurovascular structure is incised inadvertently. The incision for the osteotomy then is closed with adhesive tape, and antibiotic ointment salve is applied about each of the pins. The bone then may be lengthened from 1.5 to 2.5 cm. Currently, we prefer gradual distraction for callotasis rather than initial traction. If a spinal evoked potential reading is readily available, the distraction may be performed while the patient is anesthetized; if it is not available, the distraction may be performed while the patient is partially awakening from anesthesia. In this circumstance, the patient should dorsiflex and plantarflex the foot as the distraction occurs to ensure neurovascular stability. The previously injected lidocaine in the periosteum offers some pain relief during the distraction process.

When the tibia and fibula are to be lengthened, the aforementioned procedure is modified. The Shanz pins are inserted anteromedially approximately 1 to 2 cm along the diaphyseal side of the physis. The distraction device is placed medially to the Shanz screws, which allows adequate space anterolaterally. The osteotomy of the tibia is performed through an anterolateral incision approximately 1.5 cm in length. The osteotomy of the fibula is performed posterolaterally superior to the lateral intermuscular septum through approximately a 2-cm incision. The cortex of the fibula is exposed and osteotomized. Two cortical transfixation screws (one proximal and one distal to the osteotomy) are inserted from the fibula to the tibia. The screws secure the fibula to the tibia to prevent subsequent distraction of the ankle joint or the proximal tibiofibular joint with subsequent distraction during lengthening. To place the transfixing screws from the fibula to the tibia, the bones are drilled from the fibula to the tibia 1 cm from the osteotomy superiorly and inferiorly. Selecting the appropriate length of the screw is achieved by observing the length along the shaft of the drill as the tip of the bit penetrates the medial cortex of the tibia. When the cortical screw is inserted from the fibula to the tibia, caution must be exercised in properly guiding the screw into the tibia because the posteromedial cortex is triangular, and frequently the screw tip will try to skirt posteriorly or anteriorly to the desired position. If the screw was to skirt posteriorly or anteriorly, the torque could fracture the fibula at the area of the screw. The screw from the fibula to the tibia should not be overtightened, thereby narrowing the interosseous space. The point of the screw should not protrude past the medial cortex of the tibia because this area is subcutaneous and may be painful.

Osteosynthesis and Bone Grafting

After lengthening has been achieved, osteosynthesis is performed. Radiographs are taken 2 weeks after the termination of lengthening to determine the need for bone grafting and osteosynthesis. If there is satisfactory callus formation in the lengthened area of the bone and this callus shows progressive thickening and organization, it is sometimes unnecessary to perform bone grafting and plate fixation. In this event, the patient is allowed to start partial and gradually full weight-bearing on the lengthened extremity as the bony callus gradually thickens and becomes organized. However, if the intervening callus in the lengthened area of the bone is deficient and narrow, especially if there is a tapering of the callus to a narrow segment in the central area of the lengthened portion, it is necessary to perform plate fixation and bone grafting.

At the time of surgery, adhesive drapes are used to exclude the distraction apparatus from the surgical field. This draping is necessary to prevent contamination of the operative site. The authors have found it useful to suture the surgical drapes in place along the border of the surgical site, using a continuous nonabsorbable suture.

The patient is placed on the operating table with the posterolateral aspect of the femur or the anterolateral aspect of the tibia exposed for surgery. Preoperative and postoperative antibiotic prophylaxes are used. The bone graft is taken from the posterior iliac crest prior to making the surgical incision over the osteosynthesis site. Using careful surgical technique, the site of the osteosynthesis is exposed with as little tissue damage as possible. The fibrous tissue that lies between the bone ends is incised longitudinally. This tissue sometimes has the appearance of an elongated tubular structure occasionally containing serous fluid in the central portion. The medullary cavity of the proximal and distal ends of the bone also is exposed carefully. Minimal tissue excision is performed. An appropriate osteosynthesis neutralization plate is applied to the fragments after the plate has been contoured, if necessary, by the use of bending irons or a press. It is important that the screws at the ends of the plate do not overlap or abut against the Shanz distraction screws in order to reduce the risk of bacterial contamination from the preexisting Shanz screw pin tracts. The screws at the ends of the plate are inserted first, anchoring them firmly to cortical bone on both cortices. The more central screws then are inserted sequentially. After the plate has been affixed firmly to the bone, copious amounts of cancellous and corticocancellous bone graft material are placed circumferentially around the central elongated or lengthened area. Closure is affected in layers and dry dressings are applied.

The distraction apparatus, which should be kept in place until after the plating is complete, is now removed. The patient is not allowed to ambulate until satisfactory bone formation is seen. Removal of the neutralization plate is performed once adequate osteosynthesis has occurred; this may take several years.

Care of Pin Sites

After application of the external distraction apparatus, the screw tracts are protected by antibiotic ointment and dry sterile bandages during the first few days. Later the entry sites are cleaned every 2 or 3 days with dilute hydrogen peroxide or other noniodine-containing antiseptic solutions. The sites are then dressed with antibiotic ointment and covered with gauze dressings. The patient may be allowed to take a whirlpool bath twice weekly, as desired.

The presence of inflammatory changes, such as redness, swelling, or drainage around the pins, requires antibiotic treatment to be instituted after cultures have been taken. The authors have not found routine periodic cultures of the pin sites to be helpful. However, pin-site cultures may help in the selection of an antibiotic to be used initially for any overt infection.

Ilizarov Technique

In recent years, the Ilizarov method (also called "bloodless tranosseous distraction osteosynthesis") has become popular.[20,33–39,45] The basic principles of the technique include: (1) distraction osteogenesis; (2) corticotomy; and (3) circular external fixation with crossed transfixation wires (Fig. 11.7). Ilizarov has demonstrated with his technique that tensile stress in tissue during distraction (lengthening) can stimulate and maintain bone regeneration, which allows healing without bone grafting or internal fixation. An important and demanding aspect of this technique is performing a corticotomy, which preserves the periosteum as well as bone marrow structures. The uninterrupted periosteum produces intramembranous bone, and the bone marrow vasculature and marrow cells form endosteal osseous tissue at the distraction site.[38] The circular external fixator with crossed transfixation wires allows a versatility that includes correcting angulation deformities, correcting of rotational deformities, and performing of distraction by epiphysiolysis or corticotomy in the metaphysis or metaphysio-diaphyseal area.

Preoperative planning prior to Ilizarov lengthening is essential and possibly the most crucial step in achieving good results. The Ilizarov technique and fixator have the advantage of being exceedingly versatile. The authors prefer to list preoperatively the components of the deformity, to make a cutout of the osteotomies, and to construct the fixator to correct the deformity. Issues in planning the osteotomy include the following: (1) osteotomy should be performed preferably at the metaphysis or metaphyseal-diaphyseal region, which facilitates osseous healing; (2) angulatory, rotational, and displacement deformities (malalignment) may be corrected slowly by the external fixator or immediately for minor deformities at the time of surgery; and (3) immediate displacement of the osteotomy destroys the endosteal blood supply, which possibly impedes osseous healing.

In designing the external fixator, the authors find it helpful to consider the bony segments created by the osteotomy as requiring "stable unit" fixation to rings and to consider the interval between the stable ring units (area of osteotomy) to be available for angulation, rotation, displacement, and lengthening. To establish the stable ring unit, wires are placed as near as possible perpendicular to the bone and 90° to each other, pending the anatomy of vessels and nerves. Beaded wires are available to offer traction along the wire. The proper ring diameter allows about 2.5-cm clearance between the skin and the ring. Several connected rings or perpendicular extension posts from a ring may be necessary to secure the number of necessary wires to establish a stable unit between the bone and the external fixator. If the Ilizarov external fixator spans joints, hinges are helpful to protect the joint from excessive stress. The authors consider the hinged joint to be a portion of a stable ring unit of the fixator. The

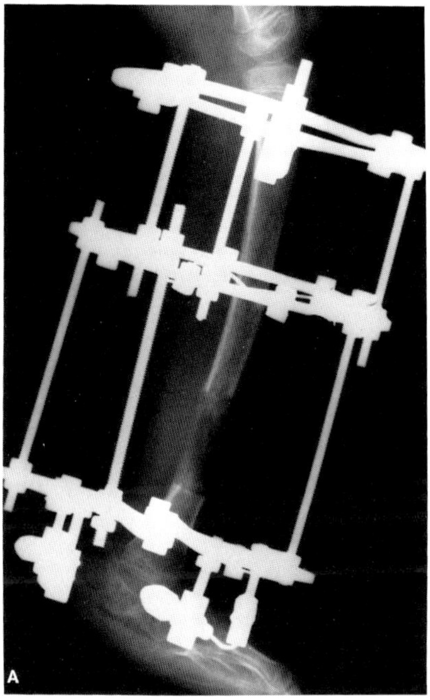

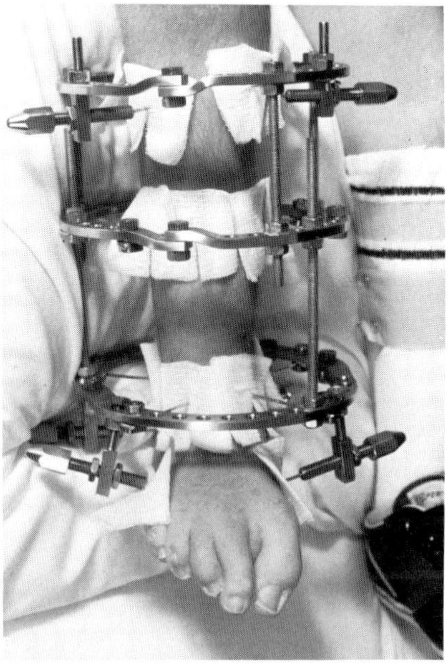

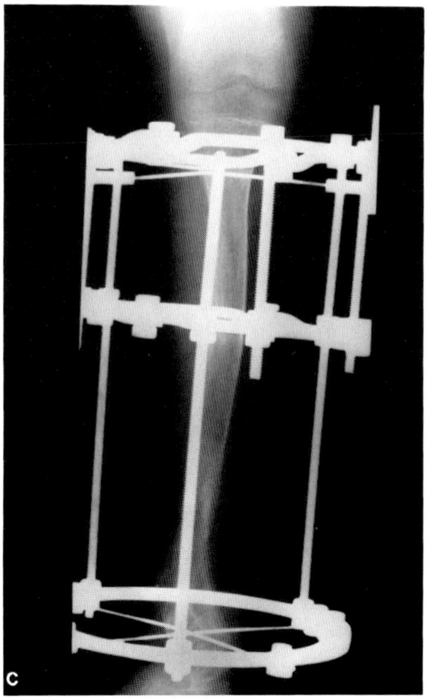

FIGURE 11.7. **A:** Tibial lengthening using Ilizarov apparatus in a 9.5-year-old-boy with congenital fibular hemimelia. In this patient distal corticotomy was performed to correct ankle valgus deformity and to obtain leg lengthening. Seventy-two days after corticotomy, osteogenesis was evident in the distraction gap (5.5 cm). Notice the calcaneal and metatarsal pin fixation. **B:** Anteroposterior view of the patient in the Ilizarov device. **C:** Five months later, consolidation of distraction osteogenesis is evident; however, the cortex is not fully matured.

construction of the external fixator is completed by linking the "stable ring units" with expandable rods, hinges, or plates to allow gradual correction of deformity.

Tibial Lengthening by the Ilizarov Method

The tibial lengthening operation is divided into steps of fibular osteotomy, insertion of wires, application of rings, construction of fixator, and corticotomy of the tibia. The authors prefer the fibular osteotomy in the diaphysis and removal of a segment of diaphyseal bone to prevent premature osseous union. A 1.5- to 2.0-cm longitudinal incision is made at the midfibular area over the lateral intramuscular septum. The peroneus longus and brevis muscles are retracted anteriorly. The periosteum of the fibula is incised longitudinally, the fibular diaphysis is cut with an osteotome, 2.0 to 4.0 mm of bone is removed, and the incision is closed.

Attention is then directed toward the tibia. The authors prefer to have the external fixator prefabricated and placed over the tibia to establish the general contour and orientation of the external fixator on the leg. The external fixator is then removed. The transfixation pins (usually 1.5 to 1.8 mm in diameter Kirschner wires) are placed in pairs through the tibia. In the immature patient, the wires must not damage the growth plate. The authors recommend that the wires be at least 1.0 cm from the plate to offer some safety from pin migration during lengthening. The wires are placed as near to perpendicular as possible to each other, pending anatomical structures. Great care should be taken not to injure nerves and vessels with the wires. The first pin of the proximal pair is placed proximally from laterally through the proximal fibula into the tibia and allowed to exit the tibia on the anterior medial surface. Great care should be taken not to injure the peroneal nerve with the pin. If any uncertainty exists, the pin may be placed through a short lateral incision over the proximal fibula. The second pin of the proximal pair is placed from postmedial to anterior-lateral through the proximal tibia. During lengthening, the tibia tends to go into slight valgus and flexion (procurvatum). Ilizarov recommends the planes of these wires be about 5° higher medially and anteriorly than laterally and posteriorly to inhibit bowing of the tibia during lengthening. The pins are attached to the rings with bolts and nuts and set at 100 to 120 kg of tension using a tension device. A third pin, with a bead against the medial cortex, can be placed 1.0 to 1.5 cm below the proximal pair and incorporated to the proximal ring to offer more stability.

If the tibial osteotomy (corticotomy) is planned at a proximal metaphyseal/metaphyseal-diaphyseal area, two additional rings with their wires are added below the osteotomy. The second pins and rings are placed about 2.5 cm below the osteotomy in the diaphysis. The distal rings and pins are in the distal metaphysis. One of the distal pins should pass from the fibula to the tibia to stabilize the ankle mortis.

When inserting wires through the anterior compartment, the foot should be plantar flexed to maintain maximum length of the anterior dorsiflexor muscle groups; but once the wire tips perforate the posterior cortex of the tibia, the foot should be dorsiflexed to maintain maximum length of the plantar flex muscles.

If the osteotomy is at the distal metaphyseal/metaphyseal-diaphyseal junction, the intermediate ring is moved to about 1.5 cm above the osteotomy. Frequently, a distal tibial metaphyseal osteotomy is used when the patient has a valgus ankle deformity. Additional half rings may be added to the foot with wires in the calcaneous and metatarsals to offer additional stability. Additional rings and wires may be added to achieve additional stability or to conform to individual patient needs.

The final step of the procedure is to perform the corticotomy. A small (1 cm) longitudinal skin incision is made just lateral to the tibial crest, 2.5 to 4 cm from the proximal tibial ring. With small periosteal elevator, medial and lateral sides of periosteum of the tibia are elevated for the passage of an osteotome. The anterior, medial, and lateral cortices of the proximal tibia are osteotomized using a 1-cm osteotome, with care being taken not to extend into the medullary cavity. Under protection of this periosteal elevator, the cortex is cut down to and through the posterolateral and posteromedial corners using 5-mm straight osteotome. By using a twisting motion in the tibia, the posterior cortex can be broken. The fracture of the posterior cortex of tibia can be confirmed and facilited by outward rotation of the distal ring with counterrotation of the proximal ring. If double-level lengthening is indicated, the distal corticotomy can be made by using the same technique. As an alternative to this corticotomy, the authors sometimes perform the osteotomy by manual osteoclasis after multidirectional percutaneous drilling. In this case, it is better to wait about 10 days before the start of distraction to allow the endosteal blood vessel to regenerate. If breakage of the cortex is doubtful, it should be confirmed by fluoroscopic examination or routine radiography. After corticotomy, the threaded rods are applied between the rings. The tilt of the proximal ring to the distal ring is eliminated by making the proximal to distal rings parallel. This maneuver produces slight varus and recurvatum at the osteotomy site of the proximal tibia and prevents valgus and procurvatum tendency at the level of proximal corticotomy.

Lengthening is performed with the Ilizarov external fixator by rotating nuts on the threaded rods, which distracts the rings. Typically, lengthening can be performed at a rate of 0.5 to 1.5 mm per day. The lengthening can be at a per day schedule, but possible healing is better if one quarter of the daily rate is achieved every 6 hours. Lengthening must be temporarily halted or even reversed if neurovascular complications, contractures, or joint subluxation occur. Patients are allowed to ambulate with crutches and bear weight on the leg being lengthened. The authors prefer to apply antibiotic ointment (Neosporin) at the pin sites daily and allow whirlpool bathing as desired. Once lengthening is achieved, the lengthening device is maintained until osseous healing occurs, as demonstrated radiographically. The patient should ambulate to stimulate bone healing. Typical healing time is about 1 month per centimeter of lengthening after single-level corticotomy.

Femoral Lengthening by the Ilizarov Method

Femoral lengthening employs similar steps as tibial lengthening, which include insertion of crossed Kirschner wires, application of rings, construction of the external fixator, and corticotomy. The authors believe the femur is more difficult to lengthen and has more complications than the tibia. At the most proximal level, half rings are used; however, the Ilizarov device is still bulky around the proximal leg. The crossed wires are more difficult to place at the proximal femur because the nerves and vessels are located anteriorly and posteriorly.

For femoral lengthening, distal femoral corticotomy can be employed after inserting the first pair of pins and rings at the junction between the proximal and middle one third of femur and the second pair of pins and rings at the distal metaphysis of the femur. If an additional proximal pin fixation is required for more stability or correction of deformity, additional Ilizarov wires can be fixed at the trochanteric area using half rings.

Because of the difficulty of bone fixation of the proximal femur, some physicians are using modifications consisting of large pins (Shanz pins) that enter the lateral aspect of the femur. These pins function as cantilever rather than as transfixation wires. Typically, two or four pins are placed in the proximal femur and secured to the modified half rings.

Postoperatively, the femoral lengthening is allowed at a rate of 0.5 to 1.5 mm/d. As with the tibia, the lengthening may be performed daily, but perhaps healing is enhanced by performing one quarter of the daily at intervals 6 hours apart. The patients participate in a daily physical therapy program to prevent contractures. The lengthening is delayed or reversed if contractures or neurovascular problems develop. The postoperative care is similar to that described for tibial lengthening.

Complications of Lower Limb Lengthening

Most large series report a high incidence of complications related to limb lengthening for lower-limb length discrepancy.† The complications that occur during distraction lengthening of a congenitally shortened extremity

† References 8, 13, 14, 18, 28, 31, 43, 44.

may be conveniently grouped into those common complications associated with all lengthenings (femoral and tibial) and with those complications that are peculiar to femoral and tibial lengthenings.

Some of the general complications already alluded to are outlined as follows:

1. Infection
   a. Pin-tract contamination
   b. Osteomyelitis
2. Nerve Damage
   a. Mechanical nerve damage by pins
   b. Sensory changes
   c. Transient motor deficits
3. Vascular Damage
   a. Mechanical vessel damage
   b. Compartment syndromes
   c. Hypertension
4. Joint Abnormality
   a. Loss of range of motion
   b. Contractures
   c. Subluxation
   d. Dislocation
5. Difficulties with Bone Healing
   a. Angulation at osteotomy site
   b. Inadequate union
   c. Malunion
   d. Delayed union
   e. Nonunion
   f. Pseudarthrosis
   g. Refracture after union
6. Emotional and Psychological Complications
   a. Depression
   b. Noncompliance

Specific Complications in Femoral Lengthening

Sciatic nerve damage is uncommon as the result of direct trauma from the distraction pins, except where pins are placed vertically in the proximal femur (as in some transfixator pin techniques). If the recommended lengthening rate and proportions are exceeded, increasing difficulty with transient paresthesias or pareses may be encountered. These may be treated by slowing the rate of distraction lengthening or by temporarily ceasing the distraction process. In most instances, these changes are not permanent. Mechanical vessel damage is similarly rare, and compartment syndromes are infrequent in femoral lengthenings.

Hypertension is detected most accurately by performing recordings of the blood pressure during the lengthening phase twice daily. Any sustained increase in systolic blood pressure of more than 15 to 20 mmHg or 10 mmHg diastolically should be an indication for cessation of lengthening. The pressure elevation usually resolves in 1 or 2 days, and lengthening may continue when this occurs.

Subluxation and dislocation of the knee are preceded by a loss of range of motion and the development of contractures. More commonly, flexion contractures occur, although extension contractures also may be seen frequently. Temporary discontinuation of lengthening and increased physical therapy are usually successful in overcoming these problems, and splinting may be used in intervals.

The hip joint may show flexion and adduction contractures that demand similar intensive physical therapy for their resolution. If the hip joint is grossly unstable prior to initiation of a lengthening procedure, it may be necessary to perform a pelvic osteotomy to obtain joint stability before embarking on a lengthening procedure. If stability cannot be gained, it may be better to consider lengthening of the tibia instead.

Bone healing may occur primarily after lengthening of the femur is achieved, provided there is satisfactory callus formation. Varus angulation often develops during distraction, and this may indicate the need for iliotibial band incision or lengthening. In the presence of a tight iliotibial band, valgus angulation at the knee may also develop, especially in patients with poorly developed lateral femoral condyle or lateral tibial condyle.

The pattern of periosteal callus formation often gives an indication as to the need for bone grafting. If the callus formation in the distraction gap narrows and tapers toward the center of the gap from either end, then the need for bone grafting is indicated, as it is unlikely that sufficiently strong bony healing will be achieved without bone graft. However, if there is abundant callus equal to or greater than the diaphyseal bone, then healing is likely to occur without additional bone grafting. In the authors' experience, grafting is more often necessary with a diaphyseal osteotomy in congenital deformities that affect the femur where the diaphysis of the bone is small.

After healing of the lengthened bone, refracture should be treated the same as a fracture occurring under other circumstances. Plating and bone grafting are often necessary, as it is often impossible to utilize intramedullary fixation techniques in this situation. The medullary canal may not have yet been reconstituted.

The emotional stress experienced by patients undergoing limb lengthening is severe. These patients face repeated operations and numerous, frequent complications. Their hospitalization is often prolonged and difficult, and adequate psychological goal support must be provided. The patients and parents should have frequent consultations with the physician and a positive, optimistic outlook must be maintained and encouraged. Adequate preoperative planning and consultation and identification of goals must be performed. The likely complications and their treatment and the risks of surgery must be explained carefully. The responsibilities of the patient must be emphasized, i.e., cooperation with the physician and care of the lengthened limb and the distraction apparatus. The physician must maintain good rapport with the patient and his or her family and be alert to any early signs of a deteriorating outlook or relationship, especially when complications occur. It is sometimes useful to interrupt the lengthening process and allow the patient to be discharged home for a few days to boost his or her morale.

Specific Complications in Tibial Lengthening

Osteomyelitis may be somewhat more frequent in tibial lengthening than in femoral lengthening because of the lesser soft-tissue coverage of the bone and its relatively poor blood supply. Nerve damage and transient neurological changes are infrequent. Vascular compromise is likewise rare, and hypertension is less of a problem with tibial lengthening than with femoral lengthening. Equinus deformity of the ankle and the knee, flexion contractures, valgus deformity of the subtalar joint, and valgus deformity of the tibia sometimes occur.

Physical therapy usually corrects the joint deformities if they are mild and treated early. Occasional Achilles tendon lengthening or tenotomy may be necessary, and triple arthrodesis rarely is needed for subtalar valgus deformity. The ankle tends to be more affected than the knee in the tibial lengthening.

Bone grafting and plating most often are required in diaphyseal osteotomy to obtain union. Careful use of the distraction apparatus, along with the use of splints and weight-bearing, may encourage strengthening and consolidation of the lengthened areas.

References

1. Abbott LC: The operative lengthening of the tibia and fibula. J Bone Joint Surg 25:128–152, 1927.
2. Achterman C, Kalamchi A: Congenital deficiency of the fibula. J Bone Joint Surg 61B:133–137, 1979.
3. Agerholm J: The zig-zag osteotomy. Acta Orthop Scand 29:63–70, 1960.
4. Altongy JF, Harcke HT, Bowen JR: Measurement of leg-length inequalities by Micro-Dose Digital radiographs. J Pediatr Orthop 7:311–316, 1987.
5. Amstutz HC: Natural history and treatment of congenital absence of the fibula. J Bone Joint Surg 54A:1349, 1972.
6. Anderson M, Green WT, Messner MB: Growth and predictions of growth in the lower extremities. J Bone Joint Surg 45A:1–14, 1963.
7. Anderson WV: Leg lengthening, abstracted. J Bone Joint Surg 34B:150, 1952.

8. Armour PC, Scott JH: Equalization of leg length. J Bone Joint Surg 63B:587–592, 1981.
9. Barr JS Ober FR: Leg lengthening in adults. J Bone Joint Surg 15:674–678, 1933.
10. Baumann F, Harms J: The extension nail. A new method for leg lengthening of the femur and tibia. Arch Orthop Unvallchir 90:139–146, 1977.
11. Bliskunov AI: Intramedullary distraction of the femur. Preliminary report. Orthop Travmatol Protez 10:59–62, 1983.
12. Bost FC, Larsen LJ: Experience with lengthening of the femur over an intramedullary rod. J Bone Joint Surg 38A:567–584, 1956.
13. Brockway A, Fouter SB: Experience with 105 leg-lengthening operations. Surg Gynecol Obstet 75:252–256, 1942.
14. Codivilla A: On the means of lengthening in the lower limbs, the muscles and tissues which are shorter through deformity. J Orthop Surg 2:353–369, 1905.
15. Coleman SS: Current concepts of tibial lengthening. Orthop Clin North Am 3:201–211, 1972.
16. Coleman SS: Lower limb length discrepancy, in Lovell WW, Winter RB (eds): *Pediatric Orthopaedics,* vol 1, Philadelphia, JB Lippincott Co, 1978, pp 805–880.
17. Coleman SS: Simultaneous femoral and tibial lengthening for limb length discrepancies. Arch Orthop Trauma Surg 1985, pp 359–366.
18. Compere EL: Indications for and against the leg-lengthening operation. J Bone Joint Surg 18:692–705, 1936.
19. Coventry MB, Johnson EW: Congenital absence of the fibula. J Bone Joint Surg 34A:941-956, 1952.
20. Dal Monte A, Donzelli O: Tibial lengthening according to Ilizarov in congenital hypoplasia of the leg. J Pediatr Orthop 7:135–138, 1987.
21. De Bastiani G, Aldegheri R, Renzi-Brivio L, et al: Limb lengthening by callus distraction (callotasis). J Pediatr Orthop 7:129–134, 1987.
22. De Pablos J: Bone lengthening by physeal distraction. An experimental study, thesis. University of Navarra, Pamplona, 1984.
23. Gill GG, Abbott LC: Practical method of predicting growth of the femur and tibia of the child. Arch Surg 45:286–315, 1942.
24. Gotz J, Schellmann WD: Continuous lengthening of the femur with intramedullary stabilization. Arch Orthop Unfallchir 82:305–310, 1975.
25. Green WT, Anderson M: Experiences with epiphyseal arrest in correcting discrepancies in length of the lower extremities in infantile paralysis. J Bone Joint Surg 29:659–675, 1947.
26. Green WT, Wyatt GM, Anderson M: Orthoroentgenography as a method of measuring the bones of the lower extremities. J Bone Joint Surg 28:60–65, 1946.
27. Greulich WW, Pyle SI: Radiographic analysis of skeletal development of hand and wrist. Stanford, Cal, Standford University Press, 1950.
28. Gross RH: An evaluation of tibial lengthening procedures. J Bone Joint Surg 53A:693–700, 1971.
29. Hass SL: Longitudinal osteotomy. JAMA 92:1656–1658, 1929.
30. Helms CA, McCarthy S: CT scanograms for measuring leg-length discrepancy. Radiology 151:802, 1984.
31. Hood RW, Riseborough EJ: Lengthening of the lower extremity by the

Wagner method. A review of the Boston Children's Hospital Experience. J Bone Joint Surg 63A:1122–1131, 1981.
32. Hootnick D, Boyd HA, Fixsen JA, et al: The natural history and management of congenital short tibia with dysplasia or absence of the tibia. J Bone Joint Surg 59B:267–271, 1977.
33. Ilizarov GA: New principles of osteosynthesis by means of crossing pins and rings—from collection of scientific publications. Kurgan, 1954, pp 146–160.
34. Ilizarov GA: The main principles of transosseous compression and distraction osteosynthesis. Ortop Travmatol Protez 11:7–15, 1971.
35. Ilizarov GA, Deviatov AA: Operative elongation of the leg. Ortop Travmatol Protez 32:20–25, 1971.
36. Ilizarov GA: Experimental, theoretical, and clinical aspects of transosseous osteosynthesis developed in KNIIEKOT Institute. Proc 2nd Int Conf 1986, pp 18–20.
37. Ilizarov GA, Makushin VD: Compression and distraction osteosynthesis in the treatment of congenital malformations of the lower limbs, in: *Materials of the YIY Congress of Traumatologists and Orthopaedists of the Ukranian SSR*. Kiev, Zdorovje, 1977, pp 115–118.
38. Ilizarov GA, Palienko LA, Shreiner AA: The bone marrow hematopoietic function and its relationship with the activity of osteogenesis upon reparative regeneration under the conditions of crus elongation in dogs. Ontogenez 15:2, 146–152, 1984.
39. Ilizarov GA, Trohova VG: Operative elongation of the femur. Ortop Travmatol Protez 34:11, 51–55, 1973.
40. Kalamchi A, Cowell HR, Kim KI: Congenital deficiency of the femur. J Pediatr Orthop 5:129–134, 1985.
41. Kawamura B, Hosono S, Takahaski T, et al: Limb lengthening by means of subcutaneous osteotomy; experimental and clinical studies. J Bone Joint Surg 50A:851–878, 1968.
42. MacKenzie WG, Bowen JR: Distraction myogenesis: An experimental study in the rat, to be published.
43. McCarroll HR: Trials and tribulations in attempted femoral lengthening. J Bone Joint Surg 32A:132–142, 1950.
44. Mahlis TM, Bowen JR: Tibial and femoral lengthening: a report of 54 cases. J Pediatr Orthop 2:487–491, 1982.
45. Mezhenina EP, Roulla EA, Pechersky AG, et al: Methods of limb elongation with congenital inequality in children. J Pediatr Orthop 4:201–207, 1984.
46. Monticelli G, Spinelli R: Distraction epiphysiolysis as a method of limb lengthening: I. Experimental study. II. Morphologic investigations. III. Clinical applications. Clin Orthop 154:254–285, 1981.
47. Moseley CF: A straight-line graph for leg-length discrepancies. J Bone Joint Surg 59A:174–179, 1977.
48. Paley D: Current techniques of limb lengthening. J Pediatr Orthop 8:73–92, 1988.
49. Putti V: The operative lengthening of the femur. JAMA 77:934–935, 1921.
50. Schollner D: New ways of operating to lengthen the femur. Z Orthop 110:971–974, 1972.
51. Schapiro F: Developmental patterns in lower-extremity length discrepancies. J Bone Joint Surg 64A:639–651, 1982.

52. Tanner JM, Whitehouse RH, Marshall WA, et al: Assessment of skeletal maturity and prediction of adult height (TW2 Method). London, Academic Press, 1975.
53. Wagner H: Surgical lengthening or shortening of femur and tibia; technique and indications, in Hungerfords DS (ed): *Progress in Orthopaedic Surgery,* vol 1. New York, Sprienger-Verlag, 1977, pp 71–94.
54. Wagner H: Operative Beinverlangerung. Chirurg 42(6):260–266, 1971.
55. Wagner H: Operative lengthening of the femur. Clin Orthop 136:125–142, 1978.
56. Westin GW, Sakai DN, Wood WL: Congenital longitudinal deficiency of the fibula. J Bone Joint Surg 58A:492–496, 1976.
57. Westin GW: Femoral lengthening using a periosteal sleeve; report on 26 cases. J Bone Joint Surg 49A:836–854, 1967.
58. Wilk LH, Badgley CE: Hypertension, another complication of leg lengthening. Report of a case. J Bone Joint Surg 45A:1263–1268, 1963.
59. Witt AN, Jager M, Hilderbrandt JJ: An implantable femur distractor for operative leg lengthening. Arch Orthop Traumat Surg 92:291–296, 1978.
60. Witt AN, Jager M, Hilderbrandt JJ: Results of animal experiments with an implantable femur distractor for operative leg lengthening. Arch Orthop Unfallchir 88:273–279, 1977.
61. Yosipovitch ZH, Palti Y: Alterations in blood pressure during leg-lengthening. A clinical and experimental investigation. J Bone Joint Surg 49A:1352–1358, 1967.

12 Prosthetic Management

George H. Thompson and
Jon P. Leimkuehler

Introduction

Prosthetic management of children with congenital lower-limb deficiencies can be a very complex process and is best carried out in special clinics offering comprehensive care for juvenile amputees. Comprehensive care is usually essential for children with multiple limb deficiencies. Approximately 70% of juvenile amputees have congenital limb deficiencies and most of these are of the lower extremities.[13] The problems confronting the orthopaedist and prosthetist in the child with a congenital lower-limb deficiency include corrective and revision surgery, the effects of growth on the involved extremity, prosthetic fitting and revisions, prosthetic training, extremity function, and psychological adaptation and acceptance. The goals of prosthetic replacement of an extremity include optimum function, comfort, and cosmesis. It is important that functional restoration be compatible, whenever possible, to the non-limb-deficient child of the same age.

Prosthetic fitting in a child is typically quite different from an adult amputee. Juvenile amputees lack systemic illnesses and have durable skin and soft tissues. As a consequence, they prefer simple, comfortable, functional, and durable prostheses. They usually do not respond well to, or accept, complex or overgadgeted prostheses. Emphasis should be placed on early prosthetic fitting and habilitation. If surgery can improve the involved limb and if there are procedures that can enhance function, they should be performed. If not, then the deformity should be accepted and compensated for prosthetically. The basic principles of surgical intervention have been discussed by Kruger.[18] These include: (1) maintenance of muscular development of the residual limb; (2) prevention of progressive deformity; (3) retention of long-bone growth plates; (4) preservation of proximal joints; and (5) stabilization of proximal joints when necessary. These principles will be emphasized throughout this chapter.

Basic Principles of Prosthetic Restoration

Body contours, movement patterns, and functional requirements of children are different than that of adults and are constantly changing throughout growth and development. These factors must be continually reevaluated in the amputee clinic. Setoguchi and Rosenfelder showed that the basic principles of prosthetic replacements in children vary according to anatomy and growth and level of neuromuscular maturation.[26] These factors are unique and must be considered in prosthetic fitting of infants and children.

Anatomy and Growth

Limb size, shape, and contours can vary considerably in the child with a congenital lower-extremity amputation and have a significant effect on prosthetic design and suspension. Typically, normal anatomic landmarks are absent or distorted by the limb malformation and when present, they are obscured by abundant adipose tissue. A prosthesis must be designed to allow relief in the socket for the soft tissue and alternative methods for suspension. As an infant or child grows, continued alterations to accommodate changes in limb shape and length as well as developmental function must be provided. The prosthesis should fit well when the child receives it. With proper maintenance and appropriate designs to accommodate revisions for both longitudinal and circumferential growth, the lower-extremity prosthesis should fit well for approximately 1 year.

Neuromuscular Maturation

The child's functional and intellectual development can also have a significant effect on prosthetic design and manufacturing. An understanding of the child's functional capabilities and needs at different ages and stages for development can guide the orthopaedic surgeon and prosthetist in selecting components and socket design. In general, the child with a congenital lower-extremity amputation is fitted when he attempts to pull to a standing position rather than at a specific age.[8,18,27] This is usually between 9 and 15 months of age. The level of amputation, the presence of bilateral amputations, associated upper-extremity involvement, and the child's general health can result in a wide variation in the age at the time of first prosthetic fitting.

In an infant, the first prosthesis is designed to simulate a toddler's stance and gait pattern. Infants typically stand with the hips flexed, abducted, and externally rotated; the knees are slightly flexed; and the feet are flat on the floor. In the infant with an above-knee amputation, further stability can be obtained by omitting the knee joint. The latter is usually added to the prosthesis at approximately 3 years of age. The school-aged child requires frequent adjustments in prosthetic fit and length, a prosthesis that can be easily applied and removed, and one that can withstand considerable abuse. Adolescents can usually be fitted in a manner similar to that of adults. Cosmesis as well as function becomes important in adolescents.

Prosthetic Restorations

There are five basic prosthetic restorations necessary in the management of congenital lower-limb deficiencies.[19] These include: (1) partial foot restorations; (2) Syme's-type prostheses; (3) below-knee prosthesis; (4) above-knee prosthesis, including knee disarticulation types; and (5) hip disarticulation and hemipelvectomy prostheses. Each of these restorations must be customized, as well as individualized, for each child because of the wide variations and complexities of the deficiencies encountered. In forming a prescription for a child, one should be principally interested in functional restoration, with cosmesis being of secondary importance. The activity levels of the child must be considered as well as the type of activity. A prescription chart for lower-extremity prostheses in children is presented in Table 12.1.

Partial Foot Restorations

Congenital absence of the toes rarely has an adverse affect on function or walking whereas partial or complete loss of the metatarsals frequently do and may require prosthetic replacement such as a shoe insert. The insert may be fabricated either from an impression or from a cast of the affected foot, and it is constructed to fit closely to the plantar surface of the foot. The toe section is fit to the shape of the patient's shoe. Distal deficiencies can be managed with an insert of this type whereas more proximal midfoot deficiencies may require a socket that extends up to or above the ankle malleoli for suspension. The Chopart "shoe within a shoe" prosthesis is frequently used when the amputation level is through the tarsal bones or more proximal.[19] In these designs, the toe section is made from a semi-rigid material that provides resistance during push-off in the gait cycle. The use of the Chopart prosthesis usually allows for adequate shoe wear and prevents the foot remnant from drifing into an equinovarus position. An ankle-foot orthosis (AFO) with foam toe extension can be considered an alternative, as it provides better toe-off than the Chopart prosthesis.[19]

When a hallux amputation occurs, an insert or prosthesis is often not required. In some cases, however, owing to the loss of support of the large toe, the shoe tends to curl up, leaving the amputee with inadequate push-off. In this case a spring steel shank can be inserted in a shoe with a

TABLE 12.1. Prescription chart.

Amputation Level	Basic Description of Prosthesis	Suspension	Foot	Knee
Hallux	1. Nothing 2. Spring steel shank in shoe			
Transmetatarsal	Molded shoe insert, toe filler			
Tarsometatarsal	Molded socket, ankle height with toe filler			
Midtarsal	Molded socket, tibial tubercle height	Self-suspending		
Syme's	Syme's prosthesis with medial or posterior opening or soft inner socket	Self-suspending	SACH	
Below the knee	Below-knee prosthesis with soft insert	1. Cuff strap, waistbelt 2. Latex, neoprene, or elastic knee sleeve suspension 3. Supracondylar suspension (SCSP)	1. SACH 2. SAFE 3. Seattle 4. Carbon Copy II	
	Below knee prosthesis with soft insert and knee joints and thigh corset	Waistbelt	1. SACH 2. SAFE 3. Seattle 4. Carbon Copy II	
Knee disarticulation	End-bearing knee disarticulation prosthesis socket options: 1. With or without soft insert 2. Medial opening socket	1. Self suspending 2. Silesian belt 3. Hip joint and pelvic belt	1. SACH 2. SAFE 3. Seattle 4. Carbon Copy II	Outside knee joints
Above the knee	Above-the-knee prosthesis socket options: 1. Quadrilateral 2. Narrow ML	1. Suction socket 2. Silesian belt 3. Hip joint and pelvic belt	1. SACH 2. SAFE 3. Seattle 4. Carbon Copy II	Single axis

Hip Disarticulation	Hip disarticulation prosthesis 1. Endoskeletal 2. Exoskeletal		1. SACH 2. SAFE 3. Seattle 4. Carbon Copy II	Single axis
Hemipelvectomy	Hemipelvectomy prosthesis: 1. Endoskeletal 2. Exoskeletal		1. SACH 2. SAFE 3. Seattle 4. Carbon Copy II	Single axis
Special Prosthesis				
Short leg	Insert in shoe or shoe buildup on sole			
When shortness exceeds end of foot in plantar flexion	Extension prosthesis encompassing foot and extending to knee	Self-suspending	1. SACH 2. SAFE 3. Seattle 4. Carbon Copy II	
PFFD (infant)	1. Shoe Lift 2. Shoe lift with double upright AFO			
PFFD (moderate shortage; stable hip and knee	Extension prosthesis encompassing foot and extending to knee or hip	1. Self-suspending 2. Silesian belt	1. SACH 2. SAFE 3. Seattle 4. Carbon Copy II	
PFFD (fused knee, Symes amputation)	Above-the-knee prosthesis, end-bearing with or without soft insert	1. Self-suspending 2. Silesian belt	1. SACH 2. SAFE 3. Seattle 4. Carbon Copy II	Single axis
Van Ness Rotational Osteotomy	Socket to fit foot with outside knee joints and socket up to hip	Self-suspending	1. SACH 2. SAFE 3. Seattle 4. Carbon Copy II	Outside knee joint

PFFD = profimal femoral focal deficiency;
AFO = ankle-foot orthosis;
ML = Mediolateral;
SCSP = supracondylar, suprapatellar;
SACH = solid ankle cushion heel.

leather sole. The shank will extend the full length of the shoe and provide the support required.

Syme's-Type Prosthesis

Children with a complete transverse deficiency of the foot, partial tarsal deficiency, fibular hemimelia, or other congenital deformities may require a Syme's or Boyd amputation. These procedures provide an end-bearing stump and preservation of the distal tibial epiphysis; they also avoid bone transection and the associated problems of bony overgrowth. A Syme's prosthesis, or modification thereof, will allow excellent restoration of function. The typical Syme's prosthesis features a hard plastic long below-knee socket with partial end-weight-bearing and a solid ankle-cushion heel (SACH) foot (Fig. 12.1). The major problem with the use of this type of prosthesis is the shape of the residual limb and the resultant problems of socket construction. The very young child with a Syme's amputation may have a very bulbous distal stump due to abundant adipose and soft tissue. Because of this discrepancy, it is usually necessary to have either a posterior or a medial opening panel or a flexible liner to allow for easier application and removal of the prosthesis. With growth, the soft tissues and ankle malleoli atrophy and thereby facilitate prosthetic fitting.

Knee flexion and valgus deformities occasionally encountered with Syme's amputation can result in a poor gait, since the swing of the prosthesis follows the alignment of the knee axis. To achieve maximum function and appearance, it is important that the prosthetic foot be accurately centered.

Syme's amputation prosthesis can also be modified to accommodate tibial deformities such as anterior bowing and excessive shortening (Fig. 12.1). The latter is corrected by simply extending the prosthesis. There are many deisgns of prosthetic feet. When choosing a foot for a growing child, the design should allow for easy lengthening of the prosthesis. Lengthening can be easily accomplished when a foot with a flat ankle surface is used. A wood spacer can then be put between the foot and ankle to lengthen the prosthesis. The SACH foot is the lightest weight and the most common foot used to accomplish this. Other feet that can be used but are somewhat heavier are the stationary attachment flexible endoskeleton (SAFE) and Seattle feet. Recently, the carbon copy II foot has been introduced. This foot is similar to the Seattle foot but is lighter and has variable firmness and toe resistance. All these feet are held on with a single bolt and allow the prosthesis to be lengthened while the patient waits.

Usually a Syme's prosthesis is self-suspending because of the bulbous distal end. However, a supracondylar strap may be necessary in very young children.

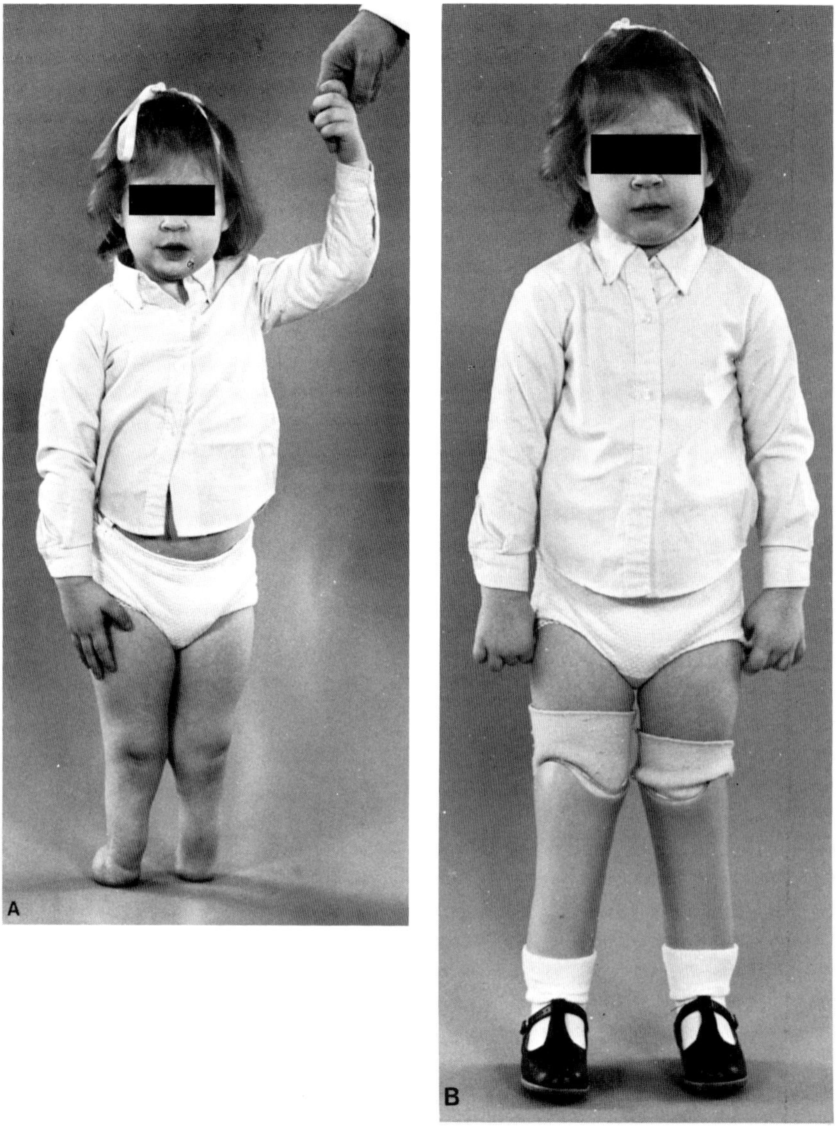

FIGURE 12.1. **A:** Four-year-old girl with bilateral complete paraxial fibular hemimelia. Syme's ankle disarticulations were performed at 9 months of age. She is able to weight-bear and ambulate without discomfort on her retained heel pads. Observe the associated tibial shortening and disproportionate appearance. **B:** Prosthetic restoration was achieved with bilateral patella tendon-bearing (PTB) laminated prostheses with soft liner and SACH feet. The prostheses were extended to restore her height and body proportions.

Below-Knee Prosthesis

The basic prosthesis for a child with a congenital below-knee amputation is the total contact patellar tendon-bearing (PTB) prosthesis and its variations.[19,28] These prostheses are generally used with a soft insert, SACH foot, and supracondylar cuff suspension strap. A removable soft insert is recommended for all below-knee prostheses for growing children. This insert can be easily modified to accommodate growth. It makes application of the socket easier and acts as a shock absorber; it also makes the prosthesis more comfortable.

McIvor and Gillespie observed an increased incidence of patella alta, lateral subluxation, and hypoplastic patellae in traumatic and congenital below-knee juvenile amputees, especially the latter, who used a PTB type of prosthesis.[23] They attributed these abnormalities to the effects of high pressure on the growing patellar tendon resulting in elongation and patella alta. They recommended that serious consideration by given to fitting young children with below-knee or Syme's amputation with a prosthesis that extends proximally around the patella, thereby decreasing pressure on the patella tendon.

A variety of supracondylar suspension are available, depending on the age of the child, the length of the stump, and the desired functional activities. The patellar tendon-supracondylar (PTS) prosthesis that extends over the femoral condyles to provide supracondylar suspension is not recommended for a growing child because of the difficulty in maintaining a proper fit. It may be useful in adolescents with mediolateral socket instability or genu recurvatum.[28] Strap suspension is required for sports activities, although wedge suspension can be utilized to improve both the appearance of the prosthesis and the elimination of soft tissue compression above the patella. Side hinges and a thigh corset are frequently used in infants and young children or in children with very short stumps or ligamentous laxity of the knee (Fig. 12.2). Another alternative method of suspension is the use of a knee sleeve (Fig. 12.3). It can be either elastic, neoprene, or latex rubber. The knee sleeve in many cases may eliminate the supracondylar cuff strap and provide good suspension. The sleeve extends part way on the outside of the prothesis and is pulled up onto the thigh after the prosthesis is in place. The latex rubber sleeve is worn against the skin on the thigh and forms a complete seal to hold the prosthesis. With this sleeve, however, perspiration can be a problem. The elastic sleeve does not hold the prosthesis as well, but it is much cooler and easier to use. Many adolescents and young adults with short stumps prefer a cuff strap in conjunction with the elastic suspension sleeve, as it will frequently eliminate the need for the waistbelt.

For cosmetic purposes in the older child and adolescent, an endoskeletal prosthesis may be used. An endoskeleton has a metal pylon between the socket and SACH foot and is covered with a soft-foam material. The

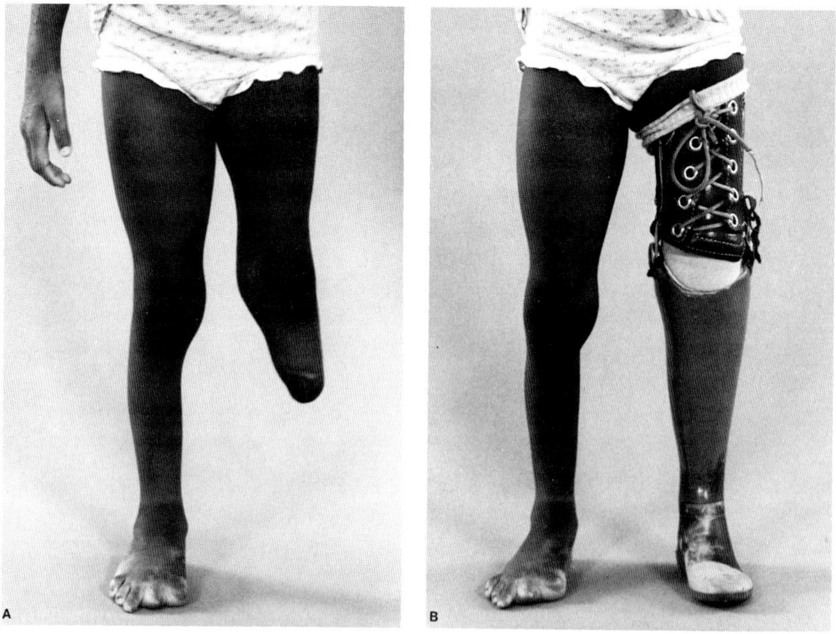

FIGURE 12.2. **A:** Six-year-old girl with amniotic band syndrome and left below-knee amputation and loss of the right great toe and second toe. The stump is moderately short and there is 10 degrees of genu valgum. **B:** Prosthetic restoration included a below-knee prosthesis with a laminated socket and soft liner, outside single axis knee hinges, leather thigh lacer, and SACH foot. The socket was designed to accommodate and correct the mild knee genu valgum.

exoskeleton is fabricated from laminated mylon stockinette and polyester resins for extra durability. Endoskeletons are too heavy and have poor durability to be used in young children.

Above-Knee and Knee Disarticulation Prostheses

Knee Disarticulation Prostheses

The basic prosthesis for a child with an absent lower leg at knee level is a plastic-laminated total contact socket with outside knee hinges, SACH foot, and a Silesian belt suspension. Young children can usually be fitted with either a quadrilateral socket or one that incorporates partial end-bearing. Most children over 3 years of age can manage a prosthetic knee joint. If there is a problem with extension or buckling of the knee, then an inverted Y-strap may be applied. It is unusual to require a knee lock even in a young child. The four-bar linkage knee may be used in larger children, as it allows swing phase frictional or hydraulic knee control while

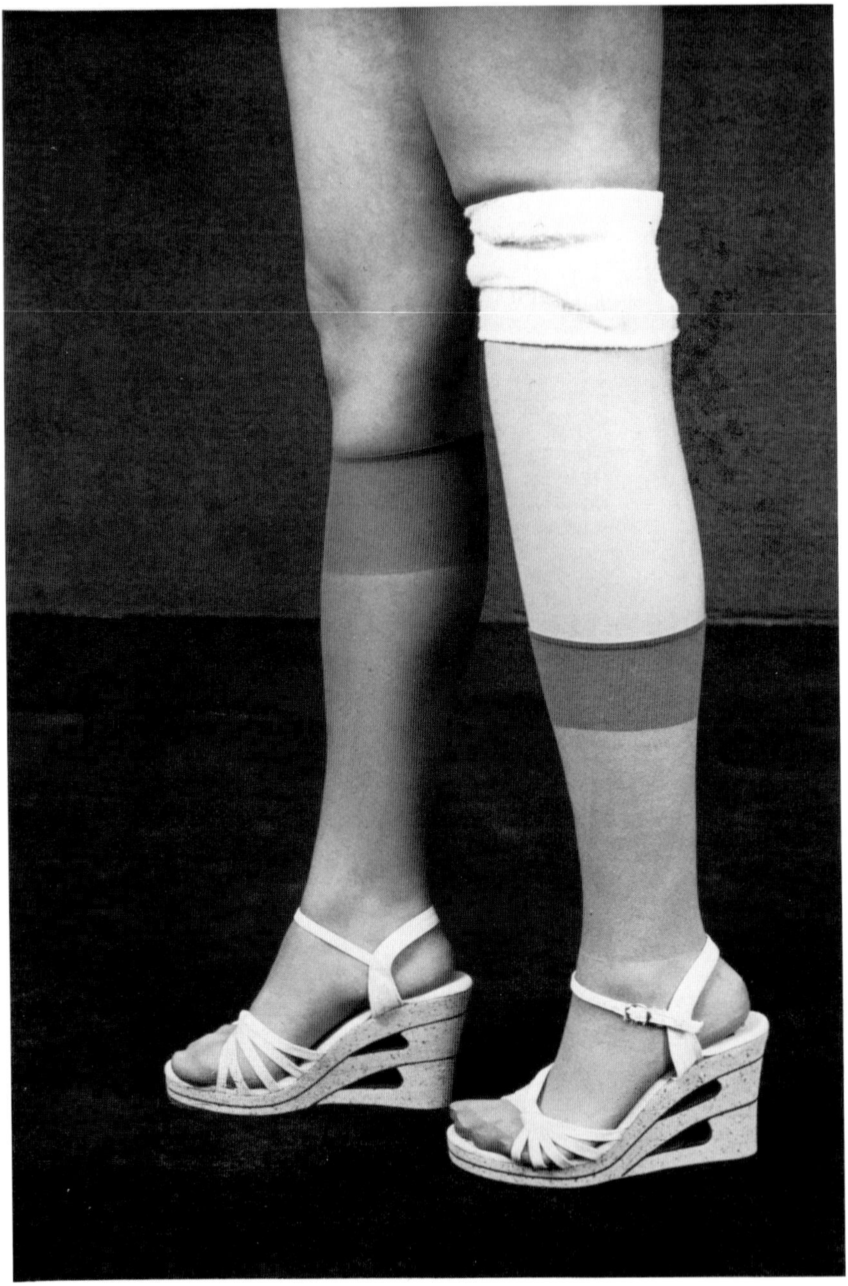

FIGURE 12.3. Adolescent female with a complete left paraxial fibula hemimelia previously treated with a Boyd amputation. She is using a below-knee prosthesis with an elastic sleeve for suspension. The SACH foot is in an equinus position to allow for shoes with increased heel height. These variations provide improved suspension, cosmesis, and increased acceptability.

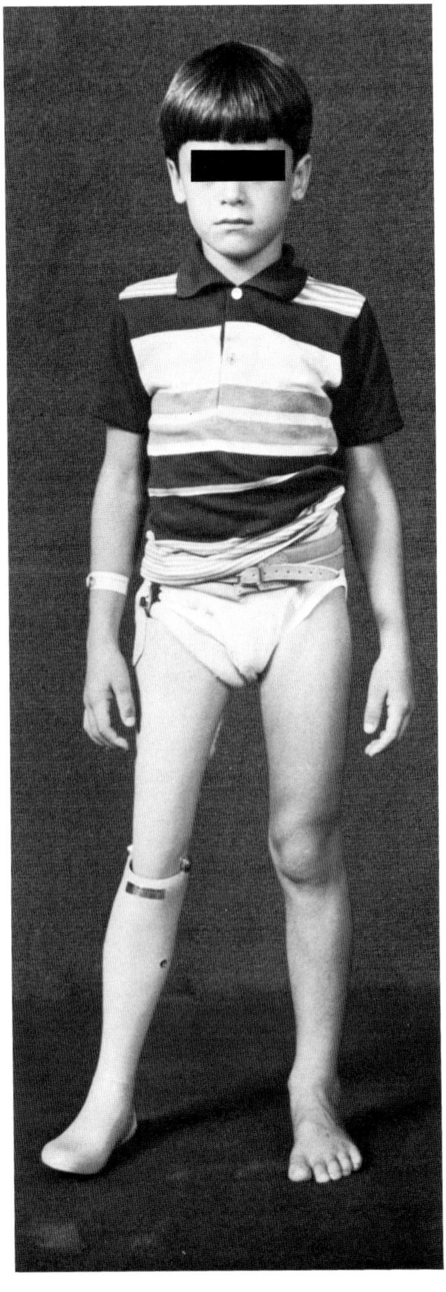

FIGURE 12.4. Six-year-old boy using an above-knee prosthetic with a plastic quadrilateral socket,single axis knee joint, SACH foot, and Silesian belt for suspension. The prosthesis is ideal for young, active children.

properly positioning the knee axis of rotation in relation to the normal limb.[28]

Above-Knee Prostheses

In children with long above-knee stumps, the prosthesis most commonly used is a plastic-laminated quadrilateral socket with a single axis knee joint, SACH foot, and Silesian belt for suspension (Fig. 12.4). Perhaps the most frequent problem in socket design for the child is failure to provide adequate preflexion of the socket, which in turn causes the child to walk with an exaggerated lumbar lordosis. For the child with a very short stump it may be necessary to use a pelvic belt with a hip joint to provide improved stability.

For the older child, conversion to a suction prosthesis may be considered (Fig. 12.5). This is usually not before 6 or 7 years of age. The addition of suction suspension prior to this age is difficult, and the child is usually not able to pull the stump into the socket by himself. Since socket fit with suction suspension is more critical, frequent socket replacement is necessary to accommodate the child's growth.

Most children 3 years of age or older can handle the prosthetic knee joint well when the prosthesis is properly aligned. If knee instability is significant, then a knee lock may be necessary until the child demonstrates adequate control of the prosthetic knee. This is best accomplished by a strap and buckle device over the anterior aspect of the prosthetic knee. The strap is gradually loosened to allow more flexion as the child develops knee control. As the child approaches adult size, a variety of knee-control mechanisms are available. The most common options are the stance-phase-controlled knee and the hydraulic-swing-phase control. The stance phase control is the design that swings freely; however, on weight-bearing, with the knee in full extension, it locks in place and will not buckle until it is unweighted. This knee is especially appropriate for a short residual limb or a hip disarticulation amputee. The hydraulic swing phase control provides varying resistance to adjust automatically from walking slow to walking fast, whereas the constant friction knee is adjusted basically for one speed of walking.

In the older child changing the SACH foot may also be a consideration. The SACH foot simulates anterior or posterior and minimal medial lateral motion at the ankle. There are now available a wide variety of feet that provide multiaxis motion for more vigorous activities, either on uneven surfaces or in sports. Usually these feet are somewhat heavier in weight. As a result, they are not recommended for the smaller child.

As the child grows older, consideration should be given to the use of endoskeletal prosthesis, especially in the female patient in whom cosmesis is important. An endoskeletal prosthesis is constructed of aluminum tubing connecting the foot to the knee joint with a covering of soft foam that can be shaped to the size of the natural leg. All the basic knee designs are available with the endoskeletal prosthesis and all the designs of feet can also be used. The foam cover is solid at the knee so that it is particularly cosmetic in appearance because no part of the internal mechanism shows. This design of prosthesis is much easier on clothing than the rigid structure of the exoskeletal with its hard laminated outer surface. Careful consideration must be given to the needs of the individual child.

Hip Disarticulation and Hemipelvectomy Prosthesis

Hip Disarticulation Prostheses

Prosthetic components at this level are the same as for an above-knee prosthesis except that a pelvic socket is used instead of an above-knee quadrilateral socket. In the very young child, age 1 to 2 years, the prescription will include a plastic-laminated pelvic bucket with a soft interface, hip joint, no knee joint, and a SACH foot. Requirement for auxillary shoulder strap suspension is frequent because of the small pelvis of the child and the critical nature of the socket fit may be inadequate to provide suspension. As the child grows older and gains in height, the prosthesis can be modified to include a single axis knee joint (Fig. 12.6). The hip joint is placed inferior and anterior to the axis of rotation of the anatomic hip joint to provide prosthetic stability in midstance.[28] As the child approaches the adolescent years, an endoskeletal hip disarticulation prosthesis may be considered. The advantage of this prosthesis is reduced weight and improved cosmetic appearance. The socket of this type of prosthesis encompasses the entire pelvis and usually has an opening in the anterior portion over the abdomen and Velcro straps for the closure. In most hip disarticulations, some weight can be carried on the ischium.

Hemipelvectomy

The hemipelvectomy prosthesis is essentially the same as the hip disarticulation prosthesis except that appropriate modifications are necessary in the pelvic bucket to accommodate the increased anatomic loss. In some cases it may be necessary to distribute weight over the entire remaining pelvis and occasionally up onto the abdomen and chest.

Special Problems

Although all prostheses for congenital lower-limb deficiencies must be individualized, there are certain disorders that present special problems. These include: (1) tibial agenesis; (2) paraxial fibular hemime-

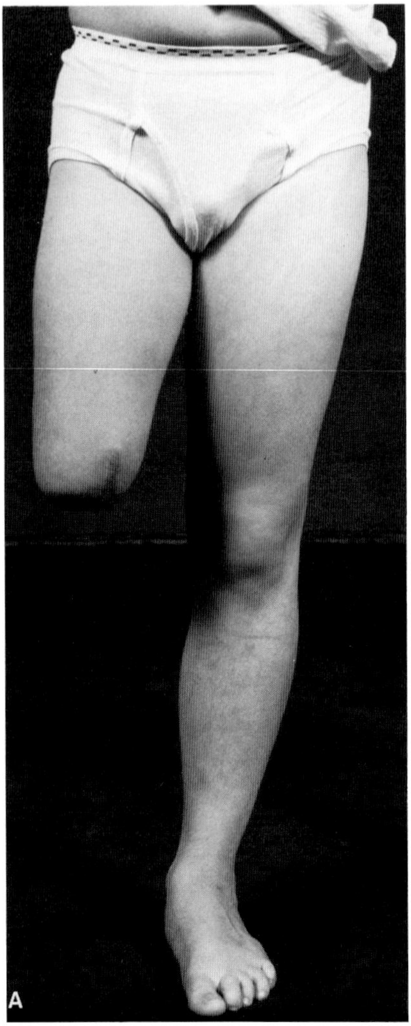

FIGURE 12.5. **A:** Nine-year-old boy with right tibia hemimelia and failed fibula centralization procedure who required a knee disarticulation amputation. **B:** Suction socket allows for a more stable fit. Additional suspension may still be necessary in older children if they are extremely active. This can be achieved with the addition of a Silesian belt as demonstrated here. **C:** Posterior view of the suction prosthesis demonstrating the padding of the proximal aspect to decrease noise during sitting and the single axis knee joint.

lia; (3) proximal femoral focal deficiency; (4) phocomelia; (5) amelia; and (6) multiple limb deficiencies.

Tibial Agenesis

Congenital deficiencies of the tibia, including hemimelia, aplasia, and dysplasia, are very rare. The prosthetic requirements depend on the type of reconstruction performed on the deficient lower leg. Kalamchi and Dawe[15] recently classified congenital deficiencies of the tibia into three groups based on clinical and radiographic findings: Type I, total absence of the tibia; Type II, distal tibial aplasia; and Type III, dysplasia of the

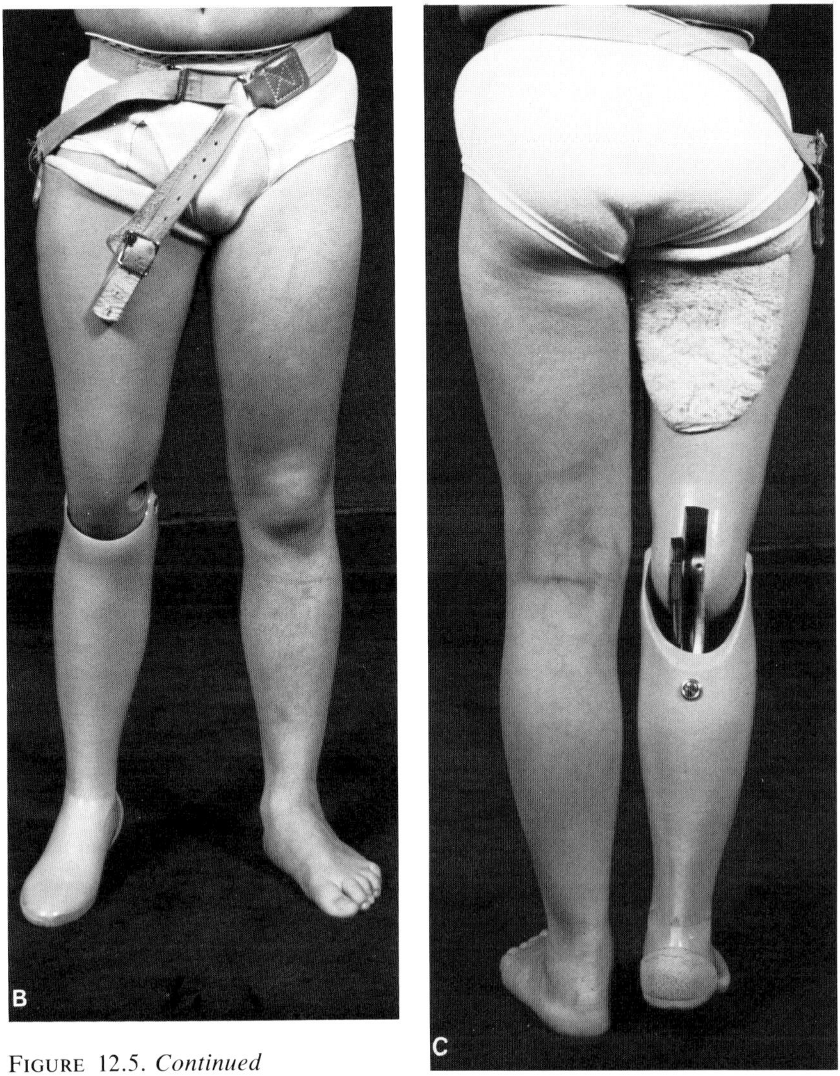

FIGURE 12.5. *Continued*

distal tibia with diastasis of the tibiofibular syndesmosis. Type I deficiencies are best managed by early knee disarticulation and early fitting with end-bearing above-knee prosthesis. Type II deficiencies are best managed by fusion of the fibula to the proximal tibial remnant. The extremity can then be managed with a below-knee prosthesis. The associated foot deformities are frequently present and best managed by either a Syme's or possibly a Boyd amputation. Kalamchi and Dawe[15] recommended a modified Boyd amputation in which the os calcis is fused to the distal fibula. This allows for a broader weight-bearing area for end-weight-

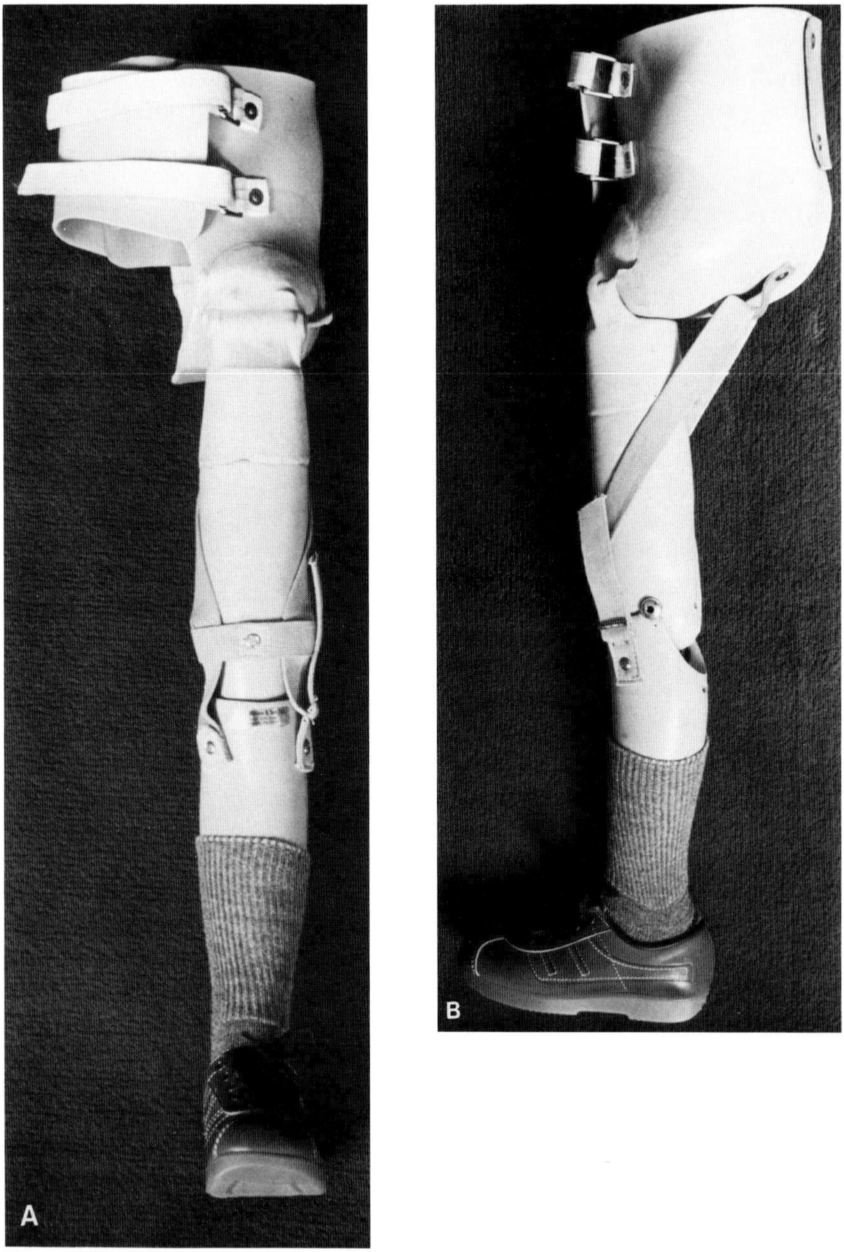

FIGURE 12.6. **A:**Hip disarticulation prosthesis with a plastic pelvic bucket, single axis hip and knee joints, and SACH foot. **B:** Side view demonstrating anterior and inferior placement of the prosthetic hip joint. Hip and knee extension is achieved by elastic strap attached to the pelvic bucket.

bearing in the prosthesis. Type III deficiencies are exceedingly rare and were demonstrated to have adequate function following a calcaneofibular fusion with a modified Boyd amputation. These children have excellent function using below-knee prosthesis with supracondylar suspension straps.

Paraxial Fibular Hemimelia

Paraxial fibular hemimelia is one of the most common congenital deficiencies of the lower extremities.[24,31] It occurs most frequently as a complete terminal deficiency with loss of one or more of the lateral rays of the foot. The distal tibial epiphysis is abnormal, the tibial is markedly shortened with an anteromedial bow, and the foot is fixed in an equinovalgus position. In more than half of the cases there is also femur involvement ranging from mild shortening to proximal femoral focal deficiency.[28] Thus, the major problems encountered in paraxial fibular hemimelia are lower extremity length unequality and foot deformity.[1,28,31] Currently, the preferred method of management for most children is ablation of the foot by the Syme's ankle disarticulation amputation between 6 and 12 months of age.[2,6,10,17,19,30]

Syme's amputation produces a sturdy end-bearing stump that can be fitted with an end-bearing below-knee PTB prosthesis. This prosthesis is fabricated to accommodate the anteromedial tibial bowing and correct the lower extremity length inequality. Because the fibula is absent, the stump is not excessively bulbous and prosthetic fitting is easily accomplished. Supracondylar suspension straps are frequently used during the first several years following the development of independent ambulation.

In bilateral cases, Syme's ankle disarticulate amputation and prosthetic fitting remains the procedure of choice. This allows optional function and correction of disproportionate dwarfism (Fig. 12.1).

Proximal Femoral Focal Deficiency

Children with proximal femoral focal deficiency have an affected thigh that is short and bulky and typically flexed, abducted, and externally rotated. Fibular hemimelia and foot deformities are present in 20% to 70% of involved children.[3] This deficiency has been classified by several authors according to the anatomic features of the proximal femur and acetabulum. The most common classifications are those described by Aitken,[3] Amstutz,[5] and Amstutz and Wilson.[4] Proximal femoral focal deficiency, depending on the severity of involvement, results in four lower-extremity biomechanical deficiencies: (1) leg length inequality; (2) malrotation; (3) inadequate proximal musculature; and (4) hip instability.[3] Surgical correction or reconstruction may be beneficial in some patients, although most will require prosthetic restoration to achieve maximum habilitation and function.[9]

Nonoperative Treatment

When surgical intervention is not permitted or planned, prosthetic restoration alone is used. If only mild femoral shortening is present a simple shoe lift may be sufficient when a child first begins to walk. If the leg length inequality is moderately severe, then a below-knee extension prosthesis is needed.[7] The first fitting is done when a child begins to show interest in standing or crawling. The foot is casted into equinus. The degree of equinus depends on the overall length requirements, although most will need 90 degrees. The initial prosthesis has the appearance of a ''ship's funnel,'' as the proximal socket is enlarged to accommodate the flexion, abduction, external rotation deformity of the thigh. The prosthesis is designed to provide weight-bearing to the plantar surface of the heel and the metatarsophalangeal area of the toes. A SACH foot is typically used. The prosthesis does not have a knee joint. The knee is added at approximately 3 years of age. This usually consists of a single axis, rigid knee hinges at the level of the anatomic foot.[9]

Operative Treatment

The surgical options available in proximal femoral focal deficiency are numerous and depend upon hip stability, the severity of femoral and lower extremity shortening, and the presence of associated foot deformities. The fitting of a below-knee extension prosthesis may be improved cosmetically as well as functionally by correcting the proximal deformities of flexion, abduction, and external rotation. This is usually accomplished through a subtrochanteric osteotomy. Other surgical options include femoral lengthening, Syme's or Boyd amputation and knee fusion with conversion of the lower extremity to a single bone, and the van Nes rotation-plasty.

When a Syme's or Boyd amputation and knee fusion are performed, it is important that the ultimate leg length inequality be calculated so that an appropriate epiphysiodesis can be performed concomitantly with the latter procedure. It is preferable to have the involved extremity approximately 5 cm shorter than the contralateral femur, as this allows space for the prosthetic knee joint. The prosthesis is an end-bearing above-knee prosthesis (Fig. 12.7). The bulbous heel pad created by the Syme's or Boyd fusion is advantageous because of its weight-bearing capabilities; it also aids in suspension of the prosthesis. The knee joint is added at approximately 3 years of age when the child is mature enough to control the knee.

In the van Nes rotation-plasty it is important that the hip be stable and that the femur places the ipsilateral ankle at the level of the contralateral

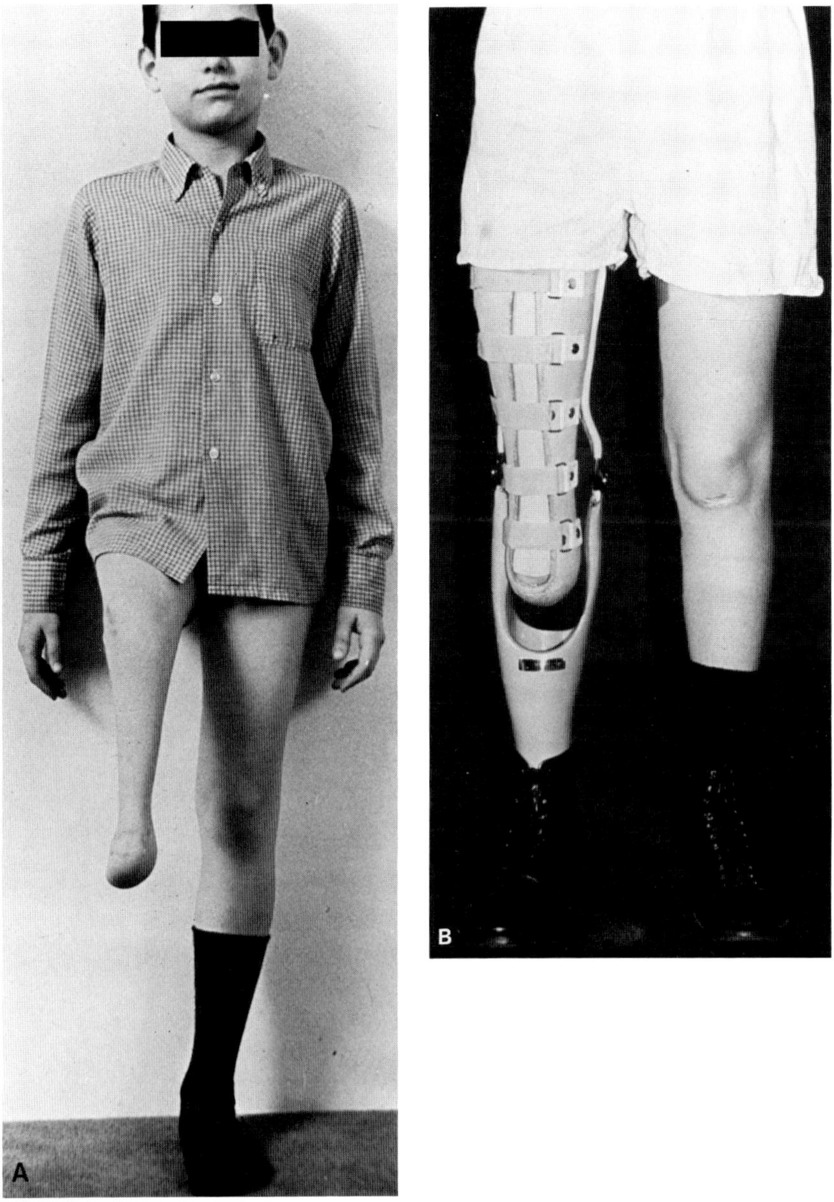

FIGURE 12.7. **A:** Twelve-year old boy with right proximal femoral focal deficiency managed by knee fusion and a Boyd foot amputation. Currently, the end-bearing stump is longer than the opposite femur, creating uneven knee levels. **B:** Above-knee end-bearing prosthesis with anterior opening, outside single axis knee hinge, and SACH foot. The knee hinges are at the same level of the opposite normal knee. This enhances function and gait. Surgical correction of the limb length inequality will allow for adequate space for a hydraulic knee as well as even knee levels.

knee.[16,29] The ankle of the involved extremity should be normal and capable of an arch of approximately 90 degrees of motion. This consideration excludes most patients with fibular hemimelia and foot deformities. If the 90-degree flexion position is not possible, the patient will have difficulty flexing the knee when seated. Bochmann described the details of fabrication alignment of the prosthesis to fit rotation-plasty.[7] The van Nes prosthesis resembles a below-knee prosthesis. The foot simulates a below-knee stump and the ankle acts as a knee joint. A thigh lacer is provided for children with stable hips whereas a quadrilateral ischial–weight-bearing socket is required for unstable hips. Outside knee hinges provide medial and lateral stability and prevent hyperextension.[8] The advantage of the van Nes procedure is that the foot and ankle joint can activate the prosthetic knee and propel the lower leg. Disadvantages, however, include poor cosmesis of the limb, some loss of function with the prosthesis off, and repeat derotation osteotomies, especially when performed in young children.[7,13]

Phocomelia

In complete lower limb phocomelia, all proximal portions of the limb are absent and the foot attaches directly to the pelvis. It is bilateral in 20% to 30% of cases.[12] Functionally, phocomelia is the equivalent of a hip disarticulation and is treated prosthetically in a similar manner. The socket must be appropriately modified to accommodate the foot. Preservation of the foot is important because it allows end-bearing in the socket, aids in prosthetic suspension, and provides sensory feedback concerning the position of the prosthesis.[2] Prosthetic management for children with bilateral phocomelia is discussed in the section on multiple limb deficiencies.

Amelia

Complete absence of the lower limb, including the foot, is termed amelia. It is a transverse terminal deficiency and is bilateral in approximately 50% of cases.[12] It, too, is the functional equivalent of a hip disarticulation, and unilateral cases are managed with a standard hip disarticulation prosthesis. Bilateral amelia, as in phocomelia, is difficult to manage and is discussed in the section on multiple limb deficiencies.

Multiple Limb Deficiencies

Children with multiple limb deficiencies, especially both lower extremities, require specialized prostheses that are designed to allow the child to achieve the maximum possible function and ambulatory potential.[20,21] Each prosthesis is custom designed and fitted to the involved extremity

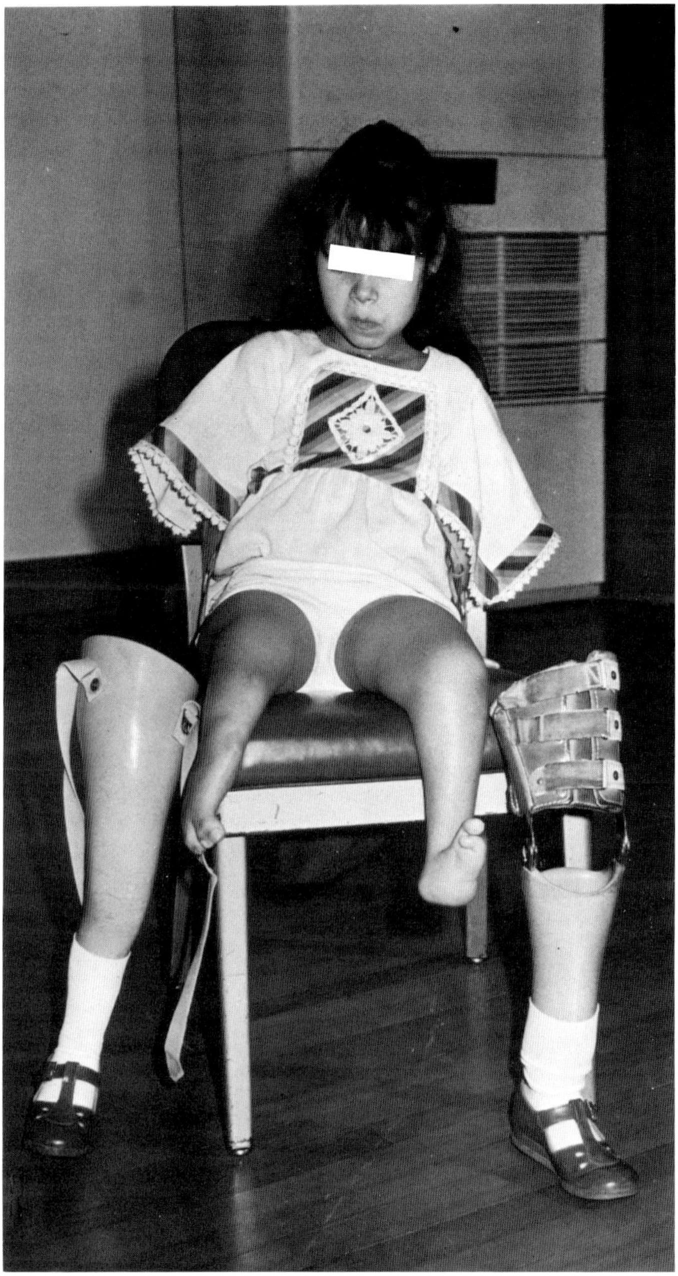

FIGURE 12.8. Seven-year-old girl with multiple congenital limb deficiencies including bilateral upper extremity phocomelia, right proximal femoral focal deficiency, bilateral complete paraxial fibular hemimelia with absent lateral rays of the feet. The right lower extremity has been fitted with a funnel end-bearing extension prosthesis while on the left an end-bearing below-knee prosthesis, single axis outside knee hinges and thigh cuff have been used.

(Fig. 12.8). Children with bilateral lower-limb deficiencies usually develop walking ability with their arms and residual lower extremities.[14] If the arms are also deficient (quadrilateral amputations), then prosthetic fitting and gait training will be very challenging.[21] In general, children with bilateral lower-limb deficiencies should be fitted as soon as possible based on the child's muscular development and ability to manage prosthetic devices. Prosthetic fittings may need to be staged or delayed, pending surgical reconstruction of one or both limbs. Children with bilateral Syme's ankle disarticulation should be able to ambulate independently without external support and to participate in all normal activities, including athletics. Similarly, children with bilateral below-knee amputations should have high rehabilitation potential (Fig. 12.9). As the amputation levels progress proximally, the rehabilitation potential becomes more dependent on functional upper limbs. In young children with bilateral above-knee amputations, initial fitting with "stubbies" may be beneficial.[14,18] Stubbies are modified quadrilateral sockets with either rocker or rubber-soled bottoms. The use of stubbies allows the child to develop balance and to learn to ambulate. The stubbies are lengthened as balance and gait progress. Ultimately, the child is fitted with articulated above-knee prostheses (Fig. 12.9B).

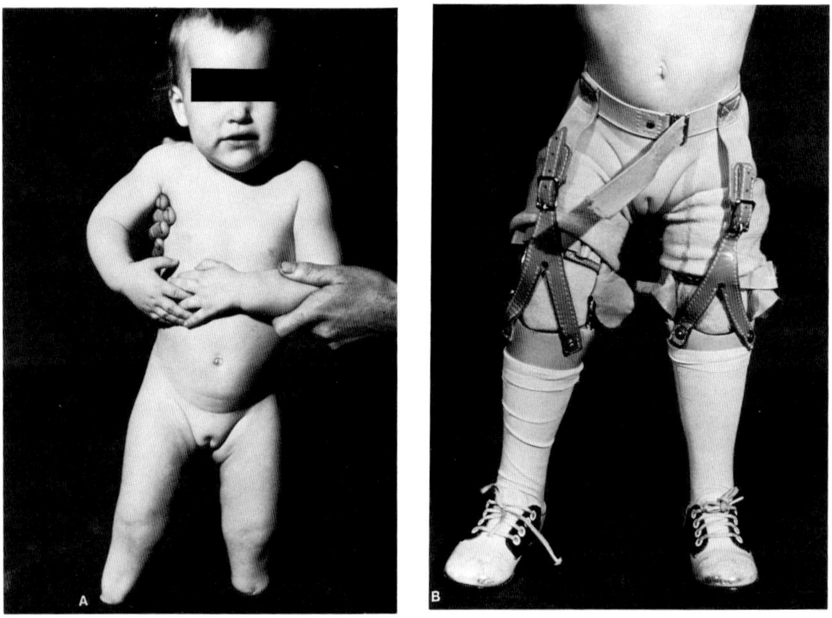

FIGURE 12.9. **A:** A four-year-old boy with bilateral congenital below-knee amputations. **B:** Prosthetic replacement with bilateral below-knee prostheses with strap suspension from a selesian belt allowed restoration at normal height and independent ambulation.

Infants with bilateral phocomelia or amelia will require a plastic-laminated "bucket-type" prosthesis attached to a firm base to facilitate head and trunk control and to achieve sitting balance. Usually 3 to 4 months later, an Ontario Cripple Children Centre (OCCC) swivel rocker can be substituted.[14,22,25] This device allows limited ambulation by converting lateral sway motion of the child's trunk to forward progression. Initially, the pylons of the swivel rocker are kept short to maintain the child's center of gravity close to the floor. As balance and coordination increase, the pylons are gradually lengthened. Children with normal upper extremities are fitted with standard or modified bilateral hip disarticulation prostheses between 2 and 4 years of age and are trained to walk with crutches.[7,18] Children with abnormal upper extremities may be fitted with articulated prostheses with swivel walker ankle joints for short distance ambulation. These children usually require some form of electrically powered wheelchair for independent mobility in the community.

Considerations for Growth in a Prosthesis

There are two areas of concern when allowing for growth in a prosthesis. The first and primary concern is length. The second concern is the fit circumferential of the socket.

For amputaion through midshaft of tibial or higher, the child amputee should have leg lengths checked in standing position every 3 months. At about every other visit, a check of the prosthesis will usually demonstrate it to be about 1 to 1.5 cm too short. The prosthesis can be lengthened by the prosthetist while the amputee waits,a shim of the appropriate thickness being placed between the foot and ankle. These shims can be added to a total of 5 to 7 cm.

Recently, Fishman et al reported on their experience with a flexible socket, rigid frame above-knee prosthesis that could accommodate both longitudinal and circumferential limb growth.[11] This type of prosthesis is beneficial because it decreases cost while maintaining comfort and function.

In a Syme's amputation, or in a similar case where there is minimal shortage and the normal epiphyses are intact, the prosthesis will probably not have to be lengthened. However, in fibular hemimelia this may not be true, and periodic adjustments for length may be necessary. This is easily accomplished by inserting spaces between the socket and SACH foot.

The fit of the socket does not usually change as quickly as the length in a growing child. Stump circumference variation can usually be accommodated with the use of stump socks. The first socket is designed to fit when the child is wearing a three-ply sock. Shrinkage and enlargement are managed by varying the thickness and number of socks. As the child grows circumferentially in the residual limb, the socket must be enlarged to accommodate this. Use of soft inner sockets as well as stump socks provides more room and makes these adjustments easier. It is also desirable to have extra distal end pads built into the socket of the prosthesis. These pads can then be removed as the child's residual limb increases in length.

Children amputees will tolerate a poor-fitting prothesis much easier than will an adult. Generally, children are not aware of any problems they are having. It is therefore especially important that the child's parents or guardian be aware of the necessity to have the prosthesis checked by their prosthetist regularly.

The useful life of prostheses for children depends, of course, on how quickly they grow. The average time a prosthesis can be used is 2 to 3 years. However, occasionally a child will outgrow his or her prosthesis in 1 year.

References

1. Achterman C, Kalamchi A: Congenital deficiency of the fibula. J Bone Joint Surg 61B:133, 1979.
2. Aitken GT: Amputation as a treatment for certain lower extremity congenital abnormalities. J Bone Joint Surg 41A:1376, 1959.
3. Aitken GT: Proximal femoral focal deficiency—definition classification and management, in Aitken GT (ed): Proximal Femoral Focal Deficiency. A Congenital Anomaly. National Academy of Sciences, 1969, pp 1–22.
4. Amstutz HC, WIlson PD Jr: Dygenesis of the proximal femur (coxa vara) and its surgical management. J Bone Joint Surg 44A:1–23, 1962.
5. Amstutz HC: The morphology, natural history and treatment of proximal femoral focal deficiency, in Aitken GT (ed): Proximal Femoral Focal Deficiency. A Congenital Anomaly. National Academy of Sciences, 1969, pp 50–76.
6. Amstutz HC: Natural history and treatment of congenital absence of the fibula. J Bone Joint Surg 54A:1349, 1972.
7. Bochmann D: Prosthetic Devices for the Management of Proximal Femoral Focal Deficiency. Orthop Prosthet 12(1):4–29, 1980.
8. Bochmann D: Prostheses for the limb-deficient child, in Kostuik JP (ed): Amputation Surgery and Rehabilitation. The Toronto Experience, Chapter 27. New York, Churchill Liningstone, 1981, pp 293–310.
9. Epps CE Jr: Current concepts review. Proximal femoral focal deficiency. J Bone Joint Surg 65A:867–870, 1983.
10. Farmer AW, Laurin CA: Congenital absence of the fibula. J Bone Joint Surg 54A:1349, 1972.
11. Fishman S, Edelstein JE, Drebs DE: Icelandic-Swedish—New York above-knee prosthetis sockets: Pediatric experience. J Pediatr Orthop 7:557–562, 1987.
12. Frantz CH, O'Rahilly R: Congenital skeletal limb deficiencies. J Bone Joint Surg 43A:1202, 1961.

13. Gillespie R: Congenital limb deformities and amputation surgery in children, in Kostuik JP (ed): Amputation Surgery and Rehabilitation. The Toronto Experience, Chapter 13. New York, Churchill Livingstone, 1981, pp 105–136.
14. Hamilton EL: Gait training part 2: Children, in Kostuik JP (ed): Amputation Surgery and Rehabilitation. The Toronto Experience, Chapter 29. New York, Churchill Livingstone. 1981, pp 331–346.
15. Kalamchi A, Dawe RV: Congenital deficiency of the tibial. J Bone Joint Surg 67B:581–584, 1985.
16. Kritter AE: Tibial rotation-plasty for proximal femoral focal deficiency. J Bone Joint Surg 59A:927–933, 1977.
17. Kruger LM: Recent advances in surgery of lower limb deficiencies. Clin Orthop 148:97, 1980.
18. Kruger LM: Congenital limb deficiencies. Part II. Lower limb deficiencies, in Atlas of Limb Prosthetics. Surgical and Prosthetic Principles, Chapter 38. American Academy of Orthopaedic Surgeons. St Louis, CV Mosby Co, 1981, pp 522–552.
19. Kruger LM, Hayes R: Prosthetic management. Part II. Lower limb prosthetic management, in Atlas of Limb Prosthetics. Surgical and Prosthetic Principles, Chapter 40. American Academy of Orthopaedic Surgeons. St Louis, CV Mosby Co, 1981, pp 581–594.
20. Laboriel MM, Setogachi Y: Research in juvenile prosthetics, in Atlas of Limb Prosthetics. Surgical and Prosthetic Principles, Chapter 42. American Academy of Orthopaedic Surgeons. St Louis, CV Mosby Co, 1981. pp 641–651.
21. Marquardt E: The Multiple Limb-Deficient Children, in Atlas of Limb Prosthetics. Surgical and Prosthetic Principles, Chapter 41. American Academy of Orthopaedic Surgeons. St Louis, CV Mosby Co, 1981, pp 595–641.
22. Matlock WM, Elliott J: Fitting and training children with swivel walker. Artif Limbs 10:27, 1966.
23. McIvor JB, Gillespie R: Patellar instability in juvenile amputees. J Pediatr Orthop 7:553–556, 1987.
24. O'Rahilly R: Morphologic patterns in limb deficiencies and duplications. Am J Anat 89:135, 1951.
25. Sauter WF: Prostheses for the child amputee. Surg Clin North Am 3:483, 1972.
26. Setoguchi Y, Rosenfelder R: The Limb Deficient Child. Springfield, Ill, Charles C Thomas Publisher, 1982.
27. Swanson AB: Congenital limb defects. Classification and treatment. Clin Symp 33, 1981.
28. Toomes RE: The amputee, in Lovell WW, Winters RB (eds): Pediatric Orthopaedics, Chapter 22. Philadelphia, JB Lippincott Co, 1986, pp 979–1030.
29. Van Nes CP: Rotation-plasty for congenital defects of the femur. Making use of the ankle of the shortened limb to control the knee joint of a prosthesis. J Bone Joint Surg 32B:12–16, 1950.
30. Westin GW, Sakai DN, Wood WL: Congenital longitudinal deficiencies of the fibula. J Bone Joint Surg 58A:492, 1976.
31. Wood WL, Zlostsky N, Westin GW: Congenital absence of the fibula. Treatment by Syme amputation—indications and technique. J Bone Joint Surg 47A:1159, 1965.

13
Sports Medicine in the Congenital Lower-Limb Amputee

PETER D. PIZZUTILLO

Little has been written about children with congenital lower-limb deficiencies and their capacity to participate in sports activity. Many Health care professionals have experience with adult amputees and children with traumatic amputations, and tend to apply that to the child with congenital limb deficiency.

Amputation is usually required in the adult as treatment for arteriosclerosis, diabetes, trauma, or infection. Prior to amputation, these patients have an established body image that includes two normal lower extremities. Their vocational and recreational life-style had long been established.

The sudden physical and psychological insult imposed by amputation of a portion of the lower extremity requires the adult to grieve the missing limb. Adjustments are required not only by the individuals, but also by their family, friends, and society.

Practical problems develop and include wear and use of a prosthesis with its change in proprioception and increased energy requirements during ambulation. The seemingly effortless performance of daily activities, in the past, now assumes a degree of difficulty.

Vocational and recreational activities are altered by prosthetic constraints, and may be further restricted by the coexistence of generalized disease, such as arteriosclerosis or diabetes. Psychological adjustments can be achieved only with significant individual effort.

In the young, healthy adult, acute trauma is the most common cause for amputation. There is an abrupt change in life-style and self-image with no antecedent disease state. Great strides have been made in the immediate prosthetic fitting of young adults to speed their return to preinjury activities. However, normalization of the individual's life will require resolution of the grief process involved in the loss of a limb and the gradual adjustment in body image.

Depending on the degree of limb loss and the physical demands imposed by some occupations, many young adults are able to resume a full life with return to preinjury occupation and recreation. The added burden of a generalized disease does not exist with this group and does not further restrict recovery. The child with normal lower extremities who has a traumatic amputation suffers a similar process and has the added problem of overgrowth of bone that may require multiple surgical revisions to ensure comfortable prosthetic wear.

Children with congenital amputation of the lower extremity differ significantly from the described populations. Because the malformation of the limb existed in utero, the newborn infant does not require a period of physical readjustment. Rather, an educational process should occur over a number of years, providing supportive, honest answers to the many probing questions. These children must acquire a feeling that love and acceptance by their family and friends exist despite their physical differences. With proper guidance, the child and family will be able to accept the deformity readily and proceed with a more normal life-style.

These children do not require change in their performance of daily living or recreational activities. Training is initiated in infancy and allows a progressive accommodation to ergometric needs. In general, these patients are in good health and are not subject to physical limitations. Definitive surgical procedures do not usually require multiple stages, and revision surgery is seldom needed for overgrowth in the congenitally deficient limb.

One of the most important factors in the normal socialization of children with lower-extremity amputation is the education, psychological guidance, and support of their parents. It is in their parent's eyes that they must first gain acceptance. This is of the utmost importance if children are to manage their differences successfully and be allowed to proceed in a positive manner as creative members of society.

Congenital anomalies of the lower extremity are varied in expression. The child's ability to participate in athletic activities depends on the type of deformity and whether the deformity is unilateral or bilateral.

The most simple significant deformity noted is congenital absence of the forefoot. These patients are fully active with or without shoewear and merely require a shoe-filler in order to wear matching shoes. There is an excellent weight-bearing surface with no problems of overgrowth or breakdown and essentially no limitations in the individual's ability to participate in all normal athletic abilities. In recent years, professional football player Tom Dempsey achieved significant recognition as a kicker in the National Football League despite congenital absence of the forefoot. In his situation, this appeared to be an advantage.

Fibular hemimelia has varied expression. The hypoplastic form exhibits only mild shortening of the fibula in relation to the tibia. Mild leg-length discrepancy can be compensated for with a shoe-lift, allowing full activity and participation without impediment to normal sports activities.

Patients with partial absence of the fibula have more significant leg-length discrepancy and may have increasing problems with deletion of the lateral rays of the foot. In addition, coalition of the tarsal bones frequently occurs in this group and does not allow for normal subtalar motion. The problems of leg-length discrepancy may be treated by epiphysiodesis of the opposite limb or by leg lengthening of the involved lower limb. The foot may be positioned in severe valgus or may be deficient in its lateral rays, leading to ankle instability. Occasionally, amputation is indicated to allow the individual to ambulate more effectively with a below-knee prosthesis. A similar treatment program is required in those patients with complete absence of the fibula and marked shortening of the remaining tibia.

Patients with the latter types of fibular hemimelia are able to run and participate in land sports—baseball, football, soccer, tennis, track, and basketball, for instance—without significant problems. Water sports also may be pursued without limitations. Snow skiing has become a very popular sport for patients with unilateral amputations at all levels of the lower extremity (Fig. 13.1).

Partial absence of the tibia is usually associated with significant leg-length discrepancy and frequently requires ablation of the foot and fitting with a below-knee prosthesis. These children function very well as below-knee amputees and seldom have difficulty with knee instability or pain.

Patients with complete absence of the tibia and good muscle control of the knee are candidates for centralization of the fibula and may then use a below-knee prosthesis with fewer energy requirements. Those with poor or absent quadriceps muscle function are treated by through-knee amputation and function effectively in an above-knee prosthesis. If involvement is bilateral, the child may choose to play with no prosthesis (Fig. 13.2).

Children treated with a through-knee or above-knee prosthesis have additional ergometric demands and do not have quality control of knee motion in their prosthesis. Although involvement in running and jumping activities is not commonly observed in this group, there are motivated children who participate in track, cross-country, and soccer activities. Skiing, wrestling, and water sports, usually without a prosthesis, are popular sports in this group.

Proximal femoral focal deficiency further limits the individual's ability to become involved in recreational sports activities. Those with bilateral femoral focal deficiency suffer from the absence of articulating hip joints and severe loss of height. The inefficiency of gait in this group usually precludes their involvement in ambulatory sports activities, though wheelchair sports are an option.

With unilateral proximal femoral focal deficiency, the ability to participate in sports will depend on the presence or absence of a stable hip joint. In patients with congenitally short femur, coxa vara with a congenitally short femur, or Type I proximal femoral focal deficiency, there is an

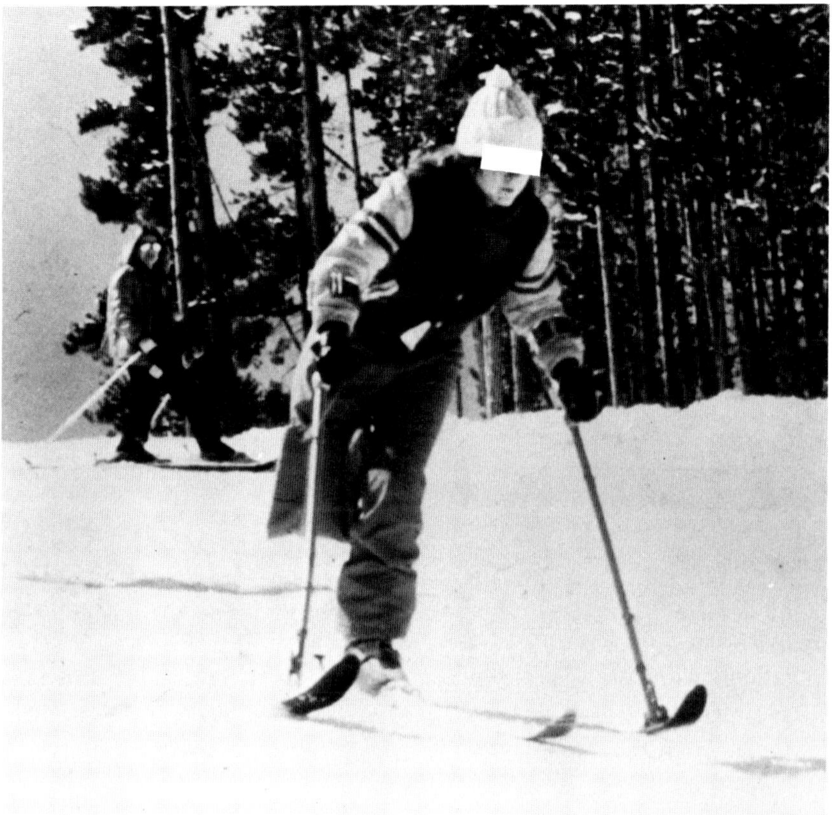

FIGURE 13.1. A teenager with unilaterally congenital lower-limb deficiency skiing without the prothesis. (The athlete is a patient of Dr. John Anthony Herring.)

articulating hip joint with efficient abductor power. Leg-length discrepancy becomes the primary problem in this group. Amputation is performed for equalization purposes and for prosthetic fitting to allow participation in hiking, soccer, wrestling, aquatics, and skiing.

Children with unilateral proximal femoral focal deficiency and no articulating hip joint suffer from marked inefficiency of the abductor mechanism and have tremendous ergometric demands during ambulation. These patients do no running or jumping. Swimming and skiing without the prosthesis have been the primary sports activities obsreved in this patient population.

A rare congenital anomaly involves disarticulation of the hip or absence of the entire lower extremity. These children are very active on one leg and, in fact, in their early childhood resist prosthetic wear because the prosthesis impedes their ability to hop at a quick rate and involve themselves in play activities, such as climbing and gymnastics. Their

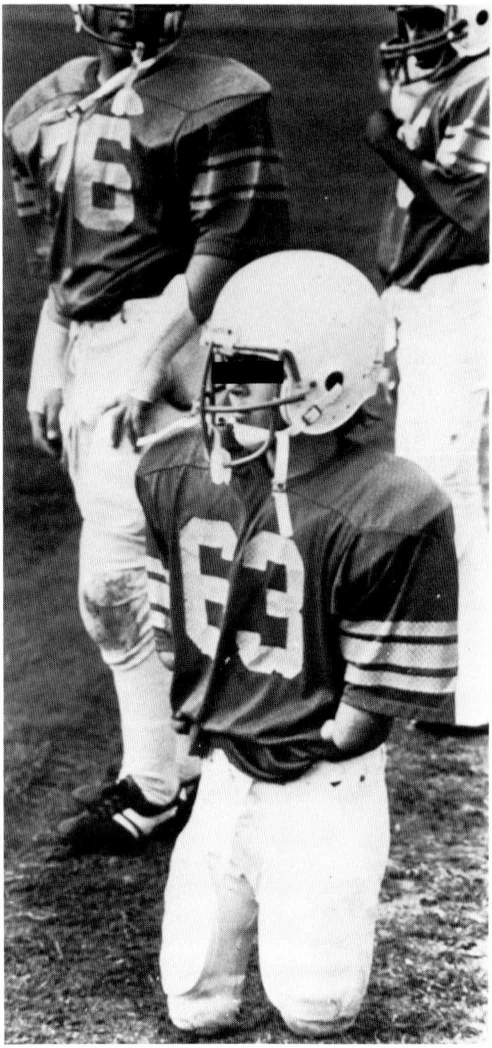

FIGURE 13.2. This individual with multiple congenital limb deficiency opted to play football without his lower-limb prothesis. (The athlete is a patient of Dr. John Anthony Herring.)

prosthetic needs require a pelvic bucket articulation, which provides stability in stance and gait and cosmetic improvement, but it is not very mobile and has increased ergometric needs.

In the author's experience, children with this deformity choose to go without their prosthesis part of the day for play activities and also prefer to ski without their prosthesis.

A good self-image, with support from family and friends, has provided a tremendous boost to children with congenital anomalies of the lower extremity to become involved in sports activity and compete with their able-bodied peers. Most of the prosthetic modifications for sports activities have been initiated by these children or their parents.

Research and development of prosthetic devices that will reduce energy demands and allow these special children to excel in their efforts is needed. Equally important is continued societal education to remove any emotional impediments to their development.

References

1. "Recreational Activities of Lower Extremity Amputees: A Survey" B. Kegel, J.C. Webster, & E.M. Burgess Arch Phys Med Rehabil 61:258–264, June 1980
2. "In What Sports Can Patients With Amputations And Other Handicaps Successfully and Actively Participate?" J.P. Smith Phys Ther 50:121–126, Jan 1970

14
The Juvenile Amputee: Physical Therapy and Sports Participation

ALAN PEOPLES

In a clinical setting dealing with a juvenile amputee, the role of the physical therapist is as a member of a team made up of an orthopedic surgeon, occupational therapist, prosthetist, social worker, adaptive physical educator, and volunteers.

Initial Management

Patients and parents who are referred to the prosthetic clinic for the first time may be apprehensive about surgery or their child's ability to function with a prosthesis. The physical therapist acts as a "social worker," helping them to adjust. The physical therapist serves as a helpful source of information for the parents. Sometimes the fear of the initial visit interferes with their comprehension. A good way to overcome this would be to invite the patient and parents to the prosthetic clinic and have them observe, ask questions, and see patients with similar problems.

The primary task of the physical therapist is instruction. Initially, this may only include the preoperative crutch training and exercises. After surgery, stump management should include wrapping the stump with an Ace bandage, plaster wrap, or stump shrinker to help shrink the stump and shape it to a rounded appearance, eliminating any "dog ears." If early ambulation is desired, an immediate postoperative-fitting prosthesis may be used, with socks being added as shrinkage occurs.

The bandage should be applied with more pressure distally than proximally, eliminating the tourniquet effect. A recurrent figure-eight pattern of application is desirable (Fig. 14.1). Avoid circular wrapping, wrinkles, or uncovering areas on the distal stump.

The child should be instructed to do his or her own wrapping to cultivate the sense of personal independence. If a child is too small to learn, then the parents must be instructed. The stump should be re-wrapped many times daily since it will loosen with movement. Daily circumferential measurements should be taken to document when the swelling has gone down and to ensure that the stump is the same circum-

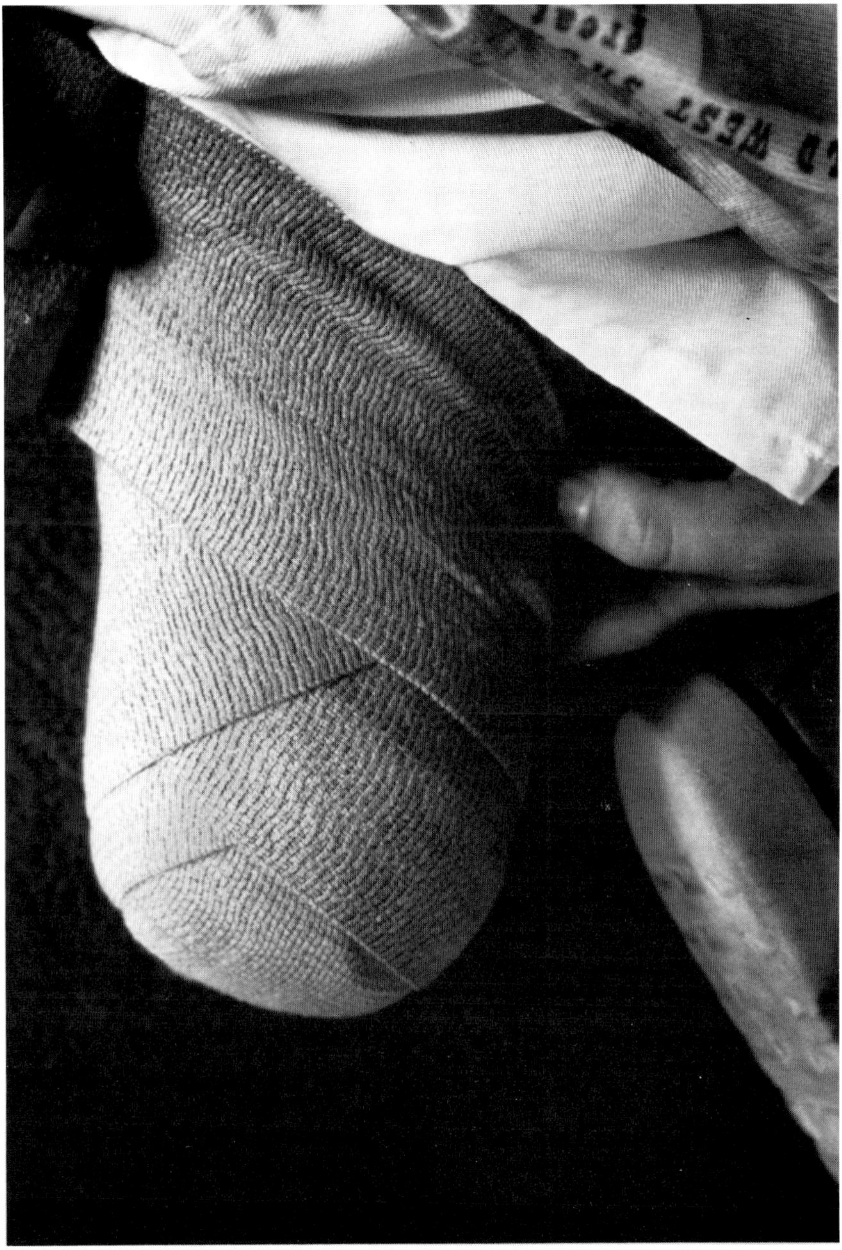

FIGURE 14.1. To help shape and shrink the stump, wrapping is applied in a recurrent figure-eight pattern with more pressure distally than proximally.

ference consistently. Casting may then begin for fitting of a permanent prosthesis. To avoid contractures of principal joints, proper positioning and exercises should be emphasized in the immediate postoperative period.

The above-knee amputee should avoid prolonged positions of hip flexion, abduction, and external rotation. These will aggravate the imbalance created by the amputation, in turn weakening the hip extensors and adductors. The patient should be checked for hip-flexion contractures and encouraged to lie prone rather than sit. The patient should also, begin postoperative hip extensor and adductor strengthening. Hip abductor strengthening is also helpful in the prevention of a Trendelenburg gait.

To prevent knee flexion contractures, a child with a below-knee amputation should avoid positioning his limb with the knee flexed for prolonged periods, and quadriceps strengthening should be started. If a contracture is present, sandbags or weights placed over the knee for extended periods of time may prove helpful (Fig. 14.2). Extension splits may be desirable for use during sleeping.

The patient and parents should be instructed to inspect the stump for any problems with skin healing, limited motion, and strength. The patient should be up and walking with crutches, with the stump always wrapped. Any areas of hypersensitivity or discomfort on the stump should be massaged by the patient, at first lightly and then with gradually increasing pressure. This helps eliminate phantom sensations and hypersensitivity.

Initial Checkout with Prosthesis

The patient and the parents are shown the new prosthesis, its care and application, the stump sock, and proper methods of hygiene for the stump. The child is asked to stand in the prosthesis for evaluation of proper length and alignment.

Assuming that this is the child's first prosthesis, his or her skin may not tolerate wearing it for long periods of time. The child must be instructed to wear the prosthesis for short intervals and to take it off and observe the redness of the stump, looking for persistent areas of skin irritation. They should not reapply the prosthesis until the redness subsides. If the redness continues, this is an indication that the fit is not ideal and adjustments must be made in the prosthesis. If there is little or no redness, the patient may wear the prosthesis for longer periods of time.

Because the child is growing, a few changes are necessary. All shoes purchased must have the same heel height as the shoe worn during the initial prosthetic fitting. Unlike many adults, children adapt to a new limb rather quickly and may need only an ambulatory aid to help accustom them to walking and weight-bearing. This will come along, with some helpful hints given to the parents such as using a walking belt, which will not interfere with the child's balance.

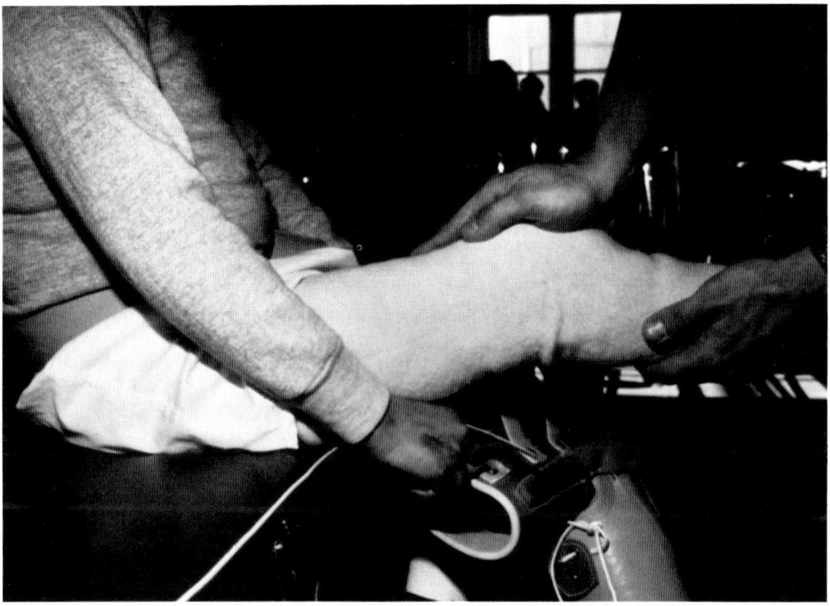

FIGURE 14.2. Prevention: Recognition and treatment of knee flexion contractures is important with below-knee amputations.

The parallel bars are usually the first device that may be needed for bilateral amputees and others who show initial difficulty and apprehension. A few patients may need to be hospitalized for gait training; however, most can be handled on an outpatient basis.

A child with a hip-disarticulation prosthesis, above-knee, below knee, Symes[7,3] or a modified prosthesis may be sent home with a rollator walker, which comes in a variety of sizes. Axillary crutches, forearm crutches, or canes may also be used to encourage weight-bearing on the prosthetic side. Crutch walking may be taught to a 3-year-old.

As a child approaches 5 years of age, training resembles that given to an adult. Initially, the child may not put much weight on the prosthesis and must be given hints, such as "keeping your nose over your toe" to promote weight shifting. As the child progresses, he or she learns the weight shift to the point that he may be able to balance on the limb. A sit-in-ring walker may be used for very small children learning to walk.

Follow-Up

The child is checked during return clinic visits approximately once every 3 to 4 months. Gait is observed and appropriate measures are taken to correct any deviations. Some gait deviations are because of differences in style. There may be nothing wrong with the patient or the prosthesis.

The most common factor that may lead to gait deviation is growth. If the prosthesis is too short, there may be flexion of the knee on the sound side to level the pelvis. Sometimes the prosthesis may appear too long when the circumferential stump growth prohibits the stump from getting down into the socket, creating an appearance of the prosthetic side being too long. There may be vaulting or toe walking on the uninvolved extremity to help equalize leg-length differences. Length is generally added or subtracted if there is one-half inch or more difference between extremities. Usually, in patients with hip problems, the length is kept short on the involved side for better stability and coverage of the hip.

A prosthesis that is too long might have the wearer holding his or her involved limb in abduction during stance and swing phase while walking. He or she may also have a high medial wall on the socket of an above-knee prosthesis that causes pain in the groin area, or it may be due to the presence of abduction contracture. The pelvic band suspension may be set in excessive abduction or there may be just the feeling of insecurity that causes an abducted gait while standing and walking.

Circumduction is seen when the patient is walking and swinging the limb out to the side during swing phase only. Usually it is because the wearer has little or no knee flexion on the swing phase of the gait, possibly owing to insecurity, weakness, incorrect alignment of the pelvic band and knee joints, or inadequate suspension.

The adjustment of knee friction is important. If the friction is stiff, circumduction will be present. If the friction is too loose, there will be excessive heel rise on walking or a terminal swing impact that presents itself as a "klunk" on knee extension. Most above-knee patients are taught to skip rather than run in their prosthesis because the friction component in the knee delays their swing phase.

Excessive lateral bending of the trunk to the prosthetic side may be from a short prosthesis, low lateral socket wall, or pain in the distal stump. Hip extensor or abductor weakness also creates lateral bending toward the weakness.

Checking alignment from the anterior and posterior view, look for excessive hip abduction, adduction, or rotation, as well as varus or valgus of the ankle. Knee valgus is commonly seen in patients with lower-limb deficiency[2] and needs to be monitored closely. In the above-knee amputee, poor fit and malalignment might result in a medial or lateral heel whip.

Observation from the lateral view may show that a child has changed heel heights on his or her shoes, exhibiting toe walking or recurvatum of the knee during heel strike. If the TKA line is malaligned in the hip disarticulation or in the above knee prosthesis, controling knee flexion or extension may be difficult.

In our monthly prosthetic clinic, patients come about once every 4 months, and sooner if need be. The prosthetic clinic fully evaluates and provides treatment with the goal of ensuring that the patient maintains his or her independence. If urgent problems are encountered, parents call the physical therapist, who will respond immediately and contact the necessary team members for a quick evaluation. Most of the problems concern skin breakdown, growth, improper fit, bony overgrowth, and prosthetic repairs.

The physical therapist serves as a vital link between the patient and the team. Serving as an instructor for the patient, guiding him or her with the prosthesis and in the proper use and care of the limb or stump. The therapist acts also as a contact and coordinator for follow-up care and scheduling of clinic appointments. He or she makes sure the patient continues to function actively and independently in the community.

Sports Participation

In any activity in which the child participates, the essential considerations are (1) what degree of success the child will have; (2) the safety of the activity; (3) the level of challenge to the child; (4) the creativity of the clinic in adapting or modifying the equipment or situations to enhance the child's performance; and (5) the level of social interaction desired.

Success. Providing a positive experience will contribute to the child's development of a healthy self-image. Observing ease of ambulation and movement skills are two simple tests to evaluate the child's ability. Is the child able to jog or run? Many children may be able to skip better than they run.

Children who have difficulty ambulating with ease should be directed to activities that may not require heavy ambulatory skills. Activities such as swimming, archery, bowling, and wheelchair sports may be more appropriate if a competitive level is desired. Team sports may be appropriate if the child is proficient at his position.

If a child feels like a second-class citizen on a team, then perhaps selecting a particular skill from a sport and using it in a recreational setting may be more suitable (e.g., playing catch in the backyard rather than on a competitive baseball team).

Evaluation of the child's ability to stand or hop on one foot, creep, crawl, and kneel is important when examining suitable activities that may require similar skills. Children with higher levels of amputation in the lower extremities should gear their activities to sports that require upper-extremity use (weight lifting, rowing, kayaking, canoeing, fishing, riflery, archery, sailing, wheelchair sports, swimming, shooting pool, and skiing.

Safety. Eliminating or managing risk factors and providing a safe environment is a must in sports. Continued skin inspection is necessary when heavy activities are engaged in.

Growth is constant when working with the child amputee. When an improper fit is encountered, excesses in pistoning may occur, leading to breakdown of the skin. If the child has lost weight, he or she may fall into the prosthesis and the leg appears shorter. Be aware of any limp due to pain from improper fits. Patients have used socks, foam,[4] artificial skin, and socket modifications when working with proper fit.

Instruct the child in the proper walking and running gait, which should not place undue stress on the prosthesis. We had a young girl who liked to decrease the amount of friction in her single-axis constant-friction, above-knee prosthesis while trying to run foot-over-foot. She constantly tore her knee apart. After teaching her to skip and increasing her friction, her repair time was significantly reduced.

The old SACH foot[5] (solid ankle cushioned heel) has been a standby for prosthetic use for several years. New developments coming up with the Seattle[6] and Carbon Copy II[1] feet are energy-saving feet, which give the patient a more natural type of gait and more of a toe-off in ambulation. Unfortunately, these modifications do not come in sizes below 6. They are much lighter than the traditional SACH foot. For those with short stumps, keeping the prosthesis on when ambulating becomes a problem; a thigh lacer or pelvic band and belt may be added. Protecting the athletes and others from possible harm when contact and limited-contact sports are encountered is always a necessity. Often a prosthesis may need to be padded for the other children's protection.

One of our patients, a young man, skiied wearing his above-knee prosthesis. However most above-knee amputees use outriggers on forearm crutches and ski without their prosthesis.

If heavy aerobic activities are undertaken, the child with congenital deformities must be evaluated for any associated congenital anomalities (heart, kidneys, etc). Guidelines for sports participation may be acquired from the American College of Sports Medicine (ACSM).

Challenge. Sports that are challenging build self-confidence in a child. Activities that are of no challenge may not hold interest. Always place activity goals that are realistic yet challenging.

Creativity. A vital ingredient for successful sports and activity participation. Suggestions such as flippers being worn on the uninvolved leg for a stronger kick may help the child adapt more easily to water activities. Assistive devices such as a crutch or crutches may be used to make ambulating easier. Sports clothing suggestions may help the child fit in more easily.

Social Interaction. A question such as, "Are you participating in physical education classes?" is always a revealing one to show how the child is dealing with his or he situation. If the child has had some problems with parental acceptance of his or her disability; their self-image and confidence may not be very high. If this is the case, a nonthreatening environment must be selected that is not as structured and is more individualized.

It should be remembered that sports are only a tool and are to be used to promote a healthy self-image. If an activity is not fun for the child, then it is the duty of the rehabilitation team to guide the family and child to successful sports and leisure-time pursuits. If the child wants to pursue a sport, there is always a way to adapt or modify the sport to meet his or her level of success.

Acknowledgment. The author would like to express his appreciation to the following individuals who shared their expertise with him during the Alfred I. duPont Institute's Prosthetic Clinic from 1971 through 1980: Robert E. Eilert, M.D.; S.S. Jaykumar; M.D., Ali Kalamchi, M.D., Harry J. Lawall, Sr., C.P.O.; G. Dean MacEwen, M.D.; Frank Malone, Sr., C.P.O.; and Peter Pizzutillo, M.D.

References

1. "Copy Cat II," Ohio Willow Wood Co, 7985 Chestnut St, Mt. Sterling, OH 43143.
2. Eilert E, Jaykumar SS: Boyd and Syme Ankle Amputation in Children. J of Bone & Joint Surg, Vol 58A, pp 1138–1141, 1976.
3. Foort J: The Canadian Type Syme Prosthesis (Series II, Issue 30) Lower Extremity Amputee Research Project, Institute of Engineering Research, University of California, Berkeley, December, 1956.
4. Prefabricated Pelite Cones for P.T.B. Liners, Durr-Fill Aver Medical, Inc, Orhopedic Div, PO Box 5189, Chattanooga, TN 37406.
5. "Sach Foot": Kingsley Manufacturing Co, 1984 Placentia Ave, Costa Mesa, CA 92627.
6. "Seattle Foot," Model and Instrument Development, 861 Poplar Place South, Seattle, WA 98144.
7. Leimkuehler Jon CPO: Symes prosthesis—a brief review and a new fabrication technique. Orthot Prosthes 34:3–12, 1980.

Index